McWhinney's Textbook of Family Medicine

McWhinney's Textbook of Family Medicine

FOURTH EDITION

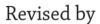

Revised by

Thomas R. Freeman, MD, MCISc, CCFP, FCFP

Professor of Family Medicine
Schulich School of Medicine and Dentistry
The University of Western Ontario
London, Ontario, Canada

OXFORD
UNIVERSITY PRESS

OXFORD
UNIVERSITY PRESS

Oxford University Press is a department of the University of Oxford. It furthers
the University's objective of excellence in research, scholarship, and education
by publishing worldwide. Oxford is a registered trade mark of Oxford University
Press in the UK and certain other countries.

Published in the United States of America by Oxford University Press
198 Madison Avenue, New York, NY 10016, United States of America.

© Oxford University Press 2016

First Edition published in 1981
Second Edition published in 1989
Third Edition published in 2009
Fourth Edition published in 2016

Library of Congress Cataloging-in-Publication Data
Freeman, Thomas, 1948–, author.
McWhinney's textbook of family medicine / Thomas R. Freeman. — 4th edition.
p. ; cm.
Textbook of family medicine
Preceded by Textbook of family medicine / Ian R. McWhinney, Thomas R. Freeman.
3rd edition. 2009.
Includes bibliographical references and index.
ISBN 978–0–19–937068–9 (alk. paper)
I. McWhinney, Ian R. Textbook of family medicine. Preceded by (work):   II. Title.
III. Title: Textbook of family medicine.
[DNLM: 1. Family Practice. WB 110]
RC46
610—dc23
2015024365

1 3 5 7 9 8 6 4 2

Printed by Sheridan, USA

To the memory of Ian Renwick McWhinney: family physician, philosopher, mentor to many.

CONTENTS

PART IV. EDUCATION AND RESEARCH

PREFACE

There are two kinds of textbooks: those that aim to cover a field of knowledge and those that aim to define and conceptualize it. This book is of the second kind. Most textbooks in clinical disciplines are structured in accordance with conventional system for classifying diseases. A family medicine text that adopts this structure faces two difficulties. Family physicians encounter clinical problems before they have been classified into disease categories. In principle, family physicians are available for any type of problem. There is thus no disease, however rare, that may not be encountered in family practice. If a text tries to cover the entire field, it risks becoming a watered-down textbook of internal medicine. More seriously, family medicine differs from most other disciplines in such fundamental ways that the conventional structure, though used in family medicine when appropriate, is at a variance with the organismic thinking that is both common and natural to our discipline.

Shortly prior to his final illness, Professor McWhinney and I were contacted by the publisher regarding preparation of a fourth edition of this textbook. His illness prevented him from taking part, but he encouraged me to undertake necessary revisions of the third edition. With the aid of the publisher, comments were sought on the third edition from leading thinkers in family medicine and, from these suggestions, revisions have been made.

Part I of the book addresses the basic principles of family medicine, beginning with the origins of the discipline. The fundamental principles are then described, along with their implications and common misconceptions. Family physicians, because of their commitment to the person, and to continuity and comprehensiveness of care, develop a unique body of knowledge. Our work contributes to and helps to define the social capital of society. The activity of family practice reflects the illnesses of the communities that practitioners serve. While communicable diseases continue to present significant challenges, noncommunicable, chronic illnesses dominate much of the clinical activity of the family physician. Families are the biological, psychological, social, and spiritual basis of our lives. While family structures evolve over time and vary from culture to culture, they have profound effects on health and illness. Although advances in genetics have been remarkable, it is perhaps the emerging knowledge of epigenetics—the influence of environment, including the social environment, on genetic expression—that will have the greatest impact on family practice. Faced with applying the principles in the context of changing social patterns, family constellations, illness patterns, and new knowledge, it is important that family physicians be aware that there is a well-defined philosophical and scientific basis to family medicine. This basis sheds light on and informs the clinical method used in family medicine as it has been defined over the past few decades. In contrast, current, conventional, allopathic medicine in its practice and organization seems animated by the ideal of curing all human ailments. This ideal has long been challenged by individuals such as René Dubos, and the constant encounter with incurable diseases and human suffering that characterizes much of family practice causes us to shift our focus from curing to helping our patients cope—to achieve a balance with their world in spite of the limitations imposed by their illnesses. Sometimes, we even witness healing taking place.

To illustrate the principles of the first section of the book, new clinical chapters have been written and are presented in Part II. As in past editions, these chapters are intended to provide a way of thinking about and approaching common clinical issues in family practice. They are all written using the same framework: prevalence in family practice; family factors, social factors, subjective experience, and clinical approach. The clinical topics are respiratory illness, musculoskeletal pain, depression, diabetes, obesity, and multimorbidity.

Part III looks at issues relevant to the family physician's daily practice. Several revisions have been made in this edition of the book. The practice of family medicine takes place in concert with other healthcare practitioners and in a network of community service providers. Care of patients in their own home has always been a part of family practice; improvements in technological supports, such as point-of-care testing, and the high cost and, in some cases, diminishing returns of in-hospital care ensure that this aspect of our work will continue to be important. A new chapter has been added entitled "Stewardship of Resources, Patient Information, and Data." The cost of health care has become a significant problem in developed as well as developing nations. All physicians have a role to play in addressing the rising costs, including the rational use of diagnostic testing and treatment. Modern medical technology plays a role in these costs. One technology, electronic health records (EHRs), is believed by many to hold some promise in identifying and reducing unnecessary expenses. However, no technology comes without consequences, and EHRs are no exception. Family physicians have always been guardians of the patient's medical record, but now, with more personal information available than ever before, many others—healthcare planners, insurers, governments, and researchers, for example—have great interest in the information in the databases that are arising in family practice. This presents new challenges for the practitioner.

Part IV turns to knowledge, at a personal level and as knowledge generation from research. As in any profession, family physicians are responsible for
ensuring their continuing education. Less often recognized is the importance
of self-knowledge. There is increasing recognition of the value of mindfulness
in our development as individuals and as practitioners. As an academic discipline, family medicine has made great strides in establishing and developing
a base of knowledge. Methods from various disciplines such as epidemiology,
the social sciences, and others have been adapted and used to address research
questions that are specific to family medicine, but that also have implications
for other branches of medicine.

Physician-philosophers are rare in any period of history and perhaps more
so in the late twentieth century than previous ones. Professor McWhinney
was such an individual. In quoting the sociologist, Daniel Bell, the author
Robert Fulford states, "The scholar . . . has an understood field of knowledge
and a tradition in which he tries to find a place. The intellectual starts his own
tradition, beginning with his personal experience, his individual perceptions
of the world, his privileges and deprivations—and judges the world by his own
standards."[1] McWhinney was such an intellectual. Despite graduating from
the best medical training that Great Britain had to offer in 1948, he was dissatisfied with the preparation for general practice that he had received. This
stimulated him to undertake a tour of the United States and Canada, supported by the Nuffield Trust. He visited with medical practitioners in all fields
of medicine and discussed the state of training for general practice. This led
to a paper, published in the journal *The Lancet* in 1966,[2] that has proved to
be seminal in the founding of family medicine as an academic discipline. In
this paper he laid out the blueprint for moving general practice, at the time
thought to be craft, to a discipline within medicine, now known as family
medicine.

Professor McWhinney provided a new map for family medicine, defining
the key places that were absent from the map that he had been provided.
He defined the pathways between these place markers and, in so doing, he
also changed the larger map of medicine, bringing into discussion such key
concepts as the central importance of the relationship between the patient
and the physician; the renunciation of the divide between the mind and the
body and of the power differential between the patient and the physician. He
taught that our commitment to patients leads to truly knowing them, not
just knowing about them. He understood that theoretical concepts cannot
become real if they do not change behavior, and that to do justice to what the
best physicians have always done, one has to change behavior at the level of
the clinical method. He was the intellectual force behind the patient-centered
clinical method as defined and studied at Western University and elsewhere.

It is rare for one person to have such an impact on so many individuals
around the world. He strongly influenced several generations of academic

family physicians, but more important, many people have unknowingly ben-
efited from caring physicians who have sought to put into practice his teach-
ings. The spirit of these lessons come to life whenever a practitioner sits at the
side of a sick or dying patient and attends—truly pays complete attention—
to the patient's suffering and, in so doing, realizes that he too suffers; whenever a clinician maintains loyalty throughout the vicissitudes of her patient's
illness; whenever scholars delve into the meaning of illness and suffering.

Although Professor McWhinney was not able to take part in the revisions
for the fourth edition, his thinking and perspective were in mind throughout.
Through the generosity of his daughters, I had access to several of the journals
that he kept over the years, and these were a frequent source of inspiration
and insight. In one of those journals he makes this entry (written in 1991 or
so), entitled "a good book shop": "The mark of a good book shop is not its size,
but the thought which goes into its display. How often have I been delighted
to find in its tables a book which is new to me and which fills a current need.
It's as if some member of the staff has been able, in some mysterious way, to
find the reader who needs it. It was this way that a book almost fell into my
hands." May this book be such a one, for you.

Thomas R. Freeman
London, Ontario
2015

NOTES

1. http://news.nationalpost.com/2011/01/29/robert-fulford-death-of-an-intellectual/.
2. McWhinney IR, General practice as an academic discipline: Reflections after a visit to the United States, *The Lancet* (1966), 1 (7434):419–423.

ACKNOWLEDGMENTS

A textbook of this type represents the efforts of many people. I wish to first acknowledge and thank Dr. Moira Stewart, who over the 40 years of our marriage has been a constant support and inspiration to me. As his first graduate student, she introduced me to Ian McWhinney when I was still a medical student and, thereby, changed the course of my career.

The Department of Family Medicine at Western has been always been a center of academic work in the field ever since Ian McWhinney founded it as the first Professor of Family Medicine in Canada. Being able to work with a wide variety of scholars at the Centre for Studies in Family Medicine (CSFM) has been an invaluable asset and I am grateful to the current Chair, Dr. Stephen Wetmore, for continuing support for academic work in the Department of Family Medicine. No less important has been the support from my clinical colleagues at the Byron Family Medical Centre. Staying grounded in clinical work is essential to understanding family medicine.

Lynn Dunikowski and her staff at the Library of the College of Family Physicians of Canada were an enormous asset in locating essential reference materials and nuggets of information.

I wish to also thank the many graduate students who, over the years, have contributed to the Theoretical Foundations of Family Medicine course in the Graduate Studies program of the Department of Family Medicine, here at Western. This program and, specifically, this course were founded by Ian McWhinney. It has attracted graduate students from around the world. The conversations that take place in this course, in seminars and online, have been a constant source of stimulation and impetus for refinement of the concepts of this book.

Many readers helped to improve various chapters and I wish to acknowledge their contributions, while emphasizing that any errors or omissions are my responsibility. Dr. Stephen Wetmore's comments on the chapters on Respiratory Illness and Musculoskeletal Pain were very helpful in improving those chapters. Dr. David Haslam provided important comments and conversations on Depression. Lauren Gurland, at the time a second-year medical student, worked diligently on the chapter on Diabetes, and Joan Mitchell

RN(EC), NP-PHC, provided very useful critical comments. Dr. Sonja Reichert provided important references and comments on the same chapter. The chapter on Obesity was critically reviewed by Dr. Helena Piccinini-Vallis and Kim Sandiland RD, and their comments provided me with greater understanding and improved the chapter. Canada is fortunate to have one of the leading researchers in Multimorbidity in Dr. Martin Fortin, who critiqued that chapter. The chapter on Stewardship of Resources, Patient Information, and Data was critically reviewed by Drs. Amanda Terry and Sonny Cejic. Dr. Moira Stewart was of great assistance in the chapter on Research.

I am very grateful to Andrea Burt for using her considerable experience and knowledge on manuscript preparation on this book.

Thank you to Rebecca Suzan, Associate Editor, Medicine, at Oxford University Press for her support in shepherding this book to fruition.

PART I

Basic Principles

CHAPTER 1

◊

The Origins of Family Medicine

The profound changes now occurring in medicine can only be fully understood if they are viewed from the perspective of history. There is nothing new about change: medicine has been changing constantly since its beginnings. Only the pace is different.

Medicine changes in response to many influences, some scientific and technological, some social. Family medicine is only one of many new disciplines that have developed in the course of medical history. New disciplines arise in a number of ways: some—such as surgery and obstetrics—have developed from ancient craft skills; some have grown up around new techniques, such as otolaryngology in the nineteenth century and anesthesiology in the twentieth; others have been formed because some area of need, such as child health, was being neglected by existing disciplines. All these influences have played their part in the recent growth of family medicine. Social changes, specialization, and a new pattern of illness have demanded a new type of physician; science has given us new insights into some old problems; and existing disciplines have tended to neglect the problems encountered in family practice.

New disciplines can begin in three ways: by transformation from an older discipline, de novo, or by fragmentation from a larger discipline. Family medicine has evolved from an older branch of medicine—general practice. The relationship, however, is not a simple one; we will be returning to it later. Let us now look in more detail at some modern trends that have influenced the development of family medicine.

CHANGES IN MORTALITY AND MORBIDITY

Epidemiology is the study of the distribution of health-related events such as diseases and death in a population for the purpose of attempting to control health problems (Porta, 2008). As human cultural, economic, and environmental changes occur, so too do morbidity and mortality patterns. These changes are referred to as epidemiological transitions (Fried and Gaydos, 2012). As human societies moved from being foraging based to agriculturally based, new diseases arose with the domestication of animals. As urbanization became more widespread, communicable diseases such as cholera, measles, smallpox, and others occurred in epidemic proportions and significantly impacted population health and longevity. This is referred to as the first epidemiological transition.

The successful control of the major infectious diseases, which ravaged even the most advanced countries until the earlier years of the twentieth century, has been followed in countries with a high standard of living by the emergence of a new pattern of disease. Instead of severe acute illnesses such as typhoid, lobar pneumonia, and diphtheria, the physician[1] is now faced mostly with chronic diseases, developmental disorders, behavioral disorders, accidents, and a different range of infectious diseases. The reduced mortality in children and adults has, with each succeeding generation, increased the proportion of elderly people in society.

This new pattern has produced a gradual change in the role of the practitioner. A person afflicted with one of the great mortal infections either died or recovered in a comparatively short period of time, usually within weeks. A person afflicted with a chronic disorder is often engaged in a prolonged struggle to adapt to his or her environment. Rather than dealing with acute life-or-death situations, therefore, today's practitioners are more likely to find themselves helping patients to achieve a new equilibrium with their environment in the face of chronic illness and disability.

Therapeutic approaches to chronic disorders call for an understanding of both the patient and the environment. Because many of the situations facing the physician are complex combinations of physical and behavioral factors, the conventional separation of physical and mental illness becomes unrealistic. The practice of preventive medicine has also changed. In a sense, we have moved from an era of public health to one of private health. The health of society depends less on new legislation than on millions of private decisions about matters as diverse as smoking, family planning, and immunization. In influencing these decisions, the physician's educational role has assumed new importance.

This is not to say that public health has ceased to be important. Clean water, a balanced diet, and good housing are still major determinants of health. There is still scope for improving public health by legislation in such areas as industrial hazards, smoking, environmental pollution, and traffic accidents. Some of our present threats to health, however, are beyond the reach of legislation.

A third epidemiological transition occurred with the re-emergence of infectious diseases facilitated by microbial resistance, rapid travel, globalization, technological change, the breakdown of public health, and consequences of ecological change brought about by deforestation, climate change, and other factors. Understanding the connection between these changes and the emergence of diseases such as Hantavirus and new strains of influenza is making plain the way in which health consists of an organism being in balance with the environment. This has necessitated moving from a mechanistic view to a more organic view of health and illness (see Chapter 6, "Philosophical and Scientific Foundations of Family Medicine").

The preceding remarks apply largely to developed, industrial societies. Much of the world's population still lives under conditions that have not existed in advanced countries since the nineteenth century. This means that the role of the family physician in such societies is different from his or her role in developed societies. These differences will be discussed in more detail later.

THE GROWTH OF SPECIALIZATION

A brief review of the development of the modern medical profession will help put our present position in perspective. The profession as we know it has existed only since the nineteenth century. Before that time, society was served by a variety of healers, only a small proportion of whom were physicians. In the seventeenth and eighteenth centuries, physicians were a small and elite group of learned men, educated in the few universities. They practiced in towns among the rich and influential, did not perform surgery or dispense drugs, and did not associate, either professionally or socially, with the craftsmen and tradesmen who ministered to the medical needs of poorer and rural people. Surgeons were craftsmen who were trained by apprenticeship; apothecaries were tradesmen who originally dispensed and sold drugs but who, in response to need, gradually took on the role of medical practitioner.

Although some physicians were among the early immigrants to North America, there were not nearly enough to meet the needs of the population. The early colonies were served, therefore, by a great variety of practitioners. Because there were no medical schools until the founding of the school at Philadelphia in the 1760s, those who wished to become physicians had to study in Europe. Their numbers were not enough for the growing population: in eighteenth-century Virginia, for example, only one in nine practitioners had been trained as a physician (Boorstin, 1958).

For a long time, graduates returning from their studies in Europe tried to maintain their distinctiveness by refusing to practice surgery or dispense drugs. The American students at Edinburgh formed the Virginia Club, one of whose articles was "that every member of this club shall make it his endeavour, if possible, for the honour of his profession, not to degrade it by hereafter mingling the trade of an apothecary or surgeon with it." However, the heavy demand for services and the breakdown of old social barriers in the new colonies soon made these aspirations impossible to fulfill. Before long, all practitioners, whether graduates or not, were practicing as general practitioners. Thus was the general practitioner born in eighteenth-century America.

In Britain, meanwhile, the same historical process was occurring. By the beginning of the nineteenth century, the status of surgeons and apothecaries had risen substantially and their work had become increasingly medical. Edward Jenner (1749–1823), the discoverer of vaccination, was a country surgeon in the west of England. By the nineteenth century, surgical training had been improved, and surgeons took the examination for membership in the Royal College of Surgeons (MRCS) after a combination of apprenticeship and hospital training.

In 1815, the Apothecaries Act gave legal recognition to the right of apothecaries in Britain to give medical advice as well as to supply drugs. The Act made it compulsory for apothecaries to undergo a five-year apprenticeship and to take courses in anatomy, physiology, the practice of medicine, and *materia medica*. It also established a qualifying examination, the Licentiate of the Society of Apothecaries (LSA). It soon became customary for practitioners to take the double qualification (LSA and MRCS) and, when an examination in midwifery was added, the graduate was qualified to practice medicine, surgery, and midwifery.[2] The term "general practitioner" was first used in the *Lancet* early in the nineteenth century. Thus, the general practitioner, born in eighteenth-century America, was named in nineteenth-century Britain. By a slow process of response to social demands, surgeons and apothecaries were gradually integrated with physicians to form the modern medical profession. The process took many years to complete, and even in Victorian times, remnants of the old distinctions were clearly evident. George Eliot's *Middlemarch* and Anthony Trollope's *Dr. Thorne* provide fascinating glimpses of the life and work of a general practitioner in nineteenth-century England.

These historical events are not irrelevant to the position of the medical profession today. There are two lessons we would do well to ponder:

1. If the profession is failing to meet a public need, society will find some way of meeting the need, if necessary by turning to a group outside the profession.[3]
2. Professions evolve in response to social pressures, sometimes in ways that conflict with the expressed intentions of their members.

THE AGE OF THE GENERAL PRACTITIONER

In Europe and North America, the nineteenth century was the age of the general practitioner. On both continents, most members of the profession were general practitioners, and there was little differentiation of function, even among the faculties of medical schools. Toward the end of the century, however, the major specialties began to emerge. Osler's address "Remarks on Specialism" (1892) was given to mark the origin of pediatrics as a separate discipline. At the same time, progress in the sciences—chemistry, physics, physiology, and bacteriology—was beginning to have an impact on medicine. Medical education, especially in North America, was divorced from the scientific foundations of medicine, and much of it was of very poor quality. In his report in 1910, Abraham Flexner described appalling conditions in many of the hundreds of small medical schools that existed in the United States and Canada. Even the time-honored apprenticeship system had fallen into abeyance. North America had an ample supply of doctors, both in town and country, but they were little prepared for the technological revolution that was about to transform medicine.

The founding of Johns Hopkins in 1889 was a landmark in the development of medicine in North America. The aim of its founders—Osler, Halsted, Hurd, Welch, and Kelly—was to place medical education on a firm scientific foundation. From the beginning, the faculty consisted entirely of specialists. In his proposals for reform, Flexner used Johns Hopkins and the German medical schools as his models. The Flexner reforms in the years between 1910 and 1930 paved the way for the next stage: the age of specialization.

THE AGE OF SPECIALIZATION

The first half of the twentieth century saw the emergence of the major specialties of medicine, each with its defined training program and its qualifying examination. Technological progress was rapid, and investment in research produced good dividends. Medical education became increasingly oriented toward laboratory science and the technology of medicine. The increasing prestige accorded to specialists and the valuation of technical and research skills over personal care made general practice unpopular as a career.

The number of general practitioners declined steadily from the 1930s, both in absolute terms and as a proportion of the profession as a whole. The process was accelerated by the virtual disappearance of general practitioners from medical faculties after World War II and by the fragmentation of the major specialties that began to occur in the 1950s.

Since the 1960s, it has become customary to distinguish between three kinds of service provided by physicians, corresponding to three levels of health care. At the primary level, generalist or primary care physicians provide continuing personal and comprehensive care. The physicians may be general practitioners or physicians limiting their practice to adults or children. At the secondary level, specialists provide care only to patients with disorders in their field of expertise, usually by referral from primary care physicians. The tertiary level comprises highly specialized services often available only in regional centers.

The fragmentation of the profession and the emphasis on technology have had one other serious effect: a deterioration of the patient–doctor relationship. More than 60 years ago, Flexner (1930) realized that something had been lost as well as gained by the reform of medical education. In his book *Universities, American, English and German*, he wrote: "the very intensity with which scientific medicine is cultivated threatens to cost us at times the mellow judgement and broad culture of the older generation at its best. Osler, Janeway, and Halsted have not been replaced. (p. 93)" This neglect of the caring and personal aspects of medicine is now beginning to have consequences, such as the increase in malpractice suits and a growing disenchantment with technology.

As the age of specialization reaches its culmination, therefore, we can see the need for a new kind of generalist. The new generalists, however, must be different from the old general practitioners. Instead of being the undifferentiated bulk of the profession, defined chiefly by lack of special training and qualifications, they now have a well-differentiated role and a defined set of skills. In the United States, the requirements for the new generalist were set out in two key reports: *The Graduate Education of Physicians* (Millis, 1966) and *Meeting the Challenges of Family Practice* (Willard, 1966). It is no coincidence that parallel changes have taken place in Canada, the United Kingdom, Holland, Australia, and other industrialized countries.

One response to the decline in general practice was the formation in the 1950s and 1960s of colleges and academies of general practice in a number of countries. The first postgraduate training programs[4] were established and much progress was made in defining the curriculum and designing examinations. At this time, the first academic chairs were established in Britain, Canada, the Netherlands, and the United States, and family medicine was introduced into the undergraduate curriculum. In 1972 the World Organization of National Colleges and Academies of General Practice/Family Medicine (WONCA) was formed.[5]

NEW DEVELOPMENTS IN THE BEHAVIORAL SCIENCES

The study of human behavior has always been important to general practitioners. In the past, however, insights have been gained intuitively rather than by an organized approach to problems. Recent developments in behavioral and social science have been important to medicine as a whole, but particularly to family medicine.

Behavioral science has directed our attention to the process by which people seek medical care, a crucial area for all primary care physicians. It has
made physicians themselves the objects of study, thus making them more
aware of the importance of their own behavior in determining the quality of
care, for example, in decision-making and prescribing. It has increased physicians' insights into the patient–doctor relationship, family relationships, and
the behavioral aspects of illness. It has made us think about some of the fundamental aspects of medicine, such as our concepts of health, disease, and
illness, the role of the physician, and the ethics of medicine. It has brought
to our attention the large portion of the iceberg of hidden illness normally
not seen by the medical profession. Finally, it has increased our knowledge of
behavioral and social factors involved in the causation of disease.

The situation with behavioral science is analogous to that of chemistry and
physiology over a century ago. A new body of knowledge demanded integration
with medicine, and integration was eventually achieved, partly by changes in
curriculum, but mainly by changes in clinical practice introduced by clinicians
who had mastered the new knowledge. In the same way, new knowledge from
the behavioral sciences will be integrated with medicine through changes in
clinical practice. As generalist clinicians practicing a patient-centered clinical
method, family physicians are in a key position to make this synthesis.

THE CHANGING ROLE OF THE HOSPITAL

Another factor in the development of family medicine has been the resurgence of interest in health care outside the hospital. The cost of inpatient
care has become so prohibitive that criteria for admission to hospitals have
become increasingly strict. The acute care hospital seems to be evolving into
an institution where only those patients needing highly technical and specialized care are treated, either as inpatients or as outpatients in specialized
clinics. For those who need care for a variety of problems over a long period of
time, the hospital is a much less satisfactory form of care. A large institution
can hardly avoid the fragmentation of care and frequent changes of personnel
that are the antithesis of integrated, personal medicine. There are also some
risks associated with hospitalization, especially for the elderly.

The practice of medicine outside the hospital, particularly at the neighborhood level, has assumed a new importance. We can now see that the overwhelming concentration of care in the hospital during the past few decades
has been a mistaken emphasis. The need during the next few decades is for
a balanced system in which personal and continuing care will be available for
all at the neighborhood level, while the hospital provides specialized support when it is needed. In some healthcare systems, including some managed

care organizations in the United States, primary care physicians do not have responsibility for inpatient care, except in a supportive role.

MANAGED CARE AND THE AGE OF INTEGRATION

In the present age we continue to see the rapid reorganization of health care in response to economic forces. The division of services into three levels—primary, secondary, and tertiary—has proved to be highly effective, validating the work done on vocational training for family medicine in the preceding decades. At its 1978 conference in Alma-Ata, the World Health Organization recognized the fundamental importance of primary care (World Health Organization, 1978).

The well-trained family doctor has become a key figure, and often a leader, in the organization of health care. At the same time, the integration of services has become essential to conserve resources and to eliminate waste. Horizontally, integration is achieved by family doctors working as team members with other health professionals and in collaboration with community support services. Vertical integration is achieved by collaboration between the three levels of care, as in hospital discharge planning.

One form of the reorganization of health care has been managed care in its various forms. A managed care organization is one that takes on the financial budget and is responsible for coordinating a full spectrum of clinical services. Health service or maintenance organizations (HMOs) and groups organized by physicians are examples of managed care in the United States. In countries with national health services, such as Canada and Britain, the responsibility for financing and providing services rests with government. Within an organization, some of the risk may be transferred to smaller groups of physicians caring for defined populations.[6]

In the United States, the role of the family physician in HMOs is sometimes described as that of a gatekeeper. The name, unfortunately, has taken on the negative connotation of a person who tries to keep people out. There are, however, many positive aspects of the role. The gatekeeper can also be described as the person who makes others welcome, meets many of their needs, and guides them through the system. The division of function between primary- and secondary-care physicians enables both groups to do what they do best. Primary care physicians help specialists maintain their skills by allowing them to concentrate their experience on the patients whose problems come within their field of expertise.

Although managed care provides primary care physicians with great opportunities, the rapid pace of change and the loss of independence can be very unsettling. As physicians become more involved in financial management, they may find themselves in conflicts of interest between the needs of their patients and the requirements of the organization.

Dissatisfaction with some aspects of managed care, such as restricted access to services through utilization review, restrictions on what providers were covered, and capitation, has led to a turning away from some forms of managed care. In some countries, including the United States, these and other issues became intensely political as managed care tried to ". . . navigate the tensions between limited resources and unlimited expectations without explaining exactly how it was so doing" (Robinson, 2001, p. 2623). Insurance companies, the medical profession, and government all proved unable or unwilling to attempt to navigate these shoals. At the same time, an increasingly sophisticated and Internet-savvy populace began to take center stage.

Although virtually all nations encountered the same issues of cost control (made more acute by economic uncertainty following the Great Recession of 2008), rising expectations, new technology, and an aging population, the particular solutions varied, reflecting historical and cultural imperatives. In the United States, maintaining individual autonomy and choice were more essential than in some other countries with a history of greater acceptance of government influence. The social upheavals of the 1960s were reflected in the late twentieth and early twenty-first centuries in the general questioning of authority, the women's health movement, minority rights, and the popularity of complementary and alternative medicine.

The ubiquity of information easily obtained on the Internet has been another factor in shifting healthcare decisions from the medical profession, insurance companies, and government to the individual. However, this practice is not without its drawbacks, principally consisting of the variability in the quality and accuracy of information gleaned from the Internet and the challenges in integrating and acting upon it in an increasingly complex healthcare system. It is in this context that having a personal physician has taken on greater importance.

The concept of a personal physician was not new (Fox, 1960; Folsom, 1966), but as the shortcomings of specialist care became more apparent, so too did the need for a trusted confidant with the knowledge and skills necessary to assist individuals in integrating medical knowledge with their own personal circumstances and values. The personal physician is the basis of many versions of healthcare reform, such as the Patient-Centered Medical Home model in the United States (see Chapter 19). These factors, combined with rising hospital costs and the availability of mobile technology, mean that more health care takes place in the community.

Because clinical education must follow the patient, this shift toward care in the community must lead eventually to a change in the clinical curriculum.

Logically, medical students should be based in primary-care institutions, where they can experience the long-term care of patients near where they and their families live and work. Some of their specialty experience can be obtained in the same setting, where family physicians, specialists, and other health professionals are increasingly collaborating. For other aspects of their education in the specialties, students can be seconded to the acute care hospital.[7]

GENERAL PRACTICE OR FAMILY MEDICINE

At the time of the revival of general practice, there was a move to change its name to "family practice" or to "family medicine," and to refer to general practitioners as family physicians. Thus, the new Board in the United States was named the Board of Family Practice. The Academy of General Practice became the Academy of Family Practice. In Canada, the College of General Practitioners changed its name to the College of Family Physicians.

The reasons for this change were mixed. On the one hand, there was the feeling that the name "general practice" had become associated with an obsolete type of medicine. On the other hand, there was a wish to emphasize that family practice was something new and different from general practice. Also, there was the need to find a name for the body of knowledge, the new clinical discipline, that was being defined.

The change of name did have some repercussions. Many general practitioners had been providing exemplary care and were functioning in precisely the way expected of the new family physicians. Family medicine was based on the best of general practice. It was sometimes difficult to explain exactly what was different about family medicine. Some existing general practitioners also felt offended by the implication that what they were doing was somehow inferior.

In the new academic departments, the change of name was viewed differently by different people. To some, using the term "family" meant that the new body of knowledge was about the family and health, and that this was what made family practice unique among clinical disciplines. To others, "family physician" was the revival of a time-honored title, used for many years as an alternative to "general practitioner." The term "family medicine" then became the name of the body of knowledge on which family practice is based, a body of knowledge that includes the family, but much else besides. The latter is the point of view we have taken, and in this book we have used the terms "family physician" and "general practitioner" interchangeably. "Family medicine" is the term we use for the body of knowledge on which their practice is based.

FAMILY MEDICINE AS A CLINICAL
AND ACADEMIC DISCIPLINE

Clinical disciplines in medicine are based on a number of factors, some epistemological, some practical and administrative. An epistemological basis for a discipline is a consensus among its members about the important problems confronting the discipline, and the knowledge appropriate for dealing with them (from the Greek *episteme*, meaning "knowledge"). In a clinical discipline this will include a common experience of clinical problems and an agreed-upon clinical method, as well as an agreement about an agenda for research. For a discipline to be truly independent, there should be some research questions that can only be addressed from inside the discipline. Even if methods are borrowed from other disciplines, only a practitioner inside the discipline can know the context in which the methods are applied, especially the methodological pitfalls. An epistemological basis also implies an agreement about what knowledge of the discipline is, and how it is acquired. As Kuhn (1970) has observed, members of a discipline also share a worldview, much of it at the unconscious level.

We believe that family medicine is a clinical discipline as we have described it. It would not be true to say that there is complete agreement on all the questions noted in the preceding section. As Kuhn, again, has observed, disagreements do occur at certain stages in a discipline's development. Psychiatry has become a major clinical discipline without ever having resolved some fundamental issues. Even allowing for these disagreements, we are impressed, in talking to family physicians from many parts of the world, the extent to which they do share the same worldview, molded by the same experience of medicine.

Some have doubted whether family medicine is a discipline in its own right, because it shares so much with other primary-care disciplines, notably primary-care internal medicine. These doubts have prompted a search for uniqueness in the idea of "the family as patient." The fact that we share a worldview with another discipline need not concern us. If an internist is providing primary, comprehensive, and continuing care to adult families, with the same epistemological base as a family physician, then he is, for all intents and purposes, a family physician. We must not confuse things with the names we call them by. Our own view is that primary-care internal medicine and family medicine in the United States are now so close that they could come together as a single discipline. The obstacles to this are not epistemological, but administrative and political. It is not unusual in medicine for divisions between disciplines to be administrative rather than epistemological. Whether pediatric cardiology belongs to pediatrics or cardiology and whether psychogeriatrics belongs to psychiatry or geriatrics are questions likely to be resolved on administrative grounds, perhaps differently in different institutions. We should not make too much of the divisions between disciplines, in medicine or in any other field. On this subject Karl Popper (1972), the philosopher of science, has written:

> But subject matter, or kinds of things, do not, I hold, constitute a basis for distinguishing disciplines. Disciplines are distinguished partly for historical reasons and reasons of administrative convenience . . . and partly because the theories we construct to solve our problems have a tendency to grow into unified systems. But all this classification and distinction is a comparatively superficial affair. We are not students of some subject matter but students of problems. And problems may cut right across the borders of any subject matter or discipline (p. 112).

Family medicine could have developed as a division of internal medicine. The reasons that it did not are as much historical and administrative as they are epistemological. By the early decades of the twentieth century, internists had ceased to see children and to do gynecology. At the same time, in many countries, internal medicine had become functionally differentiated from general practice. By the 1950s, when family medicine began to develop as a discipline, the leadership of academic internal medicine, with few exceptions, did not see the problems raised by family medicine as important. Internal medicine at that time was focusing its attention on the laboratory, rather than on purely clinical observation or on behavioral and population studies. There is no reason for thinking that this direction for internal medicine was inappropriate. It did, however, leave an entire range of problems unattended to, and family medicine was the appropriate discipline to attend to them.

As an academic discipline, family medicine has made exceptional strides in the past 50 years. Journals devoted to family medicine began in the 1950s with the advent of national colleges of general practice. Academic departments arose in many medical schools in the late 1960s and early 1970s, and with that more journals were published, so that by 2010, there were 19 in the English language alone and many more in other languages. Textbooks, too, proliferated; by 2010 there were at least 400 devoted to family medicine or primary care published in English. In addition to the research found in these sources, many family physician researchers publish in other medical journals and books. Collectively, these writings represent the evolving knowledge base of the discipline.

Since its founding as an academic discipline, family medicine has made many unique contributions to both the theory and practice of medicine in general (Freeman, 2012). Among these contributions are the following:

1. Emphasizing the importance of understanding the subjective experience of illness in the patient.
2. Drawing attention to the role played by context, both proximal (such as family and occupation) and distal (such as neighborhood and environment) in health and illness.
3. Emphasizing the humanities in medicine. Of course, family medicine is not alone in this, but many faculty members of departments of family medicine have made great contributions to raising the issue of a more humane approach to medicine to counterbalance the increasingly technological or instrumental approach to health care.
4. Family medicine pays attention to the marginalized in society. Perhaps because they practice in the community, family physicians are more aware of the effects of unmet needs. Family medicine faculty are often the leaders in schools of medicine in establishing and maintaining equity in the universities and surrounding communities.
5. Discussion of healing takes place in family medicine, a concept that too often feels alien in academic health sciences centers, where curing is more often the unspoken and utopian goal.
6. The patient-centered clinical method (Stewart et al., 2014) arose in and from family practice. It was defined, its effects on outcomes were investigated, and methods for teaching it were developed all within academic family medicine. Its principles and practice have been widely adopted throughout medicine and other healthcare disciplines, and a rich literature has developed to refine and advance its use.

NOTES

1. In Britain, Australia, New Zealand, and South Africa, the term "physician" is equivalent to "internist" in North America. In the United States and Canada, "physician" is a generic term for all medical practitioners. In this book we have used it in its generic sense.
2. The gradual absorption of apothecaries into the medical profession could conceivably have a modern parallel. If nurse practitioners assume more functions at present regarded as "medical," they may eventually be redefined as physicians.
3. The growing use of alternative medicine could be interpreted as a response to some of medicine's shortcomings.
4. An early pioneer of postgraduate training for general practice was Dr. Andrija Stamper of the former Yugoslavia.
5. WONCA has advanced the international development of family medicine and primary care in projects such as the International Classification of Primary Care (1987) and its Statement on the Role of the Family/General Practitioner in Health Care Systems (1988).
6. For a more detailed discussion of managed care, see Chapter 19.

7. A vision of the medical school is provided by the report of the Pew-Fetzer Task Force (Tresolini CP and the Pew-Fetzer Task Force, *Health Professions Education and Relationship-Centered Care*, San Francisco, CA: Pew Health Professions Commission, 1994).

REFERENCES

Boorstin DJ. 1958. *The Americans: The Colonial Experience*. New York: Random House.

Flexner A. 1910. *Medical Education in the United States and Canada: A Report to the Carnegie Foundation for the Advancement of Teaching*. The Carnegie Foundation for the Advancement of Teaching. New York.

Flexner, A. 1930. *Universities, American, English and German*. New York: Oxford University Press.

Folsom MB. 1966. *National Commission on Community Health Services: Health Is a Community Affair*. Cambridge, MA: Harvard University Press.

Fox TF. 1960. The personal doctor and his relation to the hospital. *The Lancet* 2:743–760.

Freeman T. 2012. Family medicine's academic contributions. *Turk Aile Hek Derg* 16(4):181–198.

Fried BJ, Gaydos LM (eds). 2012. *World Health Systems: Challenges and Perspectives*, 2nd edition. Chicago: Health Administration Press.

Kuhn TS. 1970. *The Structure of Scientific Revolutions*. Chicago, IL: University of Chicago Press.

Millis JS (chairman). 1966. *The Graduate Education of Physicians: Report of the Citizens Committee on Graduate Medical Education*. American Medical Association. Chicago, Illinois.

Osler W. 1892. Remarks on specialism. *Archives of Paediatrics* 9:481.

Popper KR. 1972. *Conjectures and Refutations*, 4th edition. London: Routledge and Kegan Paul.

Porta M. 2008. *A Dictionary of Epidemiology*, 5th edition. Oxford; New York: Oxford University Press.

Robinson JC. 2001. The end of managed care. *JAMA* 285(20):2622–2628.

Stewart M, Brown JB, Weston WW, McWhinney IR, McWilliam C, Freeman TR. 2014. *Patient-Centered Medicine: Transforming the Clinical Method*, 3rd edition. Oxford: Radcliffe Press.

Willard RD (chairman). 1966. *Meeting the Challenges of Family Practice: Report of the Ad Hoc Committee on Education for Family Practice of the Council on Medical Education*. American Medical Association. Chicago, Illinois.

World Health Organization. 1978. *Alma-Ata 1978: Primary Health Care*. Geneva: World Health Organization.

CHAPTER 2

☙

Principles of Family Medicine

Family medicine can be described as a body of knowledge about the problems encountered by family physicians. This is, of course, a tautology, but then so are the descriptions of all applied subjects. As in other practical disciplines, the body of knowledge encompassed by family medicine includes not only factual knowledge but also skills and techniques. Members of a clinical discipline are identifiable not so much by what they know as by what they do. Surgeons, for example, are identifiable more by their skill in diagnosing and treating "surgical" diseases than by any particular knowledge of anatomy, pathology, or clinical medicine. What they do is a matter of their mindset, their values and attitudes, and the principles that govern their actions.

In describing family medicine, therefore, it is best to start with the principles that govern our actions. We will describe nine of them. None is unique to family medicine. Not all family physicians exemplify the entire nine. Nevertheless, when taken together, they do represent a distinctive worldview—a system of values and an approach to problems—that is identifiably different from that of other disciplines.

1. Family physicians are committed to the person rather than to a particular body of knowledge, group of diseases, or special technique. The commitment is open-ended in two senses. First, it is not limited by the type of health problem. Family physicians are available for any health problem in a person of either sex and of any age. Their practice is not even limited to strictly defined health problems: the patient defines the problem. This means that a family physician can never say, "I am sorry, but your illness is not in my field." Any health problem in one of our patients is in our field. We may have to refer the patient for specialized treatment, but we are still responsible for the initial assessment and for the coordination and continuity of care. Second, the commitment has no defined endpoint. It is not

terminated by the cure of an illness, the end of a course of treatment, or the incurability of an illness. In many cases the commitment is made while the person is healthy, before any problem has developed. In other words, family medicine defines itself in terms of relationships, making it unique among major fields of clinical medicine. The full implications of this difference are discussed in the section "The Doctor's Work" later in this chapter.

2. The family physician seeks to understand the context of the illness. "To understand a thing rightly, we need to see it both out of its environment and in it, and to have acquaintance with the whole range of its variations," wrote the American philosopher William James (1958). Many illnesses cannot be fully understood unless they are seen in their personal, family, and social context. When a patient is admitted to the hospital, much of the context of the illness is removed or obscured. Attention seems to be focused on the foreground rather than the background, often resulting in a limited picture of the illness.

3. The family physician sees every contact with his or her patients as an opportunity for the prevention of disease or the promotion of health. Because family physicians, on the average, see each of their patients about four times a year, this is a rich source of opportunities for practicing preventive medicine.

4. The family physician views his or her practice as a "population at risk." Clinicians think normally in terms of single patients rather than population groups. Family physicians must think in terms of both. This means that patients who have not attended for such procedures as immunization, Papanicolaou smears, or blood pressure tests are as much a concern as those who are attending regularly. Electronic records make it very easy to maintain up-to-date attendance records of the entire practice population.

5. The family physician sees himself or herself as part of a community-wide network of supportive and healthcare agencies. All communities have a network of social supports, official and unofficial, formal and informal. The word *network* suggests a coordinated system. Until recently, this has often not been the case. Too often, family physicians, hospital doctors, medical officers of health, home care nurses, social workers, and others have worked in watertight compartments without a grasp of the system as a whole. At the time of writing, many jurisdictions are in the process of reforming family practice as a key link in the network, which will enable patients to benefit from whichever provider they require.

6. Ideally, family physicians should share the same habitat as their patients. In recent years, this has become less common, except in rural areas. Even here, the commuting doctor has made an appearance. In some communities, notably the central areas of large cities, doctors have virtually disappeared. This has all been part of the recent trend toward the separation of life and work. To Wendell Berry (1978), this is the cause of many modern ills: "If we

do not live where we work, and when we work," he writes, "we are wasting our lives, and our work too." The Love Canal disaster in Niagara Falls provides a vivid illustration of what can happen when physicians are remote from the environment of their patients. This abandoned canal had been used by a local industry for the disposal of toxic waste products. The canal was then covered over and, some years later, houses were built on the site. During the 1960s, householders began to notice that chemical sludge was seeping into their basements and gardens. Trees and shrubs died, and the atmosphere became polluted by malodorous fumes. About the same time, residents in the neighborhood began to suffer from illnesses caused by the toxic chemicals. It was not, however, until a local journalist did a health survey in the area that an official health study was done. This showed rates of illness, miscarriage, and birth defects far in excess of the norm (Brown, 1979). How did the cluster of illnesses in an obviously polluted environment escape the notice of local physicians? One can only assume that they treated patients without seeing them in their home environment. It is difficult to believe that a neighborhood family physician, visiting patients in their homes and interested in their environment, would have remained unaware of the problem for so long. To be fully effective, a family physician still needs to be a visible presence in the neighborhood.

7. The family physician sees patients in their homes. Until modern times, attending patients in their homes was one of the deepest experiences of family practice. It was in the home that many of the great events of life took place: being born, dying, enduring or recovering from serious illness. Being present with the family at these events gave family doctors much of their knowledge of patients and their families. Knowing the home gave us a tacit understanding of the context or ecology of illness. *Ecology*, derived from two Greek words, *oikos* (home) and *logos*, means literally "study of the home." The rise of the modern hospital removed much of this experience from the home. There were technical advantages and gains in efficiency, but the price was some impoverishment of the experience of family practice. The current redefinition of the hospital's role is now changing the balance again, and we have the opportunity to restore home care as one of the defining experiences and essential skills of family medicine. The family physician should be a natural ecologist (see Chapter 17). At the time of writing, a shortage of general practitioners (GPs) has made it difficult for practices to visit their patients in need. At the same time, there are new reasons for attending housebound patients. Hospitals are dangerous for the elderly, who are susceptible to hospital infections and rapid deterioration from the change of environment. Attending patients with short-term illnesses prevents patients from spreading or acquiring diseases in emergency rooms and doctors' offices. Advances in technology have made point-of-care diagnosis and therapy much easier than before.

8. The family physician attaches importance to the subjective aspects of medicine. For many years, medicine has been dominated by a strictly objective and positivistic approach to health problems. For family physicians, this has always had to be reconciled with a sensitivity to feelings and an insight into relationships. Insight into relationships requires knowledge of emotions, including our own emotions. Hence, family medicine should be a self-reflective practice (see Chapter 6).

9. The family physician is a manager of resources. As generalists and first-contact physicians, they have control of large resources and are able, within certain limits, to control admission to hospital, use of investigations, prescription of treatment, and referral to specialists. In all parts of the world, resources are limited, sometimes severely limited. It is, therefore, the responsibility of family physicians to manage these resources for the benefit of their patients and for the community as a whole (for more on stewardship of resources, see Chapter 18). In certain cases, the interests of an individual patient may conflict with those of the community as a whole, and this can raise ethical issues.

IMPLICATIONS OF THE PRINCIPLES

Defining our discipline in terms of relationships sets it apart from most other fields of medicine. It is more usual to define a field in terms of content— diseases, organ systems, or technologies. Clinicians in other fields form relationships with patients, but in general practice the relationship is usually *prior* to content. We know people before we know what their illnesses will be. It is, of course, possible to define a content of general practice, based on the common conditions presented to family physicians at a particular time and place. But strictly speaking, the content for a particular doctor is whatever conditions his or her patients happen to have. One of the consequences of this is that family physicians' practices frequently have a low prevalence of many rare diseases (e.g., Charcot-Marie-Tooth disease, myasthenia gravis). This means that sometimes an individual practitioner will become knowledgeable about individual rare diseases, especially in the way that they affect his or her patients. Other relationships also define our work. By caring for members of a family, the family doctor may become part of the complex of family relationships, and many of us share with our patients the same community and habitat.

Defining our field in these terms has consequences, both positive and negative. Not to be tied to a particular technology or set of diseases is liberating. It gives general practice a quality of unexpectedness and flexibility in adapting to change. On the other hand, it is poorly understood in a society that seems to place less and less value on relationships and that emphasizes brief episodic encounters. In current society, many equate the idea of specialization with progress itself, though this concept is not without its critics. According to Wright, "As cultures grow more elaborate, and technologies more powerful, they themselves become ponderous specializations—vulnerable and, in extreme cases, deadly."[1] One major consequence of the family medicine worldview is that we cannot be comfortable with the mechanical metaphor that dominates medicine, or with the mind/body dualism derived from it. Another is that the value we place on relationships influences our valuation of knowledge. Those who value relationships tend to know the world by experience rather than by what Charles Taylor (1991) calls "instrumental" and "disengaged" reason. Experience engages our feelings as well as our intellect. The emotions play a very significant part in family practice.

Long-term relationships lead to a buildup of particular knowledge about patients, much of it at the tacit level. Because caring for patients is about attention to detail, this knowledge of particulars is of great value when it comes to care. On the other hand, it can make us somewhat ambivalent about classifying patients into disease categories. "Yes," we might say, "this patient has borderline personality disorder but he is also John Smith, for whom I have cared for fifteen years." On the whole, our tendency to think in terms of individual patients more than abstractions is a strength, though it can lead us astray if it diverts us from the appropriate pursuit of diagnostic precision. Our valuation of particular knowledge, however, can make it difficult for us to feel comfortable in the modern academic milieu, where diagnosis and management are more usually seen in terms of generalizations than particulars. The risk of living too much in a world of generalizations and abstractions is detachment from the patient's experience and a lack of feeling for his suffering. Abstraction produces accounts of experience that, for all their generalizing power, are stripped of their affective coloring and are far removed from the realities of life. The ideal for all physicians is an integration of the two kinds of knowledge: an ability to see the universal in the particular.

The most significant difference between family medicine and most other clinical disciplines is that it transcends the mind/body division that runs through medicine like a geological fault line. Most clinical disciplines lie on one side or the other: internal medicine, surgery, and pediatrics on one side; psychiatry, child psychiatry, and psychogeriatrics on the other. Separate taxonomies of disease lie on either side: textbooks of medicine and surgery on one, the *Diagnostic and Statistical Manual of Mental Disorders* on the other. Therapies are divided into the physical and the psychological. In clinical practice, internists and surgeons do not normally explore the emotions, psychiatrists do not usually examine the body. Because family medicine defines itself in terms of relationships, it cannot divide in this way.[2]

One of the legacies of the mind/body division is a clinical method that excludes attention to the emotions as an essential feature of diagnosis and management. Another is the neglect in medical education of the emotional development of physicians. A contemporary writer has referred to the "stunted emotions" of physicians (Price, 1994). We may be seeing the consequences of this neglect in the alienation of patients from physicians, the widespread criticism of medical care, the turning to alternatives to allopathic medicine (see Chapter 23), and the high levels of emotional distress among physicians.

Because family medicine transcends the "fault line," the conventional clinical method has never been well suited to family practice. Perhaps this is why the initiatives to reform the clinical method have often come from family medicine. The most important difference of the patient-centered clinical method is that attention to the emotions is a requirement. Family medicine has also emerged as one of the most self-reflective of disciplines.

With developments in cognitive science and psychoneuroimmunology, and the high prevalence of illness that does not lie on one side or the other, the fault line is likely to become increasingly redundant. As medicine strives to achieve a new synthesis, it could learn much from our experience.

CONFLICTING ROLES

Hidden among the principles are some potential conflicts between the family doctor's roles and responsibilities. The first principle is one of commitment to the individual patient, to respond to any problem the patient may bring. It is the patient who defines the problem. According to the third principle (responsibility for prevention), it is usually the doctor who defines the problem, often in situations where the patient has come for an entirely different purpose. It may be argued that anticipatory medicine is part of good clinical practice. Taking the blood pressure is part of the general clinical assessment, and if the diastolic pressure is 120 mm Hg, good preventive and clinical practice requires that the problem be attended to, even if the patient has no symptoms related to high blood pressure and has only come because of a tension headache.

The issue becomes more complex as one moves along the continuum from the presymptomatic detection of disease to the identification of risk factors arising from a patient's habits and way of life. The number of risk factors increases and the reduction of risk involves behavioral changes that may be very difficult to attain. All this may be successfully integrated with clinical practice, and may actually be demanded by a public who are educated to expect anticipatory care. At some point, however, an emphasis on anticipatory care may compete for time and resources with care based on responding to problems identified by patients. Striking the right balance may be difficult if physicians are constrained either by requirements of managed care or by funding arrangements designed to emphasize anticipatory care.

The fourth principle (the practice as a population at risk) adds another dimension. Here, the focus is switched from the individual to the group. The measure of success is statistical. The motivation may be to extend effective care to all patients in the practice, especially those who may not be aware of its availability. The other extreme, however, is to judge success by the magnitude of adherence in the practice population. If funding is dependent on certain targets, outreach to the practice population may compete for time and resources with other practice services, and there may be pressure on patients to adhere to recommendations. The demand on practice resources may be increased by approaches aimed at identifying unmet needs in the geographic area of the practice, and of conducting audits requiring expensive epidemiological methods. Too much emphasis on the population approach, at the expense of meeting the needs of individual patients, may, as Toon (1994) suggests, have an effect on the orientation and thought patterns of the physicians. Rather than thinking about their patients, they may find themselves preoccupied with their figures.

The ninth principle (management of resources) may also become the source of conflict if a practice becomes responsible for managing and paying for all the services needed by its enrolled patients. The time necessary for management may reduce the time for patient care, and conflicts of interest may arise when an individual patient's interest conflicts with the interests of the group, or if the doctor stands to gain from economies in expenditure.

Conflicting ideas on the roles of the family physician can make it difficult to agree on criteria of quality, especially at times of rapid social change like the present. Toon (1994) suggests that where there is already a strong tradition of general medical practice there may be an intuitive concept of good general practice that will eventually lead to a synthesis. The path to a synthesis will be easier if administrators and managers tread lightly in making changes that alter the balance between the doctors' responsibilities, especially those changes that can divert us from our traditional responsibilities to individual patients.

CONTINUITY OF CARE

For a discipline that defines itself in terms of relationships, continuity—in the sense of an enduring relationship between doctor and patient—is fundamental. Hennen (1975) has described five dimensions of continuity: interpersonal, chronological, geographic (continuity between sites: home, hospital, office), interdisciplinary (continuity in meeting a variety of needs, e.g., for obstetric care, surgical procedures), and informational (continuity through the medical records). We use *continuity* here in the sense of overall, direct, or coordinative responsibility for the different medical needs of the patient

(Hjortdahl, 1992a). The key word here is *responsibility*. Obviously the physician cannot be available at all times, nor can he or she carry out all the care a patient may need. The doctor is responsible for ensuring continuity of service by a competent deputy and for following through when some aspect of care is delegated to a consultant. Responsibility is the key in all important relationships.

On the basis of a sequence of studies from a number of perspectives, Veale (1995, 1996)[3] has described four types of general practice utilization. In the first, a consumer visits only one GP. In the second, all the visits are to one practice. In the third type, the consumer visits a variety of GPs for different purposes. One doctor may be seen because of proximity to place of work, another for proximity to home, or the selection of GP may depend on the nature and severity of the problem and the doctor's expertise. This type of utilization appeared to work well for consumers who take responsibility for coordinating their own care. In the fourth type of utilization, the consumers decide which doctor they will see on a visit-by-visit basis, with no expectation that there will be continuity of care from any of them.

There was strong preference, by both consumers and doctors, for the first type of utilization. Three benefits were associated with visits to one GP: coordination of care, familiarity and openness in the therapeutic relationship, and the opportunity for monitoring of treatment and mutual agreement about management. However, consumers who had all their visits to one GP did not necessarily reap the benefits of continuity. Nor did visits to several GPs in the same practice, or to GPs in different practices, preclude continuity.

Brown et al. (1997) have shown that continuity of care can be experienced by patients even in a university group teaching practice with frequent changes of trainees.[4] Long-term patients of the practice, recruited to focus groups, identified four factors contributing to their experience of continuity: the sense of being known as a person by the doctors, nurses, and receptionists; the relationship with a team of doctor–nurse–trainee–receptionist; the sense of responsibility demonstrated by the physicians, including their openness and honesty in dealing with uncertainty; and the comprehensiveness and availability of the services provided, including a 24-hour on-call service and willingness to see patients at home and in the hospital.

Continuity in the patient–doctor relationship is a mutual commitment. Veale (1996) concludes that it is best understood, "not as an entity provided by doctors, but rather as an interaction over time, constructed jointly by consumers and their G.P.s." Continuity "cannot be delivered to a passive recipient by the G.P., however skillful." The essential preconditions of continuity were ready access, competence of the doctor, good communication, and a mechanism for bridging from one consultation to the next. There was a tendency for young and healthy people to prefer the visit-by-visit approach, for people with young children to have continuity with a practice, for those with several distinct problems to visit a variety of GPs, and for the elderly and people with serious illness to prefer continuity with one doctor. Attitudes to continuity may therefore change as people grow older and experience different needs (Veale, 1996).

It is difficult for a doctor to feel continuing responsibility for a patient who does not value it. Some experience of a continuing commitment is required for a sense of responsibility to grow. Hjortdahl (1992a) found that duration of the relationship and frequency of contacts (density) were important in developing the sense of responsibility. After 1 year, the odds of the doctor feeling this sense doubled, and after 5 years they increased 16-fold. If there were four or five contacts over the previous year, there was a 10-fold increase in the sense of continuing responsibility, compared with only one visit.

Once this mutual commitment has developed, failure to honor the commitment may be seen as a betrayal of trust: if, for example, the doctor terminates the relationship when a patient develops AIDS or is too ill to leave home.

A commitment of this nature carries with it a sense of loyalty. Spiro, quoting Royce, reminds us that loyalty is "the willing and practical and thoroughgoing devotion of a person to a cause. A man [or woman] is loyal when, first, he has some cause to which he is loyal; when, secondly, he willingly and thoroughly devotes himself to this cause; and when, thirdly, he expresses his devotion in some sustained and practical way, by acting steadily in the service of his cause" (Spiro, 1998, p. 221). Loyalty is a virtue if it is directed at something greater than self-interest or group interest. The proper application of any virtue such as loyalty requires constant attention to the ever-changing context and a sense of proportionality. It is tied to the old concept of justice as the sense of giving anything or anyone their just "due" (Grant, 1986, p. 56). This exercise requires self-discipline and sometimes is referred to as mindfulness. "If I am loyal, my cause must from moment to moment fascinate me, awaken my muscular vigor, stir me with some eagerness for work, even if this be painful work. I cannot be loyal to barren abstractions. I can only be loyal to what my life can interpret in bodily deeds." (Royce, 1909, p. 130). In the words of George Grant, "In the traditional teaching about justice it was recognized that human nature was so constituted that any desire which has not passed through the flesh by way of actions and settled dispositions appropriate to it is not finally real in the soul." (Grant, 1986, p. 56).

The value placed on the continuity of personal care is reflected in the way a practice is organized. Reception staff can make every effort to book patients with their chosen physician. The practice's philosophy of continuity can be clarified and conveyed to staff and patients. Individual patients' preferences with regard to continuity can be noted and, if possible, accommodated. The on-call system can be organized so that patients see a doctor who communicates with their own doctor, has access to their medical record, and can make a home visit when required. Dying patients, and others with special needs, can be kept out of the on-call system. Continuity can be enhanced by having the patient's record available at all times to those providing care.

THE DOCTOR'S WORK

Continuity of care is based on the idea that physicians cannot be substituted for one another like replaceable parts of a machine. What kind of people will physicians become if they treat themselves as replaceable parts? In his book *The Transformations of Man*, Lewis Mumford (1972) describes work as an educative process. He quotes Le Play as saying, "The most important product that comes out of the mine is the miner." In his book *Good Work*, Schumacher (1979) describes work as "one of the most decisive influences on (a person's) character and personality." Yet, he writes, "The question of what the work does to the worker is hardly ever asked."

Hannah Arendt differentiated between three types of activity: action, work, and labor (Graner, 1987). Action, the highest of human activities, is self-expression; it has no product to which it is secondary; the activity is good in its own right. Work has an end or product, but still has an element of self-expression in that the worker—a craftsman or artist—can put something of himself or herself into the product. The products are not standardized; each one is unique. In his book *Akenfield*, about the changing life of an English village, Ronald Blythe (1969) describes how plowmen used to work in the old days:

> Each man ploughed in his own fashion and with his own mark. It looked all the same if you didn't know about ploughing, but a farmer could walk on a field ploughed by the different teams and tell which bit was ploughed by which. Sometimes he would pay a penny an acre extra for perfect ploughing. . . . The men worked perfectly to get this, but they also worked perfectly because it was their work. It belonged to them. It was theirs.

In labor, man has the least opportunity for self-expression and he produces nothing that is his own. The production line is a modern example of labor, but history has many others. (One laborer is indeed replaceable by any other.) Even labor can be redeemed, but only by making it an opportunity for fellowship, as when laborers share danger, or sing together as they work.

Some historic trends have been moving medicine away from action toward labor. The whole aim of technology is to turn out a standardized product of high quality and consistency. This is not an ignoble aim and, wherever it is attainable in medicine, is to be welcomed. Sometimes new technologies replace human activities that have become drudgery. At the time when the printing press was introduced, hand copying had become a standardized, repetitive activity. In medicine, however, the opportunities for standardization are limited. Human variability is such that for a seriously ill person, the physician cannot be entirely replaced by a machine. If we insist on treating ourselves as such, we should not be surprised if society treats us as laborers rather than as professionals. We should also not be surprised if it does something to us as people. As we withdraw from our patients, we will be the poorer for it. Our professional lives will be less satisfying and we will lose much of the depth of experience that medicine can give us.

Changes in the organization of the practice can interfere with the patient–doctor relationship. Difficulty in getting appointments can divert patients with acute illness to the Emergency Room or walk-in clinic, or to another doctor in the practice. Keeping some gaps in the schedule for patients with acute illnesses does not take much time and will maintain the doctor's experience in this branch of medicine. A practice that opts out of home or hospital visits, or -afterhours service, will cut itself off from many of its patients.

Robert Louis Stevenson thought that the physician, like the soldier, the sailor, and the shepherd, stood above the common herd. In all generations up to our own, the people who followed these callings were brought face to face with the fundamental data of human existence. For the physician, it was the daily confrontation with disease and death. Our technology now makes it possible to experience disease more as a computer printout, a scan, or a monitor reading, and to distance ourselves from the dying. Because our work has a great influence on the kind of people we become, the implications for our profession are profound. Susanne Langer (1979) also wrote of how we find meaning in our work:

> Men who follow the sea have often a deep love for that hard life. . . . Waters and ships, heaven and storm and harbour, somehow contain the symbols through which they see meaning and sense in the world . . . a unified conception of life whereby it can be rationally lived. Any man who loves his calling loves it for more than its use; he loves it because it seems to have "meaning." (Langer, 1979, p. 288).

Unfortunately, we do not always have the choice of how we will work. There is a strong trend toward managed care, either in the form of large corporations, or in state-controlled health services. Much of this is the inevitable result of the increasing complexity of medicine, the need to control costs, and the desire for equality of access to care. The drive by managers for efficiency can place stresses on relationships between doctors and patients and between professional colleagues. The rigid application of clinical guidelines, and the enforcement of sharply defined professional roles, can be a threat to clinical judgment and professional morale. The fragmentation of medicine makes it necessary to distinguish the roles of primary care physician and referral specialist. But the types of collaboration between family physician and specialist vary from patient to patient and from condition to condition. It is better to leave room for clinical judgment and some flexibility of professional roles. Tight control can become soul destroying, with an ultimate reduction, rather than improvement, in efficiency and quality.

CUMULATIVE KNOWLEDGE OF PATIENTS

Continuous and comprehensive care allows the family physician to build up, piece by piece, a "capital" of knowledge about patients and families. This is one of the family physician's most precious assets. Hjortdahl (1992a) found a strong link between continuity of personal care and accumulated knowledge. Knowledge accumulates slowly during the first few months of the relationship, increases sharply between 3 and 12 months, then flattens out somewhat, but still increases steadily during the next few years. The frequency of contact also contributes to the accumulation of knowledge, the major impact being at four to five visits a year. Much of this knowledge is at the tacit level. Prior knowledge reduced the duration of the consultations in 40% of visits and was associated with fewer tests, more use of expectant management, fewer prescriptions, more use of sickness certification, and more referrals (Hjortdahl and Borchgrevink, 1991; Hjortdahl, 1992b). Doctors felt that prior knowledge contributed more to management than diagnosis, and more to chronic problems than to minor infections and injuries. The contribution of personal knowledge to our work accounts for the nakedness we feel when seeing a patient for the first time and, most poignantly, when we leave our practice and find that there is a whole body of knowledge we cannot take with us. It is a fallacy to assume that we have a comprehensive knowledge of all our patients, however, even after many years. The knowledge is acquired only as the opportunity arises and when it is needed. Often it is acquired only when the patient is ready to give it. Only in a minority of patients does this knowledge amount to a full picture.

THE ROLE OF GENERALIST

The family physician is, by nature and function, a generalist. If any organization is to remain healthy, it must have a balance between generalists and specialists. If this seems like a statement of the obvious, let us remember that until very recently, many influential voices in medicine questioned the value of a medical generalist. The explosion of knowledge, this argument ran, has made it impossible for any individual to cover the entire field: it is inevitable, therefore, that medicine will fragment into specialties as it advances. The fallacy in the argument is the assumption that knowledge is a quantity—a lump of material that grows by accretion. We call it "the lump fallacy." The naivete of the assumption can be demonstrated by following the argument to its conclusion. Let us assume that the knowledge of one branch—pediatrics, for example—is at present of a quantity that can be covered by one physician. If knowledge is exploding, then after *n* years, it will have to fragment into pediatric subspecialties, and after another interval each subspecialty will have to fragment again, and so on. If the original assumption is correct, then there is no reason that the process should stop at any time, for further fragmentation is always possible. What we end with, of course, is a *reductio ad absurdum*. Nevertheless, the prospect of being a generalist is one that many students and residents find daunting. It may be helpful, therefore, to examine the role of generalist in medicine and other walks of life, for the generalist/specialist problem runs through the whole of modern society.

The role of generalists in any organization—whether it be a business, a university, or an orchestra—can be described as follows. They have a perspective of the entire organization—its history and traditions, its general structure, its goals and objectives, and its relationships with the outside world. They understand how each part functions within the whole. They act as a communication center: information flows to them from all parts of the organization and from the outside world; information flows from them in both these directions. They help the organization adapt to changes, both internal and external. Problems arising within the organization, or between the organization and its environment, come to the generalist for assessment. Having defined the problem, the generalist may either deal with it or refer it to a specialist.

Once the problem has been defined as lying in his or her field, the specialist may then take on a decision-making role, with the generalist maintaining overall responsibility for ensuring that the problem is dealt with in the best interests of the whole organization. If the specialist finds that the problem is not in his or her field, it is referred back to the generalist. If we substitute the word *organism, person,* or *family* for *organization,* it is not difficult to see how these functions are carried out by the family physician.

Much of the apprehension about becoming a generalist is based on six misconceptions about the roles of generalist and specialist in medicine:

1. *The generalist has to cover the entire field of medical knowledge.* The generalist's knowledge is just as selective as the specialist's. Like specialists, generalists select the knowledge they need to fulfill their role. In subarachnoid hemorrhage, for example, the family physician needs to know the presenting symptoms and the cues that enable him or her to make an early diagnosis and referral. The neurosurgeon, on the other hand, needs to know the detailed pathology and the techniques of investigation and surgical treatment. We have chosen as an example a condition in which the generalist's

role is chiefly early identification of the problem. In other conditions, of course, the generalist will retain total responsibility for management, and the knowledge required will differ accordingly.

2. *In any given field of medicine, the specialist always knows more than the generalist.* This statement expresses the feeling of generalists that when they survey the field of medical knowledge, there is no area they can call their own. Wherever they look, there is some specialist whose knowledge is greater than theirs. But this is not true. We become knowledgeable about the problems we commonly encounter. Specialists become knowledgeable about rarer variants of disease because they are selected for them by generalists. Generalists become knowledgeable about the common conditions that rarely reach the specialists. Family physicians sometimes encounter this when, under pressure from a patient or his family, they consult a specialist even though they know that they are in full command of the situation. They then find to their surprise that the specialist is out of his or her depth, because it is a common variant of the disease that he or she has rarely encountered. Note that the two domains complement each other. Specialists can become knowledgeable about the rare variants only because their experience is concentrated for them by generalists.

3. *By specializing, one can eliminate uncertainty.* The only way to eliminate uncertainty is, as Gayle Stephens (1975) pointed out, to reduce problems to their simplest elements and isolate them from their surroundings. Any clinical specialty that did this would soon cease to be of value.

4. *Only by specializing can one attain depth of knowledge.* This fallacy confuses depth with detail. Depth of knowledge depends on the quality of the mind, not on its information content. The difference between depth and detail is illustrated in a story told of the Vietnam War by Peer de Silva (1978). De Silva was listening to a briefing for Robert McNamara during one of his visits to Saigon. McNamara was bombarding the briefing officers with questions about yards of barbed wire and gallons of gasoline. "I sat there amazed," wrote de Silva, "and thought to myself, what in the world is this man thinking about? This is not a problem of logistics. . . . This is a war that needs discussion of strategic purpose and of strategy itself. What is he talking about?" (de Silva, 1978, p. 210). McNamara was, of course, a generalist and an able one. But in this case he was confusing depth with detail, thus failing to identify the main problem.

5. *As science advances, the load of information increases.* The contrary is true. It is the immature branches of science that have the greatest load of information: "The factual burden of a science varies inversely with its level of maturity," wrote Sir Peter Medawar (1967). "As science advances, particular facts are comprehended within, and therefore, in a sense annihilated by, general statements of steadily increasing power and compass—whereupon the facts need no longer be known explicitly, that is, spelled out and kept

in mind." (Medawar, 1967, p. 114). Imagine what it must have been like to learn about infectious diseases before the days of Koch and Pasteur! It is true, of course, that information, as measured by publications, is increasing exponentially. We must not make the mistake, however, of equating this information with knowledge. Much of it is of little value, much of it ephemeral, much of technical interest to specialists only, and much of it related to the testing of hypotheses that will eventually be rejected or incorporated into the main body of medical knowledge.

6. *Error in medicine is usually caused by lack of information*. Very little medical error is caused by physicians being ill informed. Much more is caused by carelessness, insensitivity, failure to listen, administrative inefficiency, failure of communication, and many other factors that have more to do with the attitudes and skill of the physician than his lack of factual knowledge. Naturally, we want physicians to be well-informed, but this will not guarantee medical care of high quality. The physician must also know how to obtain information and how to use it.

Society's attitude to generalists, like its attitude to work, has implications for the development of the human personality. In his book *The Conduct of Life*, Lewis Mumford (1951) describes the effects of the fragmentation produced by our mechanistic culture: "In accepting this partition of functions and this overemphasis of a single narrow skill, men were content, not merely to become fragments of men, but to become fragments of fragments: the physician ceased to deal with the body as a whole and looked after a single organil. . . ." (Mumford, 1951, p. 185).

"As a result," Mumford goes on, "the apparently simple notion of the balanced person . . . almost dropped out of existence: repressed in life, rejected in thought. Even groups and classes that had once espoused the aristocratic ideal of living a full and rounded life, . . . dropped their traditional aspirations and made themselves over into specialists, those people Nietzsche called *inverted cripples*, handicapped not because they have lost a single organ, but because they have over-magnified it." (Mumford, 1951, p. 185).

To Alfred North Whitehead (1926), wisdom is the fruit of a balanced development of the personality. His criticism of professional education in his day (the 1920s) was that it lacked balance. The student was expected to master a set of abstractions, but there was no balancing emotional and moral development. If anything, professional education in our own day is even more unbalanced. Perhaps this explains the decline of wisdom that has been a notable feature of the last century.

Many of us live in societies that value excellence. The idea of excellence, however, is the development of a single talent to its utmost limit, whether it is in sports, business, or professional life. Little attention is given to the price that may be paid for this excellence in stunted, one-sided personalities, or to the effects on society as a whole of fostering in its members only one type of excellence. In deciding to be generalists, family physicians have renounced one-sided development in favor of balance and wholeness. They do pay a price for this: in lack of recognition by a society that is itself unbalanced; and in sacrificing special talents in favor of overall excellence. The personal rewards, however, are great. "Only men who are themselves whole," wrote Mumford, "can understand the needs and desires and ideals of other men." (Mumford, 1951, p. 186).

Two final points should be made. Because the family physician is a generalist, this does not mean that all family physicians have identical knowledge and skills. All of them share the same commitment to patients. By virtue of special interest or training, however, a physician may have knowledge that is not shared by colleagues. In any group of family physicians, this can be a source of enrichment. One may be skilled in reading ECGs, another may have a special interest in child health or the care of elderly patients. This distinction sometimes becomes blurred in debates between rural and urban physicians, whose workloads differ. Both have become adapted to the needs of their patients and the resources available in the community in which they practice. The rural family physician may be required to do more procedures, including surgery, while the urban family physician may develop greater knowledge and expertise in the management of drug dependency, for example. Though their practice profiles differ, they are both family physicians who are attending in a comprehensive way to their practice population and the needs of their community. The important point is that this should not lead to fragmentation. Family physicians may be differentiated, but family medicine should not fragment. If it were to do so, the role of generalist would be lost.

The family physician acts not only across clinical boundaries, but across that very difficult one: the boundary between medical and social problems. The boundary is difficult because it is seldom clear-cut. Patients' problems have a way of bestriding it. To the family physician, therefore, falls the responsibility of managing the interface between clinical practice and the counseling professions.

THE HUMAN SCALE

General practice has traditionally been based in small, widely dispersed units rather than large institutions. This has been important in providing an environment on the human scale, where patients can feel at home in familiar surroundings, close to their own neighborhood. If this sense of intimacy is to be preserved, it is important that these small units continue to be the basic organization of general practice. In former times, the office or surgery was often in the doctor's home, which itself was part of the community served by the practice. Now, the more usual setting is a medical center where family physicians work in a team with other professions. There are many benefits to this type of organization, but there are also risks. The larger the organization, and the more people involved, the more difficult it becomes to preserve the sense of the practice as a welcoming and familiar place.

One disadvantage of the dispersal of general practice in small units is the difficulty we have in organizing ourselves for activities that go beyond the individual practice. This may be needed, for example, when tackling some community-wide health problem, negotiating shared care with specialized services, or arranging deputizing services. The funding of Divisions of General Practice by the Australian government is an approach to meeting this need. Grants are provided to groups of GPs who wish to organize themselves to address issues in their local health services. In the United States, the growth of managed care stimulated the development of primary care physicians' organizations. The patient-centered medical home is currently under development, as are various versions of family health teams. In the developed world there are many new versions of primary care renewal. One characteristic common to many of them is the concept of a team approach to delivery of care in the community (Institute of Medicine, 2001). Teams that function effectively have been found to improve access to care, continuity of care, patient satisfaction, and better processes of care for specific diseases (Grumbach and Bodenheimer, 2004). Nevertheless, organizing interdisciplinary teams for the family medicine setting is a challenging task and may involve some drawbacks. The family physician may feel that some of the most important positive interactions with their patients are taken away from them and delegated to other team members, thereby reducing satisfaction with work. The optimal makeup of teams that meet the variety of problems common in family medicine will differ from one area to another. There is a move toward a disease-management approach in primary care, but patients do not come with a single disease, nor do physicians "manage" them as one might do with an employee.

IS FAMILY MEDICINE UNIVERSAL?

If the principles set out in this chapter have an enduring value, they should be applicable to all cultures and all social groups. If family medicine were to become a service available only to the affluent members of industrialized societies, it would soon lose adherents. Yet there are those who see the problems of poor countries and poor communities as so different that they require a different and more basic approach. Their needs, it is argued, are for clean water, better housing, sanitation, and immunization, rather than for the type of personal care provided by family physicians.

There is some truth in this. Elementary public health measures are still the first need in many societies. But they are not the only need. Other problems will yield only to the personal, family-centered approach. Dr. Cicely Williams (1973), well known for her description of kwashiorkor, became convinced that the answer to malnutrition was family-based health care.

We believe firmly that these principles have universal application. How they are applied, however, will vary according to circumstances. If there is only one physician for 50,000 people, it is obvious that his or her role as a manager of resources, leader, teacher, and resource for difficult problems will be predominant. The application of the principles on the personal level will be the responsibility of other personnel working under his or her supervision. With cities in some countries growing in population exceeding 30 million, the public health services can be overwhelmed, especially when many areas are covered with slums without sewage and garbage disposal and basic communications. In these cases, the task of maintaining health may fall on organizations with physicians who have a generalist orientation.

NOTES

1. Wright R, *A Short History of Progess* (Toronto: House of Anansi Press, 2004), p. 29.
2. For a fuller discussion of these implications, see article by McWhinney IR, The importance of being different, *British Journal of General Practice* (1996), 46:433–436.
3. Bronwyn Veale used four research methods: epidemiological surveys, interviews, focus groups, and health diaries kept by patients, combined with monthly interviews. The latter method enabled utilization by each patient to be studied along a trajectory.
4. Brown and her colleagues formed five focus groups from patients who had been with the practice for over 15 years (*n* = 55). The average age of participants was 55 and the average time as a patient of the practice was 21 years. About half the patients had made visits to both staff physicians and trainees, the remainder receiving care primarily from either staff physician or a succession of trainees.

REFERENCES

Berry W. 1978. *The Unsettling of America: Culture and Agriculture.* New York: Avon Books.

Blythe R. 1969. *Akenfield: Portrait of an English Village.* London: Allen Lane, Penguin Press.

Brown JB, Dickie I, Brown L, Biehn J. 1997. Long-term attendance at a family practice teaching unit. *Canadian Family Physician* 43:901–906.

Brown MH. 1979. Love Canal and the poisoning of America. *Atlantic Monthly*, December.

De Silva P. 1978. *Sub rosa: The C.I.A. and the Uses of Intelligence.* New York: Times Books.

Graner JL. 1987. The primary care crisis, part II: The physician as labourer. *Humane Medicine* 3:20.

Grant G. 1986. *Technology and Justice*. Toronto: Anansi Press.

Grumbach K, Bodenheimer T. 2004. Can health care teams improve primary care practice? *Journal of the American Medical Association* 291(10):1246–1251.

Hennen BKE. 1975. Continuity of care in family practice, part 1: Dimensions of continuity. *Journal of Family Practice* 2(5):371.

Hjortdahl P, Borchgrevink CF. 1991. Continuity of care: Influence of general practitioners' knowledge about their patients on use of resources in consultations. *British Medical Journal* 303:1181.

Hjortdahl P. 1992a. Continuity of care: General practitioners' knowledge about, and sense of responsibility towards their patients. *Family Practice* 9(1):3.

Hjortdahl P. 1992b. The influence of general practitioner's knowledge about their patients on the clinical decision-making process. *Scandinavian Journal of Primary Health Care* 10(4):290.

Institute of Medicine. 2001. *Crossing the Quality Chasm: New Health System for the 21st Century*. Washington, DC: National Academy Press.

James W. 1958. *The Varieties of Religious Experience*. New York: Penguin Books.

Langer SK. 1979. *Philosophy in a New Key*. Cambridge, MA: Harvard University Press.

Medawar PB. 1967. *The Art of the Soluble*. London: Methuen.

Mumford L. 1951. *The Conduct of Life*. New York: Harcourt Brace and World.

Mumford L. 1972. *The Transformations of Man*. New York: Harper Torchbooks.

Price R. 1994. *A Whole New Life*. New York: Atheneum Macmillan.

Royce J. 1909. *The Philosophy of Loyalty*. New York: Macmillan Company.

Schumacher EF. 1979. *Good Work*. New York: Harper and Row.

Spiro H. 1998. *The Power of Hope: A Doctor's Perspective*. New Haven, CT, and London: Yale University Press.

Stephens GG. 1975. The intellectual basis of family practice. *Journal of Family Practice* 2:423.

Taylor C. 1991. *The Malaise of Modernity*. Concord, Ontario: Anansi Press.

Toon PD. 1994. What is good general practice? Occasional Paper 65. Royal College of General Practitioners.

Veale BM, McCallum J, Saltman DC, Lonesgan J, Wadsworth YJ, Douglas RM. 1995. Consumer use of multiple general practitioners: An Australian epidemiological study. *Family Practice* 12:303.

Veale BM. 1996. Continuity of care and general practice utilization in Australia. Ph.D. thesis, Australian National University.

Whitehead AN. 1926. *Science and the Modern World*. Cambridge: Cambridge University Press.

Williams C. 1973. Pediatric perceptions: Health services in the home. *Pediatrics* 52:773.

CHAPTER 3

☙

Illness in the Community

S tudies of illness in the community have revealed that physicians see only a small fraction of the health problems experienced by the population at large. Green et al. (2001) brought up to date a summary of the data from a number of community surveys in a diagram reproduced in Figure 3.1. Of 1000 people in the general population over the age of 16, in a typical month, 800 will report having some sort of symptom and 327 will consider seeking medical care. One hundred and thirteen will attend the office of a primary care physician, 65 will visit a complementary or alternative care provider, 21 will go to an outpatient clinic at a hospital, and 14 will receive home care. Only 13 will go to an emergency department and 8 will be hospitalized. Fewer than 1 will be admitted to an academic health science center.

In retrospective population surveys, about 90% of adults report a symptom during the previous 2 weeks. Only one in every four or five of these have consulted a physician in that period (Wadsworth, Butterfield, and Blaney, 1971; Dunnell and Cartright, 1972).

In an interview survey in Glasgow, Hannay (1979) found that 86% of adults and children reported at least one physical symptom in a 2-week period. The most common symptoms were respiratory, with tiredness being second, and headaches being third in order of frequency. The predominance of respiratory symptoms was similar to that in surveys in Australia and the United States. Respiratory illness is also the most common diagnosis in general practice. Fifty-one percent of adults had one or more mental symptoms in the 2-week period (e.g., anxiety, depression, insomnia, obsessional thoughts, paranoid ideas). Twenty-four percent of the children were reported by parents to have behavioral problems (e.g., developmental problems, enuresis, school problems, discipline problems). Almost a quarter of the adults had at least one social problem (e.g., unemployment, financial difficulties).

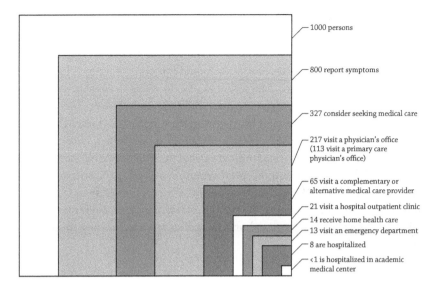

1000 persons

800 report symptoms

327 consider seeking medical care

217 visit a physician's office
(113 visit a primary care
physician's office)

65 visit a complementary or
alternative medical care provider

21 visit a hospital outpatient clinic

14 receive home health care

13 visit an emergency department

8 are hospitalized

<1 is hospitalized in academic
medical center

Figure 3.1:
Monthly prevalence of illness in the community and the roles of various sources of health care.

Reprinted with permission from Green L, Fryer GE, Yawn, BP, Lanier D, Dovey SM. 2001. The ecology of medical care revisited. *New England Journal of Medicine* 344(26):2021–2025.

Analysis of simple correlations in the Glasgow survey showed that a high prevalence of symptoms was associated with increasing age, female sex, unemployment due to illness, marital separation or divorce, passive as opposed to active religious affiliation, living on or above the fifth floor in high-rise buildings, and a high number of moves of domicile (mobility). The neuroticism score increased with all the adult symptom frequencies. Subjects with low extroversion scores had significantly more mental and social symptoms. On regression analysis, the neuroticism score, age and sex, living in high-rise buildings, passive religious affiliation, and mobility all remained significant variables.

Health diary studies have provided useful insights into the symptom burden that exists in the population. In a prospective study using the health diary method, adults recorded at least one complaint on 21.8% of days and only on 6% of these days was a doctor consulted (Roghmann and Haggerty, 1972). In a study of 107 participants extending over a 3-week period, 3.25 problems were recorded, but less than 6% of these resulted in professional care being sought (Demers, Altamore Mustin, et al., 1980). In a group of elderly people, self-treatment was found to be common, with prescription and over-the-counter medications being the most frequent interventions. The decision to seek professional help among this group of people had more to do with the level of pain or discomfort, interference with daily activities, or whether they thought it was something serious, rather than with familiarity with the symptom or causal explanations (Stoller, Forster, and Portugal, 1993). In another prospective study of women using health diaries, symptoms were recorded on 10 days out of 28 on the average. The yearly average of symptom episodes was 81. A doctor was consulted for 1 out of every 37 symptom episodes (Banks, Beresford, Morrell, et al., 1975). Women consistently report more physical symptoms than men; in a study comparing health diary entries of a group of women and men over a 4-week period, it was found that negative mood was the strongest predictor of physical symptoms, which were, in turn, the strongest predictors of illness behavior. Differences in mood states seem to mediate gender differences in symptom reporting (Gijsbers van Wijk, Huisman, and Kolk, 1999). It is clear that the occurrence of symptoms is the norm rather than the exception. The important questions, therefore, are not whether symptoms are present, but how serious or frequent they are, and how they are acted on.

THE SICK ROLE AND ILLNESS BEHAVIOR

Two concepts are helpful in analyzing the decision to consult a physician: the sick role and illness behavior. The concept of the sick role was introduced by Sigerist (1960) and Parsons (1951). According to Parsons, when a person has consulted a physician and has been defined as sick, he or she occupies a special role in society. Entering the sick role has certain obligations and privileges. The individual is exempted from normal social obligations and is not held responsible for his or her incapacity. On the other hand, the sick person is expected to seek professional help and to make every effort toward recovery. Whether a person decides to enter the sick role when he or she becomes ill is dependent on many individual and group factors that are independent of the severity of the illness.

Illness behavior is defined by Mechanic (1962) as "the ways in which given symptoms may be differentially perceived, evaluated, and acted (or not acted) upon by different kinds of persons." The illness behavior exhibited by an individual determines whether or not he or she will enter the sick role and will consult a physician. Lamberts (1984) has introduced the concept of problem behavior: the actions of a patient with a problem of living as distinct from an illness.

The importance of distinguishing between illness and illness behavior is illustrated by irritable bowel syndrome. People with functional gastrointestinal disorders (FGD), including irritable bowel syndrome, were compared to the general population with respect to psychological traits, recent life events, social support, self-rated health, and frequency of physician consultation. The FGD group had significantly worse scores than the general population for depression, emotionality, and physical symptoms. They worried more about their health and their quality of life was lower, they had more negative life events in the previous 12 months, their rating of overall health was lower, and they had fewer social supports. However, when the FGD group was divided into those who consulted a physician and those who did not, the non-consulters differed from the general population in fewer variables (somatization, emotionality, quality of life, health rating, and social support). Visits to physicians were highly correlated with depression, subjective health rating, and duration of periods with symptoms. Also important was the opinion of the healthcare system. It would seem that in people with FGD, there are two kinds of psychological conditions: those related to the illness itself, and those related to the decision to seek medical care. Importantly, in this study, life events, whether perceived as positive or negative, correlated with consultation behavior (Herschbach, Henrich, and von Rad, 1999).

An understanding of illness behavior can change the perspective of the physician. The key question may be "why did the patient come?" The aim of therapy may be not to remove the symptoms but to help the patient to live with them, as many others in the population have learned to do.

UNDERREPORTING OF SERIOUS SYMPTOMS AND CONSULTATION FOR MINOR SYMPTOMS

Variations in illness behavior are responsible for two phenomena of interest to family physicians: failure to consult with serious symptoms, and attendance with minor symptoms.

In the Glasgow survey, Hannay estimated the degree of incongruous referral, defined as either failure to consult, with symptoms being assessed by the patient himself or herself as serious, or consulting for symptoms assessed by the patient as minor. Physical, mental, and behavioral symptoms were graded for pain, disability, seriousness, and duration, using the patient's own (or for children's behavioral symptoms, the parents' own) assessment. A mean severity score was then calculated for each subject. Social symptoms were graded separately for worry or inconvenience. The extent of incongruous referral of both kinds is shown in Figure 3.2. Twenty-six percent of people with physical, mental, or behavioral symptoms did not seek professional help for serious symptoms. Eleven percent sought professional help for minor symptoms. For social symptoms, the figures were 16% and 12%, respectively. Of the medical symptoms, behavioral symptoms in children were most likely to be referred for professional help, followed by physical symptoms in all subjects, mental symptoms in adults being the least likely to be referred.

In the Glasgow survey, failure to consult for serious symptoms was associated with unemployment due to illness, passive religious allegiance, lower social class, living alone, and higher neuroticism scores. On regression

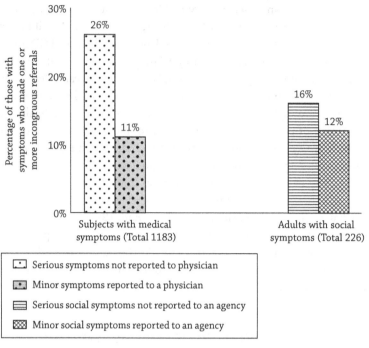

Figure 3.2:
Incidence of incongruous referral in the Glasgow survey.
Reprinted with permission from Hannay DR. 1979. *The Symptom Iceberg: A Study in Community Health.* London: Routledge and Kegan Paul.

analysis, neuroticism, poor past and present health, increasing age, female sex, and mobility were significant associated variables.

Consultation for minor symptoms was associated on regression analysis with greater number of present illnesses, separation or divorce, increasing age, female sex, few years in present residence, poor experience with doctors or hospitals, difficulty in contacting a doctor, and number of hospital stays.

Using the same definition for incongruous consultations as the Glasgow Study, Elliott and colleagues (Elliott, McAteer, and Hannaford, 2012) surveyed registered patients in 20 British general practices seeking information on their experience of a range of symptoms (from those deemed by physicians to being self-limited and minor to severe and potentially serious) in the past 2 weeks. Respondents were also asked to rate each symptom as to severity and the extent to which it interfered with daily life, as well as whether they sought a consultation with their physician for the symptom. Seventy-five percent of respondents reported at least one of the listed symptoms, with younger respondents, those with chronic conditions, or those unable to work due to illness or not in paid work more likely to have symptoms. Only 8% of symptom bearers sought a consultation with their general practitioner. Approximately one-fifth of the 7995 symptoms resulted in an incongruous consultation: 3.2% were consultations for a patient-perceived low-impact symptom, and 17.3% were for nonconsultations for symptoms perceived by patients as having a high impact. Box 3.1 lists the 10 most frequently endorsed symptoms. Symptoms such as blood in the stool, fainting, wheezy chest, shortness of breath, unintentional weight loss, and chest pain—all of which could represent a serious condition—dominated the reasons for low-impact consultations. Physicians might well conclude that patients made an appropriate decision to consult in these situations, even though the symptoms had low impact. On the other hand, the commonest symptoms that had high impact but did not result in consultation were fainting, feeling depressed, difficulty sleeping, vomiting, and coughing up blood. High-impact nonconsultations exceeded low-impact consultations for all symptoms. Respondents who initiated consultation for low-impact symptoms were more likely to have a chronic condition, have poor role physical scores, poor bodily pain scores, and a belief in the importance of reassurance from a health professional. High-impact nonconsulters tended to be younger, ex-smokers, in poor health, unable to work due to illness, and to endorse a feeling that not wasting their GP's time was important.

Other investigators have described factors affecting illness behavior. In his book *The Health of Regionville*, Koos (1954) noted that upper-class persons more often reported themselves ill than did lower-class persons, and were more likely to seek treatment when ill. Lower-class persons had more symptoms, but reported themselves to be less often ill and were less likely to visit

---

Box 3.1

THE TEN MOST FREQUENT SYMPTOMS
ENDORSED BY PATIENTS

---

1. Feeling tired/run down
2. Headaches
3. Joint pain
4. Back pain
5. Difficulty sleeping
6. Sore throat
7. Nervousness/anxiety
8. Indigestion/heartburn
9. Cough
10. Feeling depressed

Adapted from Elliott AM, McAteer A, Hannaford PC. 2012. Incongruous consultation behaviour: Results from a UK-wide population survey. BMC Family Practice 13:21.

a physician. Some of these differences in relation to specific symptoms are illustrated in Box 3.1.

In a study of women aged 20–44, Banks et al. (1975) found that those with a high level of free-floating anxiety were more likely to consult their general practitioners about their symptoms. The nature of the symptoms had a strong correlation with the decision to seek care. Table 3.1 illustrates the wide variation in response to different symptoms.

Mechanic (1962) found that persons reporting high stress levels, especially interpersonal difficulties, showed a high inclination to use medical services.

A taxonomy of illness behavior was framed by one of the authors (McWhinney, 1972) to attempt to more fully integrate the behavioral sciences with traditional medical diagnosis. This taxonomy remains relevant in understanding some incongruous consultations. In this framework, individuals will attend their physician for one or a combination of five reasons: limit of tolerance (no longer able or willing to put up with a symptom); limit of anxiety (concerned about the possible implications of a symptom); problem of living presenting as a symptom; administrative reason; attendance for reasons other than illness.

Table 3.1. PERCENTAGE OF RESPONDENTS IN EACH SOCIAL CLASS RECOGNIZING SPECIFIED SYMPTOMS AS NEEDING MEDICAL ATTENTION

Symptom	Class I ($n = 51$) (%)	Class II ($n = 335$) (%)	Class III ($n = 128$) (%)
Loss of appetite	57	50	20
Persistent backache	53	44	19
Continued coughing	77	78	23
Persistent joint and muscle pains	80	47	19
Blood in stools	98	89	60
Blood in urine	100	93	69
Excessive vaginal bleeding	92	83	54
Swelling of ankles	77	76	23
Loss of weight	80	51	21
Bleeding gums	79	51	20
Chronic fatigue	80	53	19
Shortness of breath	77	55	21
Persistent headaches	80	56	22
Fainting spells	80	51	33
Pain in chest	80	51	31
Lump in breast	94	71	44
Lump in abdomen	92	65	34

Reprinted with permission from Koos EL. 1954. *The Health of Regionville: What the People Thought and Did about It*. New York: Columbia University Press.

Zola (1966) interviewed Italian-American and Irish-American patients before they saw the physician on new visits to hospital clinics. Information on the primary diagnosis, secondary diagnosis, potential seriousness, and degree of urgency was obtained from the physician. Besides comparisons between the two groups, comparisons were also made between matched pairs of one Irish and one Italian patient of the same sex who had the same primary diagnosis, the same duration of illness, and the same degree of seriousness.

Major differences emerged. The Irish denied that pain was a feature of their illness more often than did the Italians. More Irish described their chief problem in terms of specific dysfunction; more Italians described it in terms of a diffuse difficulty. The Irish tended to limit and understate their difficulties, whereas the Italians tended to spread and generalize theirs. In the matched pairs, the Italians complained of more symptoms, more bodily areas affected, and more kinds of dysfunction than did the Irish, and more often felt that their symptoms affected their interpersonal behavior (Table 3.2).

Zborowski (1951) studied reactions to pain in patients of Jewish, Italian, and "Old American" stock. Data were collected from interviews with patients, from observation of their behavior when in pain, and from discussion with doctors and nurses involved in the care of the individual.

Jews and Italians were described as being very emotional in their responses to pain. Italians, however, were mainly concerned with the immediacy of the pain, whereas Jews focused their concern on the meaning of the pain and its long-term implications. The two groups also differed in their attitudes to analgesic drugs. The Italians called for pain relief and soon forgot their sufferings

Table 3.2. THE LIKELIHOOD OF SYMPTOM EPISODES
LEADING
TO CONSULTATION WITH PHYSICIAN

Symptom	Ratio of Symptom Episodes to Consultations
Changes in energy	456:1
Headache	184:1
Disturbance of gastric function	109:1
Backache	52:1
Pain in lower limb	49:1
Emotional/psychological	46:1
Abdominal pain	29:1
Disturbance of menstruation	20:1
Sore throat	18:1
Pain in chest	14:1

Adapted from Banks MH, Beresford SAA, Morrell DC, Waller JJ, Watkins CJ. 1975. Factors influencing demand for primary medical care in women aged 20–44 years: A preliminary report. *International Journal of Epidemiology* 4:189.

when this occurred. The Jews were reluctant to accept drugs, were concerned about their side effects, and regarded them as giving only temporary relief.

The "Old American" patients tended to have a detached and unemotional attitude to their pain. Like the Jewish patients, "Old Americans" were concerned about the meaning and future implications of their pain; but, whereas the anxieties of the Jews were tinged with pessimism about the outcome, the "Old Americans" tended to retain an attitude of optimism born of their confidence in the skill of the expert.

The interpretation of the previous two studies carries a danger in leading to stereotyping people on the basis of their perceived cultural background. Physicians must make no such assumptions. The studies have been kept in the present edition to demonstrate that one's cultural milieu can have a significant impact on how one perceives changes in health and responds to those changes. Individual differences are likely to be more important.

In summary, illness behavior is related to ethnic origin, social class, age, sex, nature of illness, religious affiliation, personality, and environmental factors. Hannay's (1979) findings challenge the widely held belief that neuroticism is strongly related to high utilization of services and to consultation about trivia. In the Glasgow study, it was the less neurotic who were more likely to seek professional advice both in general and for "trivia." It was the more neurotic who were most likely to be part of the symptom "iceberg."

SELF-CARE AND OTHER ALTERNATIVES TO MEDICAL CARE

It will be clear from the studies mentioned that the majority of symptom episodes are managed by the sufferers themselves without recourse to medical advice. Self-care refers to all the actions taken by a sufferer on his or her own behalf. These actions may replace medical advice, or they may precede consultation with a physician. Self-care can take a number of forms:

1. Studies in Britain and the United States (Freer, 1978) have shown high rates of self-medication (50%–80% of adults reported taking an over-the-counter medication in a 2- to 4-week period). The great majority of these are analgesics, cold remedies, and antacids. The pharmacist is often a source of advice on over-the-counter medication. In a study of primary care given by pharmacists in London, Ontario, Bass (1975) found that in neighborhood pharmacies, for every 100 prescriptions issued, about 19 other people asked for advice on health problems. The most common of these were upper respiratory infections, stomach and bowel complaints, pain, and inquiries about vitamins. Increasing self-care has become the norm with the widespread use of the Internet. Even medications that

normally require a prescription from a physician may be obtained by direct order over the Internet. As chronic diseases have come to dominate health care, self-management has taken on greater importance. It represents one of the components of the Chronic Care Model, and various jurisdictions have deregulated some medications and have instituted telephone helplines to support self-management, partly in the belief that it will lower healthcare costs.

2. Although most attention has been focused on medication, a large number of other remedial actions may be taken. In a study using the health diary method, Freer (1978) found that a large number of nonmedical actions were reported. Some of these were social actions, like talking to friends or relatives, attending a club, or going out for a meal; others were individual actions, like doing housework, going out shopping, or gardening. All these actions were recorded because they were viewed as being therapeutic.

3. There may be lay referral, or consultation with family members, friends, neighbors, and other nonprofessional people whose advice may be sought. Certain individuals in a neighborhood may have a reputation for being knowledgeable in health matters. Others may be valued for their advice on personal problems. All societies have resources of this kind, quite independent of the healthcare system. Kleinman (1980) called this the "popular sector," and it represents the largest sector of any healthcare system (Stevenson et al., 2003). It is likely, however, that in highly mobile societies there is less opportunity for such informal aid systems to develop. This may help explain the large number of personal problems that are presented to family physicians in industrialized societies.

4. Folk healers and practitioners of alternative medicine are widely available in most societies. This folk sector (Kleinman, 1980) may be used as the initial source of care, or as an additional resource when the healthcare system has not met the patient's expectations. Alternative medicine is widely used in Western countries (see Chapter 23).

The prudent family physician will always ask his or her patients what they have already tried before making recommendations. This is necessary for a holistic understanding of their patient and for achieving common ground in the consultation (see Chapter 8).

REFERENCES

Banks MH, Beresford SAA, Morrell DC, Waller JJ, Watkins CJ. 1975. Factors influencing demand for primary medical care in women aged 20–44 years: A preliminary report. *International Journal of Epidemiology* 4:189.

Bass M. 1975. The pharmacist as a provider of primary care. *Canadian Medical Association Journal* 112:60.

Demers RY, Altamore R, Mustin H, Kleinman A, Leonardi D. 1980. An exploration of the dimensions of illness behavior. *The Journal of Family Practice* 11(7):1085–1092.

Dunnell K, Cartwright A. 1972 *Medicine Takers, Prescribers and Hoarders*. London: Routledge and Kegan Paul.

Elliott AM, McAteer A, Hannaford PC. 2012. Incongruous consultation behaviour: results from a UK-wide population survey. *BMC Family Practice* 13:21.

Freer CB. 1978. Self care: A health diary study. Master of Clinical Science thesis, The University of Western Ontario.

Gijsbers van Wijk CM, Huisman H, Kolk AM. 1999. Gender differences in physical symptoms and illness behavior. *Social Science & Medicine* 49(8):1061–1074.

Green L, Fryer GE, Yawn, BP, Lanier D, Dovey SM. 2001. The ecology of medical care revisited. *New England Journal of Medicine* 344(26):2021–2025.

Hannay DR. 1979. *The Symptom Iceberg: A Study in Community Health*. London: Routledge and Kegan Paul.

Herschbach P, Henrich G, von Rad M. 1999. Psychological factors in functional gastrointestinal disorders: Characteristics of the disorder or of the illness behavior? *Psychosomatic Medicine* 61:148–153.

Kleinman A. 1980. *Patients and Healers in the Context of Culture: An Exploration of the Borderland Between Anthropology, Medicine and Psychiatry*. Berkeley: University of California Press.

Koos EL. 1954. *The Health of Regionville: What the People Thought and Did about It*. New York: Columbia University Press.

Lamberts H. 1984. *Morbidity in General Practice: Diagnosis Related Information from the Monitoring Project*. Utrecht: Huisartsenpers.

McWhinney IR. 1972. Beyond diagnosis: An approach to the integration of behavioural science and clinical medicine. *New England Journal of Medicine* 287(8):384–387.

Mechanic D. 1962. The concept of illness behaviour. *Journal of Chronic Disease* 15:189.

Parsons T. 1951. *The Social System*. Glencoe, IL: Free Press.

Roghmann KJ, Haggerty RJ. 1972. The diary as a research instrument in the study of health and illness behaviour. *Medical Care* 10:143.

Sigerist HE. 1960. The special position of the sick. In: Roemer MI, ed., *The Sociology of Medicine*. New York: M.D. Publications.

Stevenson FA, Britten N, Barry CA, et al. 2003. Self-treatment and its discussion in medical consultations: How is medical pluralism managed in practice? *Social Science & Medicine* 57: 513–527.

Stoller EP, Forster LE, Portugal S. 1993. Self-care responses to symptoms by older people: A health diary study of illness behavior. *Medical Care* 31(1):24–42.

Wadsworth MEJ, Butterfield WJH, Blaney MEJ, Butterfield WJH, Blaney R. 1971. *Health and Sickness: The Choice of Treatment*. London: Tavistock.

Zborowski M. 1951. Cultural components in responses to pain. *Journal of Social Issues* 8:16.

Zola IK. 1966. Culture and symptoms: An analysis of patients' presenting complaints. *American Sociological Review* 31:614.

CHAPTER 4

✣

The Family in Health and Disease

The importance of the family to family physicians is inherent in the paradigm of family medicine. Family medicine does not separate disease from person or person from environment. It recognizes the strong connection between health and disease, and personality, way of life, physical environment, and human relationships. It understands the strong influence that human relationships have on the outcome of illness and recognizes the family as the crucible of the development of the person.

Doherty and Baird (1987) describe four levels of physician involvement with families. The first is minimal involvement. The second is the provision of information and advice. To practice at this level, the physician must be open to engaging families in a collaborative way, taking care to communicate medical findings and treatment options to family members, and listening attentively to their questions and concerns. This does not require special knowledge of family development or reactions to stressful experiences.

The physician at the third level includes the preceding elements, but also has an understanding of the affective aspects of family relationships. The physician is therefore able to provide emotional support and to help family members deal with the feelings aroused by having a family member with illnesses such as cancer, schizophrenia, diabetes, and physical disability. To practice at this level, the physician needs a knowledge of family development and of how families react to stressful experiences. He or she has to be a skilled listener, responsive to the subtle cues by which emotional needs are expressed. Also needed is enough self-knowledge to be aware of how the physician's own feelings and family experiences affect his or her relationship with the patient and family.

At the fourth level, the physician can carry out a systematic assessment of family function and can plan an intervention designed to help a family deal with its problems. This will often include reframing the family's definition of the problem and encouraging family members to consider new ways of coping with their difficulties. To practice at this level, the physician needs an understanding of systems theory and the skills of convening and conducting a family conference. This may include engaging family members who are reluctant to participate and encouraging poorly communicating family members to express themselves.

Levels three and four must be distinguished from family therapy, which is based on the idea that the identified patient is presenting a "symptom" of family dysfunction. Therapy is therefore directed toward the whole family system. At levels three and four, a member of the family is sick and the physician is helping the family to care for the patient. Of course, the levels may overlap with family therapy. A family with a sick member may also be dysfunctional; but family physicians will mostly be helping ordinary families mobilize resources to improve their coping skills.

Confusion has arisen from time to time between family medicine and family therapy. In family therapy, the physician can carry out a planned course of therapy for a dysfunctional family. The physician requires the insight and skill to intervene in such a manner as to change the way the family functions. The few family physicians working at this level are trained family therapists who combine the roles of family physician and family therapist, some of them receiving referrals from other family physicians.

The therapist's aim is to change the way the family functions. He or she usually has no continuing commitment to maintain the health of individual members of the family. If change in the family is against the interests of an individual member, then the needs of the family may take precedence over the individual.

There are other differences between a family therapist and a family physician.[1] Therapists starting to work with a family are not usually influenced by previous relationships with individual members. They begin as neutral and detached observers. Family physicians, on the other hand, will often be the object of different feelings in different members of a family. The physician may be seen, for example, as an ally by the wife, as an enemy by the husband, and as an authoritarian parent by the children. Similarly, it is difficult for the family physician to avoid bias toward or against one or other member of the family. The family therapist has no other commitment to members of the family other than to conduct family therapy. The family physician, even if trying to help a family to change, still has to treat the wife's urinary tract infection, the children's respiratory infections, or the husband's depression. At the end of therapy, the family therapist usually has no further responsibility to the family. The family physician's responsibility to its individual members is open-ended. The context in which the family physician works is worlds away from the working context of a family therapist. This does not mean that family physicians do not help families to change: it means that they do it in their own way, appropriate to their own context. Failure to understand this has led to disappointment in psychiatrists and behavioral scientists who have tried to teach family therapy to family physicians, and to family physicians who have confused their mission. It is yet another example of the truth that clinical methods cannot be transferred unmodified from one context to another.

Brennan (1974) has made the important distinction between "the person in the family" and "the family in the person." The person in the family represents the interpersonal relationships in the family group. The family in the person represents the individual's incorporated experience of his or her family of origin—an experience that profoundly affects self-concept and relationships with others. A person is raised and nurtured in a family for the early years of life, but the family remains "in" the person until his or her death.

Of course, family physicians are not the only clinicians who have this understanding of the family. Other physicians, especially those providing long-term care, may work with an awareness of the family context. Family physicians cannot claim to be the sole possessors of this knowledge. Whether a physician does so, however, is largely a matter of training. A physician who has not learned to "think family" in his or her training is not likely to "think family" in practice. The experience of one of the authors (IRMcW) provides an example: "My preparation for general practice was a year as resident in internal medicine, culminating in the Membership of the Royal College of Physicians (MRCP). When I entered practice I had no concept of the importance of the family in medicine. For example, I did not even make the connection between severe headaches in a young man and the fact that his child had muscular dystrophy. It was not for many years that, under the influence of academic family medicine, I developed some capacity for 'thinking family.'" Other physicians can work with families, but the fact is that outside family medicine, few are trained to do so.

Although a clinician from another discipline may, by his ability to "think family," resemble a family physician, there remain some important differences arising from the fact that the latter often cares for several members of the family. First, this personal knowledge of individual members can give the physician the advantage of knowledge of the family context that can be obtained in no other way (Case 4.1).

It could be argued that a physician caring for any one of the individuals in Case 4.1 could, by attentive listening, have obtained the same knowledge about the family. The knowledge, however, would have been of a different quality from that obtained through personal relationship with all three members and would probably not have been applied until extensive investigations had been done.

CASE 4.1

A young married woman with no children came to see me (IRMcW) with lower abdominal pains. Because she had previously had an ectopic pregnancy, this was suspected at first. Observation in the hospital was sufficient to exclude this diagnosis. The pains continued, however, and it became clear that the patient was going through a severe marital crisis. During the same week, her husband came to see me with intercostal muscle pain and her father attended with depression, neither of them connecting their problems with the family situation. The illnesses of husband and father took on a new meaning in the context of the crisis in the family. The crisis came to a head in the same week with the separation of husband and wife.

The picture of a family obtained through the eyes of one of its members is often very different from the picture obtained from the physician's personal knowledge of other family members. This derives from the reality that the family experience is different for each member of the family. Accepting without corroboration the version given by one family member is one of the most common pitfalls for the family physician (Case 4.2).

CASE 4.2

A man who was already a patient of the practice married a woman from another town. Soon after their marriage the husband came to see me (IRMcW) because he was worried about his wife's behavior. From his description I thought she might be developing schizophrenia. I suggested that she herself should come to see me. She did not come, but soon afterward I was asked to see her at home because she was vomiting. Her husband was there when I visited. It soon became clear that she had hyperemesis gravidarum. I explained the problem and its management and arranged for follow-up. Apart from some reticence, her behavior seemed normal. Shortly after my visit, the husband told me that she had left him and had returned to her hometown. I heard no more until she came to see me one day, late in her pregnancy. She came to explain her sudden departure. Soon after her marriage she had developed a deep antipathy toward her husband because of his behavior toward her. Shortly after my visit, things had come to a head and she had decided to leave him. She had returned to her hometown and made arrangements to have the baby there. There was no evidence of mental instability.

CASE 4.3

An elderly woman who shared a house with her sister had troublesome neurodermatitis and seemed anxious and tense. Her sister was also a patient and always produced in me (IRMcW) a vague feeling of threat and uneasiness. I wondered if she was having the same effect on her sister. The response to the question, "How do you get on with your sister?" was an outburst of feeling.

When the physician does have personal knowledge of all family members, he or she may be able to form hypotheses based on this personal knowledge (Case 4.3).

Another advantage of caring for the entire family is the increase in management options available to the family physician. If, for example, the physician has determined that the problem with a crying baby is causing the mother's exhaustion and depression, attention can be turned to the mother.

Caring for more than one member of a family can lead the physician to some ethical issues that do not arise in other fields of medicine. These issues arise when the interests of different family members conflict. Dealing successfully with them requires both moral awareness and a knowledge of pitfalls.

It could still be maintained that this knowledge and these skills are not unique to family medicine. An internist could care for a family with adult members in exactly the same way. Of course he or she could, and he or she would be functioning as a family physician. The name and the academic pigeonhole are not really important. In practice, however, we still doubt whether many physicians outside family medicine are trained to think and practice in this way.

FAMILY NORMS

In Western countries, we tend to assume that the norms we take for granted in human development and family function are universal. Western assumptions about the value of individual autonomy, and the need to raise children to be independent, are foreign to the cultures of India, Japan, and many other countries. Childrearing in India and Japan, for example, fosters dependence and interdependence. India is a "high-context" society (see Chapter 8). Roland (1988) observes that "contextualizing rather than universalising is central to Indian cognition. . . . Everything from the . . . time of day, which has its own moods and flow, to specific houses [and] landscapes . . . have their own substances, gross or subtle, which flow from their context to those around through permeable ego boundaries ... every-thing in one's environment becomes personalised." (Roland, 1988, p. 273). These characteristics are compellingly captured in contemporary Indian literature (Mistry, 2002).

Although the norms are so different between one culture and another, the importance of family relationships in health and disease is universal. Differences between cultures may have therapeutic implications. Family studies in the West and in India have shown that Indian families have a higher tolerance and acceptance of family members with schizophrenia, and are less likely to respond to them with negative emotions (Leff, 1989). While highly interdependent kinship groups may limit individual freedom, they can also provide strong support in illness and adversity. A high value placed on independence can lead to different needs in family members that are difficult to reconcile without conflict. In a culture of restrictive family relationships, individuals may be expected to sacrifice their own aspirations for the greater good of the family, and to stifle their feelings. Roland (1988) observes that Indian women who are obliged to bottle up their feelings often develop somatic symptoms. In contrast to people with similar illnesses in Western countries, however, Indians are more likely to understand the connection between their symptoms and the stresses of living in the extended family.

Among immigrant families, the first generation born in the new culture tends to adopt its values, rather than those of their parents. The stage is then set for a stressful intergenerational conflict.

WHAT IS A FAMILY?

The changing nature of the family in industrial societies has led some to question whether the idea of a family physician is still appropriate. The error here is to identify "family" with a particular kinship group, such as the so-called nuclear family of father, mother, and children. If a family is defined as a group of intimates with both a history and a future (Ransom and Vandervoort, 1973), then the actual structure of the group may vary without changing its essential function. Any general practice is likely to contain family groups of different kinds. Most families will probably represent the common kinship group in the culture from which the practice population is drawn. This will vary in different parts of the world, according to whether the practice is in North America, Latin America, the West Indies, Africa, and so on. It may also vary within the same country, for example, if the practice has an immigrant, native, or inner-city population.

Although most families in a practice will probably be conventional kinship groups, other kinds of families will almost certainly be represented. There is nothing new in this. When I (IRMcW) entered practice in the 1950s, these nontypical family groups were quite common: elderly women living together, often widowed or unmarried sisters; unmarried brothers and sisters; male or female couples living in stable relationships; elderly widowers with house-keepers who had become part of the family; and gay couples. We took it for granted that these groups functioned like families.

The decline of the extended family in many industrialized societies has been overemphasized. It is true that many families become widely scattered, but modern communications make it much easier for family members to remain in touch with each other, and to come together at times of crisis. It is not unusual today for families to come together from the ends of the earth.

RECENT CHANGES IN THE STRUCTURE AND FUNCTION OF THE FAMILY

It seems a truism to state that family structures are changing. When has it ever been otherwise? The structure of families across cultures and over time has always been changing. During the Middle Ages family structure changed very slowly, however. The onset of the industrial revolution rapidly sped up changes in families. While change is not new, the pace of change in the latter half of the twentieth century and the early years of the twenty-first has been extraordinary and is present across cultures and around the world. Older, more traditional family structures tend to last longer in rural areas, but as populations become more urbanized, these structures change as well, often producing intergenerational tensions.

Changes in family structures and function have been accelerated with the education of women in society and the availability of birth control. The changing role of women in both industrialized, urban societies and those emerging from agrarian-based economies has been a signature event in the late twentieth and early twenty-first centuries. These trends represent a challenge to traditional, patrilineal societies. The combination of education and fertility control in women has been associated with reduced family sizes. More women in the workforce has meant that women have greater economic autonomy. Declining fertility rates have been a factor in immigration policies, and new immigrant families are commonplace in many countries. Technologies such as artificial insemination, in-vitro fertilization, borrowed wombs, and surrogate mothers enable new family constellations (Segalen, 1996). Families with same-sex parents are increasingly common.

With rapid changes come some dislocation, and their impact has been felt in the kind of health problems encountered by family physicians. Fragile families, buffeted by adverse social and economic forces, have become a source of the "new morbidity" (Haggerty, 1975): spousal and parental violence, sexual abuse, parental distress, eating disorders, and premature parenthood. Domestic violence itself spawns or exacerbates many other health problems that present to family physicians (Heise, Pitanguy, and Germain, 1994; Day 1995).

In the United States, as of 2013, the poverty rate was 14.5%, down from 15% in 2012, but the rate for children living in poverty was 19.9% (US Census Bureau, 2013). This is of great importance as poverty is a powerful determinant of health.

The United States has seen an increase in the average age at marriage and in families without children younger than 18 years. There is a greater proportion of births to women older than 30 years. The rate of births to unmarried women went from 5.3% in 1960 to 40.6% in 2008. Divorce rates nearly doubled from the 1950s, reaching a peak in the 1980s and showing a slight decline since. Most divorced couples remarry, so "step-families" are more common. Single-parent families headed by women have experienced a rapid growth since 1970, and represent 29.5% of all households with children. These families report incomes that are only 31% those of married-couple families. As more women come into the workforce, there has occurred an increased demand for alternative child-care arrangements. There is a hidden cost to these arrangements, as they lead to longer days for children and more exposure to infectious diseases. Care by baby boomers of their own parents has led to the designation "sandwich generation" as they try to balance the needs of elderly family with those of the younger generation. Children are increasingly raised in a media-rich environment of television, computers, smartphones, and so on, over which there seems to be little control. Not surprisingly, many parents express concerns about their own abilities to meet the competing demands and challenges represented by these changes (American Academy of Pediatrics, 2003). Pregnant teenagers are a particularly vulnerable group, tending to come from poorer families and to have poorer education and job prospects. In 2011, 63% of children under the age of 18 lived with two married parents, 5% with two unmarried parents, and 24% with a single female parent. Five percent lived with a guardian (Laughlin, 2014). A much higher proportion of African-American families have a single parent, usually female. Fifty-nine percent of men aged 18–24 were still living in their parent's home compared with 51% of women of the same age. The number of one-person households has increased from 17.1% in 1970 to 27.5% in 2012 with the largest increase being in men living alone (Vespa, Lewis, Kreider, 2013).

There are links between economic trends and these changes in family composition and stability. High rates of unemployment and lower earning capacity among males are associated with lower marriage rates, more births to single women, and increased likelihood of marital disruption. Unmarried, unemployed adult males still living with parents have become more common.

WHAT IT MEANS TO "THINK FAMILY"

A family is a social organization or system and has features in common with other social systems. A system (see Chapter 5, "Philosophical and Scientific Foundations of Family Medicine") is defined as a number of parts and processes standing in mutual interaction with each other. The family system changes over time as its members grow older. Part of "thinking family" is an awareness of the challenges faced by a family in adapting to these changes.

Any change in one part of the family system has repercussions for the entire family. A major change—such as birth, death, marriage, divorce, disability, loss of job—has profound effects. A family physician has to be attentive to the needs of family members affected by the misfortunes of their relatives: the children of divorced couples; the siblings of a disabled adolescent; the widows and widowers; the wife of an unemployed man.

Social systems depend for their proper functioning on information and communication. Problems in the family are often due to remediable difficulties in communication, especially the communication of feelings. "Thinking family" is being aware of a physician's responsibility for providing good information, and being vigilant for communication blocks within a family.

"Thinking family" is being sensitive to the unmentioned family stresses that often lie behind depression and somatic symptoms such as headaches, dyspepsia, or recurrent abdominal pain. It is also being aware of the effects on the family system of the physician's own actions—for example, admitting somebody to the hospital, making a serious diagnosis. Case 9.1 in Chapter 9 is an example of the failure to "think family."

"Thinking family" is being aware of some of the traps that await the unwary physician: being enlisted by one side of a family conflict, accepting the family's views of a troublesome adolescent, and disclosing to other family members information that should be confidential.

THE INFLUENCE OF THE FAMILY ON HEALTH AND DISEASE

The family has six main effects on the health of its members.

Genetic Influences

Every individual is a product of the interaction between his or her genotype and the environment. Recent advances in describing and understanding the human genome make it more important that family physicians be conversant with and able to communicate the significance of the results of genetic counseling to patients and their families.

The Family Is Crucial in Child Development

Although children have a remarkable capacity for overcoming early difficulties, there is a large body of evidence supporting the relationship between family dysfunction and childhood disorders—both physical and behavioral.

Parental deprivation for prolonged periods is associated with psychological problems, including suicide, depression, and personality disorder. The relationship is by no means constant, and the outcome depends on individual factors such as the previous parent–child relationship and the availability of parent substitutes. The evidence is sufficiently suggestive, however, for the family physician to advise parents to avoid separation from the child whenever possible in the crucial stage between 3 months and 4 years. When separation is unavoidable, as in the serious illness of mother or child, care should be taken to minimize the trauma by providing a good mother-substitute or by keeping the child's time in the hospital to a minimum.

One of the most important longitudinal studies of family function and child health was the Newcastle-upon-Tyne "Thousand Families" study (Miller, Court, Walton, and Knox, 1960). A group of 1142 infants was enrolled at the beginning of the study in 1947. These children and their families were observed and examined over a 15-year period by a team of health visitors (public health nurses) and pediatricians. By 1962, 763 children remained in the study. The results are generally applicable to any industrial community, although allowances must be made for the preponderance of working-class families and the comparative poverty of the community in the early years of the study.

Respiratory disease was the most common health problem. In the first 5 years it accounted for half of all illnesses and two-thirds of all infections. The frequency and severity declined during the school years, but the ratio of respiratory to total illness remained. At all ages the incidence and severity of lower respiratory infection was strongly related to adverse family factors. In 1961, 45 children had some disability due to respiratory disease: 6 had suppurative otitis media, 11 recurrent bronchitis, 10 asthma, 6 allergic rhinitis, and 4 bronchiectasis.

Intestinal infections were strongly related to inadequate housing, overcrowding, and poor maternal care. In 20 "streptococcal families" there were repeated streptococcal infections in different family members over months or years. In 25 "staphylococcal families" there was a similar pattern of repeated staphylococcal infections. Staphylococcal infection in preschool children was strongly associated with large families, overcrowding, and poor maternal care.

Nonfebrile convulsions were significantly associated with low social class, a family history of seizures, mental illness, parental deprivation, and defective child care.

Accidents in the first 5 years accounted for 8% of the total illness and nearly 50% of noninfectious illness. The peak incidence was in the second year. In this age group, more than half the accidents occurred at home. Accidents during the school years more commonly occurred away from home. At all ages there was a significant association with poor maternal care and low intelligence in the child.

Enuresis affected 18% of children at 5 years, 12% at 10, 6% at 13, and 2% at 15. Enuretic children were smaller than nonenuretic children, had a lower mean IQ, and more of them were maladjusted. Enuresis was associated with low social class, overcrowding, poor maternal care, and absence or ineffectiveness of the father. The authors conclude that "bedwetting is seen as a developmental disability, mainly determined by the interaction of adverse social, emotional and intellectual factors" (p. 153). Dysrhythmic speech was found in 43 children, and nine still stuttered at the age of 15. Stuttering was more common in children from families with adverse factors.

Children with behavioral disturbance (nearly 20%) were below the mean in height, weight, intelligence, school attainment, and ability to communicate. Their parents were younger, more recently married, often lived with relations, and tended to be dependent on their parents. A high proportion of mothers had a history of mental illness and had experienced severe stress during pregnancy. Miller and his colleagues (1960) conclude, "At the centre of maladjustment was a deeply unsatisfactory relationship between mother and child. Separation was a contributory factor, but mainly through intensifying preexisting family instability. The extent of maladjustment suggests urgent need for a critical study of existing methods of treatment and a more intensive search for rational ways of prevention" (p. 255).

Other work has continued to demonstrate the importance of parenting and the harmful effect of parenting failure on child development. Klaus and Kennell (1976) have demonstrated the importance of early postnatal bonding between mother and child, a relationship enhanced by breastfeeding but made more difficult by some of the procedures used in obstetric units in the past. More attention is paid to skin-to-skin time immediately after birth. This refers to the length of time the newborn is in direct contact with the mother or father and is positively associated with improved physiological and cognitive control in children (Feldman, Rosenthal, and Eidelman, 2014).

Parental neglect, both physical and emotional, is considered to be the most common cause of failure to thrive. In emotionally deprived children, the secretion of growth hormone is reduced. Inadequate parenting has a range of effects on child development, from physical trauma at one end of the scale to mild behavior disorders at the other. What makes this doubly important is that children deprived of adequate parenting are likely to repeat the same pattern when they themselves become parents.

The importance of fathers to the development of children has recently received more attention. Fathers' engagement or involvement with their children has been associated with decreased behavioral problems in adolescence, better social functioning in childhood and adulthood, and better educational outcomes (Sarkadi, Kristiansson, Oberklaid, and Bremberg, 2008).

Boyce (2009) summarizes several decades of epidemiological and biomedical research on the health of children. Adverse childhood events, such as physical, sexual, or emotional abuse or loss of parent or an addicted or depressed parent, are associated with elevated risks of the major sources of adult mortality as well as respiratory infections and mental health problems. Chronic stress affects cellular aging and epigenetic and genetic expression.

A number of longitudinal studies (Smith and Joshi, 2002; Batty, 2004), along with new knowledge from the neurosciences, have provided important insights into the influence of early environment (biological, psychological, and social) and family life on later health. Life-course research has begun to emphasize that many of the chronic diseases of adult life have their roots in early childhood. The concept of developmental "windows" for the optimal establishment of various human functions is important to understanding the impact of early family life on later health.

The Early Years Study (McCain and Mustard, 1999) summarizes the literature on environmental influences on the developing neuroarchitecture of children. The first few years of life represent a window of opportunity that, if missed because of poor nutrition, or physical and psychological stress, has an enduring impact. In this early time period, as neural connections are made and nurtured, the groundwork for functions such as binocular vision, emotional competence, habitual ways of responding, and language are laid down. After age 6 it becomes much more difficult to make changes in these areas. If the child receives inadequate or inappropriate stimulation during this period, he or she will be more prone to learning difficulties and behavioral and emotional problems later in life. For some, this may include juvenile delinquency and crime. Further, poor nutrition in early life predisposes to later development of hypertension, diabetes, and obesity. The neural and endocrine responses to stress are determined during these early years and, in both animal and human studies, it has been shown that poor nurturing in this time period leads to prolonged hormonal responses, long after the original stimulation has subsided. This has negative long-term biological effects, for although stress hormones are a useful short-term adaptation, when prolonged they cause multiple deleterious effects. When there is a dysfunctional development of the limbic system and midbrain, it appears that children live in a constant state of low-grade arousal that may negatively impact on their learning capabilities. They become labeled as "learning disabled" and may resort to inappropriately aggressive behavior in order to cope with their stress.

Longitudinal studies have demonstrated that women who experience family disruption and conflict during their early years were more prone to depression and other mental health problems in adult life (Maughan and McCarthy, 1997). The advent of longitudinal studies has contributed to a new area of epidemiology called the *life history approach*. Emotional learning in early life happens implicitly, begins before birth, and is shaped in the "limbic nexus" of family life. The concept of "limbic attractors" has been borrowed from systems theory to explain the tendency of repeating certain emotional behavioral responses, even when we desire a different outcome. This has been used to explain the observation that some individuals repeatedly enter into damaging relationships, for example.

Some Families Are More Vulnerable to Illness Than Others

In one of the seminal studies in family medicine, Huygen (1982) has described and analyzed his experience with families in a rural community in Holland over a period of more than 30 years. As one part of his study, he examined family influences on morbidity in samples of 100 young families and 100 older families. In the young families there was a significant correlation between morbidity rates in members of the same family. The correlation was greatest between mothers and children. The differences between families in frequency of illness tended to be stable over the years. Families with high morbidity rates tended to be high over the whole 20-year period, and those with low rates tended to be low over the whole period. The differences between families with high and low rates were not explained by factors such as hygiene, housing, and income. There were, however, significant relationships between emotional stability in the parents and family illness rates. Illness rates were higher in families where one or both parents were emotionally unstable and where there was marital discord.

In the older families, similar relationships were found. There was a familial incidence of disorders of the skin, respiratory tract, and gastrointestinal tract, and of nervous disorders and accidents. In nervous disorders the correlations were significant only between father and mother, and there were no significant correlations between parents for accidents and gastrointestinal disorders. Further analysis showed that vulnerable families were susceptible to the entire range of these disorders, not one particular category. This is consistent with the finding of Hinkle (1974) that vulnerable individuals are susceptible to the entire spectrum of diseases "across the board," leading him to formulate the concept of "general susceptibility to illness."

Huygen found that members of the same family, although similar in their illness patterns, were not similar in their rates of patient–doctor consultations and admission to the hospital. This suggests that the similarities between family members were due to similar frequencies of illness rather than to similarities of illness behavior.

In 1970, Huygen and his colleagues carried out a cross-sectional study of 210 randomly selected families from his practice who had not been involved in the earlier studies. The children were between 12 and 22 years of age, and the parents' ages ranged from 40 to 64. Medical students visited the families and collected data on sense of well-being, symptoms, medical knowledge, readiness to seek medical help, anxiety level, and experience with serious illness in their neighborhood. These data were related to the number of contacts with the family doctor and number of diagnoses between 1967 and 1970.

There were highly significant correlations between family members in their sense of well-being and in the number of symptoms experienced. Medical help was sought for less than 10% of all symptoms. There were significant correlations between family members in readiness to seek medical help and in contacts with the family doctor. Anxiety scores, however, showed little correlation between family members.

The psychological and social characteristics of parents showed a stronger relationship with the frequency of illness in their children than with their own. Children had more illnesses when

their parents tended to avoid conflicts;
their mother was little involved in social networks outside the family;
their parents were prone to somatic complaints;
their parents had less than average sense of well-being;
their mother was strongly inclined to accept the sick role;
there was a discrepancy in their parents' knowledge of the complaints of the
    spouse.

Huygen interpreted these results as supporting Balint's concept of "the child as a presenting symptom."

In a prospective study of the relationship of family structure and functioning, and life events, to the outcome of pregnancy, Ramsey, Abell, and Baker (1986) found that abnormal family functioning was a strong predictor of low birth weight. The abnormalities of function included disengagement, enmeshment, and both rigid and chaotic families.

One of the largest studies examining the association between maltreatment in childhood and adult health is the Adverse Childhood Experiences (ACE) Study. Initiated in 1995, it involves 17,000 members of health maintenance organizations (HMOs), and it continues to gather information. Using a score of the total count of adverse childhood events (ACE score) it has been

Box 4.1

HEALTH CONDITIONS LINKED TO ACE
SCORE IN CHILDHOOD

Alcoholism and alcohol abuse
Chronic obstructive pulmonary disease (COPD)
Depression
Fetal death
Health-related quality of life
Illicit drug use
Ischemic heart disease (IHD)
Liver disease
Risk for intimate partner violence
Multiple sexual partners
Sexually transmitted diseases (STDs)
Smoking
Suicide attempts
Unintended pregnancies
Early initiation of smoking
Early initiation of sexual activity
Adolescent pregnancy

demonstrated that as the score increases, the risk for a large number of health problems also increases. These problems are listed in Box 4.1.

Infectious Disease Spreads in Families

Streptococcal and staphylococcal family infections have already been mentioned. Meyer and Haggerty (1962) showed that streptococcal infection is related to acute and chronic family stress.

Virus infections have a strong tendency to spread from the index cases to other family members. In their study of family infections in Cleveland, Dingle, Badger, and Jordan (1964) found that infections were introduced into the home, in descending order of frequency, by schoolchildren under 6, preschool children, schoolchildren over 6, mothers, and fathers. Respiratory and intestinal infections decrease in frequency with increasing age. The number of infections is directly related to family size. Preschool children are the most susceptible to infections because they have not yet acquired immunity. Children starting school are more likely to bring infections home because they are exposed to other children at a time when their immunity is incomplete.

The number of infections falls rapidly as immunity is acquired during the early school years.

The same infection may take different forms as it spreads through the family. A virus may produce sore throat in one member, diarrhea in the next, cough and coryza in another. The mumps virus may produce parotitis in one member, orchitis in another.

Tuberculosis, venereal diseases, intestinal parasites, and skin infections must be included in any list of family infections.

Family Factors Affect Morbidity and Mortality in Adults

Mortality is significantly increased in widowers and widows in the first year after bereavement. This increase in mortality is not confined to one or two causes of death: it covers the whole range of diseases.

Mortality for most causes of death is much higher among widowed, divorced, and single people than among the married. Widowers are especially susceptible. Kraus and Lilienfeld (1959) have shown that young widowers (aged 25–35) have a mortality rate 12 times higher than the comparable married group for tuberculosis, 8 times higher for vascular lesions of the nervous system, 10 times higher for hypertensive heart disease, 8 times higher for influenza and pneumonia, and nearly 5 times higher for arteriosclerotic heart disease.

Bereavement is associated with an increase in consultation rate. This probably represents both a true increase in morbidity rate and an increased utilization of medical services.

In counties of North Carolina, stroke mortality in African-American males was significantly related to family disorganization as measured by rates of divorce, separation, and single parenthood. In males between 35 and 44, mortality increased almost threefold as the level of disorganization increased from the lowest to the highest levels (Nesser, 1975).

Medalie and Goldbourt (1976) showed that males with severe family problems were three times more likely to develop angina than those with a low score for family problems. In males with high anxiety levels, the risk of developing angina was significantly lower in those who received much support and love from their wives than in those who did not.

For reasons that are little understood, husbands and wives are more often concordant for hypertension than would be expected by chance.

Family factors affect not only the occurrence of illness, but also the utilization of medical services. Utilization increases at times of family stress. Clustering of visits may be an important cue to family problems.

The Family Is Important in Recovery from Illness

Family support is an important factor in the outcome of all kinds of illness, but especially in chronic illness and disability. Pless and Satterwhite (1973) found that children with chronic disease fared better in well-functioning than in poorly functioning families.

When combined with the emerging understanding from the neurosciences, a picture is evolving that recognizes the impact of genetic endowment, and prenatal and early childhood environment, on later physical and mental health and over the course of a person's lifetime. This begins to provide a unified vision of human health and disease for family practitioners. It fits well with the fundamental assumptions in the discipline of family medicine. When we confront an adult with a new diagnosis, we need to understand the entire history of the patient, not only current and recent lifestyle choices. The physician who has attended a patient for a long period of his or her lifetime, perhaps including the prenatal period, delivery, and childhood, has an obvious advantage in coming to an insightful understanding and helping the patient cope realistically with the implications of a new diagnosis, illness, or life event. Indeed, such a physician has become an integral part of the patient's life history, and vice versa. In addition, however, this new understanding of the importance of host factors in early life requires physicians to be advocates for measures that address negative environmental influences in early life.

THE FAMILY LIFE CYCLE

An understanding of the family life cycle, together with an understanding of individual development, can help the physician form good hypotheses about the problems that patients are experiencing. In the course of its development, the family goes through a number of predictable transitions: marriage, childbirth, school years and adolescence, school graduation and starting work or further education, children leaving home, involution, retirement, and widowhood. The physician, by using his or her insight into these transitions, can help families anticipate and prepare for them, and at the same time can enrich his or her own understanding of the context of illnesses.

Families also experience unexpected crises that demand adaptive responses: illnesses, accidents, divorce, loss of job, and death of a family member.

Duvall (1977) has developed an eight-stage schema of the family life cycle. Duvall's schema is reproduced in Figure 4.1, with the number of years an American family can be expected to spend in each stage. All families, of course, do not go through the complete cycle in sequence or the time frames shown in the figure. One child may remain in the home after attaining adulthood and

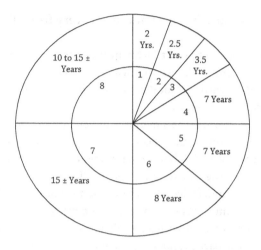

1. Married couples (without children)
2. Childbearing families (oldest child 30 months)
3. Families with preschool children (oldest child 30 months –6 years)
4. Families with school children (oldest child 6–13 years)
5. Families with teenagers (oldest child 13–20 years)

6. Families launching young adults (first child gone to last child leaving home)
7. Middle-aged parents (empty nest to retirement)
8. Aging family members (retirement to death of both spouses)

Figure 4.1:
The family life cycle by length of time in each of eight stages.
From Duvall EM. 1977. *Marriage and Family Development*, 5th ed. Philadelphia, PA: Lippincott.

may stay there until the parents die. Divorced people with children, if they remarry, go through stages one and four at the same time.

DEVELOPMENTAL TASKS

Developmental tasks are defined by Duvall as tasks that arise at a certain stage in the life of the individual or family, adaptation to which may lead to happiness and success with later tasks. Maladaptation to these tasks, on the other hand, may lead to unhappiness, disapproval by society, and difficulty with later tasks. In assuming a developmental task, an individual must (1) perceive new possibilities for his or her behavior, (2) form new conceptions of self, (3) cope effectively with conflicting demands, and (4) have the motivation to achieve the next stage in his or her development. Sometimes the developmental tasks of different family members are in harmony, as when a husband and wife are jointly learning to live in an "empty nest." Often, however, developmental tasks of family members are in conflict, and many of the tensions of family life are caused by these conflicts. The adolescent's need to achieve independence almost inevitably brings him or her into conflict with the parents' task of guiding his or her development to a responsible maturity. When husband and wife both have careers, their needs for education and career development can easily lead to conflict at some stage in the family life cycle.

Duvall's concept of the developmental tasks facing the family at each stage in its life cycle is shown in Table 4.1. The family's developmental tasks are centered on the family's most important function: the nurturing of children from birth to maturity. They obviously relate closely to the developmental tasks of individual family members.

In recommending the family life cycle and the concept of developmental tasks as a perspective for family physicians, a word of caution is necessary. Families have taken on many new dimensions, including unmarried couples, single-parent adoptions, permanent single-parent households, and same sex unions with or without children. Becoming familiar with these various family constellations and their functioning will stand the family physician in good stead (Walsh, 2012). The expectations of individuals and families vary greatly between one culture and another. Other cultural groups, elsewhere in the world and even in North America, can be expected to have different norms. Family physicians should be aware of the cultural rituals that mark the major transitions of family life in their patients—hence the importance for family physicians of learning the cultural norms of their patients. Whatever the cultural differences, however, it is probably a universal reality that family life is marked by crises and conflicts, adaptation and maladaptation.

THE TRAUMAS OF FAMILY LIFE

Besides the normal transitions, many families also face adverse conditions and go through traumatic episodes that may have profound effects on health (McEwen and Seeman, 1999; Seeman, Crimmins, Huang, 2004). The cumulative effect of genetic endowment and environmental stress, or wear and tear, is known as the allostatic load and has been linked to the long-observed negative relationship between socioeconomic status and health.

The Effects of Inadequate Parenting

In all families, the arrival of children is a major change. In some families, it produces stresses that the system is too fragile to bear. The effects on the children can range from failure to thrive to physical abuse.

Family physicians are in a very good position to identify families that are at risk for these problems, especially if they are caring for the mother during

Table 4.1. STAGE-CRITICAL FAMILY DEVELOPMENTAL TASKS THROUGH THE FAMILY LIFE CYCLE

Stage of the Family Life Cycle	Positions in the Family	Stage-Critical Family Developmental Tasks
1. Married couple	Wife/Husband	Establish a mutually satisfying marriage
		Adjusting to pregnancy and the promise of parenthood
		Fitting into a new kin network
2. Childbearing	Wife–mother	Having, adjusting to, and encouraging the development of infants
	Husband–father	
	Infant daughter or son or both	Establishing a satisfying home for both parents and infants
3. Preschool-age	Wife–mother	Adapting to the critical needs and interests of preschool children in stimulating, growth-promoting ways
	Husband–father	
	Daughter–sister	
	Son–brother	
		Coping with energy depletion and lack of privacy as parents
4. School-age	Wife–mother	Fitting into the community of school-age families in constructive ways
	Husband–father	
	Daughter–sister	
	Son–brother	
		Encouraging children's educational achievement
5. Teenage	Wife–mother	Balancing freedom with responsibility as teenagers mature and emancipate themselves
	Husband–father	
	Daughter–sister	
	Son–brother	
		Establish postparental interests and careers as growing parents
6. Launching center	Wife–mother–grandmother	Releasing young adults into work, military service, marriage, etc., with appropriate rituals and assistance
	Husband–father–grandfather	
	Daughter–sister–aunt	
	Son–brother–uncle	
7. Middle-aged parents	Wife–mother–grandmother	Rebuilding the marriage relationship
	Husband–father–grandfather	Maintaining kin ties with old and younger generations
8. Aging family members	Widow–widower	Coping with bereavement and living alone
	Wife–mother–grandmother	
	Husband–father–grandfather	Closing the family home or adapting it to aging
		Adjusting to retirement

Reprinted with permission from Duvall EM. *Marriage and Family Development*, 5th ed. Philadelphia, PA: Lippincott. 1977.

pregnancy. No single cue is a certain indication that a problem exists. It only indicates a need for extra vigilance. Some situations are known to be associated with problems of parenting:

Parents: unsatisfactory childhood experience with their parents; early marriage; single parents; psychiatric illness; immaturity; prison record in father; alcoholic background in family of origin.

Children: prematurity; handicapped children; unwanted children; babies who cry a lot.

Problems of parenting need to be understood not as the result of single causes, but rather as the result of mismatches between parent and child and to the stresses of a difficult environment. A mother who is able to cope with a normal child may become an abusing parent if her child is handicapped. The physician has to observe the interaction between parent and child, rather than individual behavior. The prenatal and postnatal periods provide opportunities for making systematic observations of maternal and child behavior. Boxes 4.2, 4.3, and 4.4, give warning signs that may be detected during pregnancy, delivery, and the postpartum period. Once a family has been recognized as vulnerable, they can be given additional support in the form of more frequent visits by doctor or nurse and extra time for dealing with problems.

Domestic Violence

Some conflict occurs in all families. The ways in which conflict is handled and resolved are a measure of how well the family functions. Continuing, unresolved conflict between husband and wife, or between parents and children, may present to the family physician as depression in an adult or child, as physical injury in the wife, as somatic symptoms in adults or children, as school behavior problems, or as acting-out behavior in adolescents. Sometimes, the presentation is a cluster of illnesses in different family members (Case 4.4). Intimate partner violence (IPV) is both common and commonly overlooked. In the United States, 35.5% of women

---

CASE 4.4

A 10-year-old boy was brought by his mother with aches and pains. No physical abnormality was found. A few weeks later his teenaged sister was admitted to the hospital with attempted suicide. On further inquiry, the mother revealed that her husband had been waking in the night and terrorizing the family by violent behavior.

Box 4.2
HIGH-RISK SIGNALS IN THE PRENATAL CLINIC SETTING

These are the indication of possible problems. A high-risk situation is created by varying combinations of these signs, the family's degree of emphasis on them, and the family's willingness to change. The interviewer must take into consideration the mother's age, culture, and education, as well as observations of her affect and the significance of her feelings. Many of these signs can be observed throughout the perinatal period; they are listed in this order because they are found most commonly at these times:

- Overconcern with the unborn baby's sex
  - Reasons that a certain sex is so important, for example, to fill the mother's needs
  - The mother's need to please the father with the baby's sex
  - The quality and rigidity of these needs
- Expressed high expectations for the baby
  - Overconcern with the baby's physical and developmental progress, behavior, and discipline
  - The parents' need to have control over the baby's actions and reactions
  - Is this child wanted in order to fulfill unmet needs in parents' lives?
- Is this child going to be one too many?
  - Is there adequate spacing between this child and the next younger child?
  - During the pregnancy, has there been evidence of a disintegrating relationship with the older child(ren), for example, physical or emotional abuse for the first time?
- Evidence of the mother's desire to deny the pregnancy
  - Unwillingness to gain weight
  - Refusal to talk about the pregnancy in a manner commensurate with the reality of the situation
  - Not wearing maternity clothes when it would be appropriate
  - No plans made for the baby's nursery, layette, and so forth, in the home
- Great depression over the pregnancy
  - Date of onset of depression to this pregnancy
  - Report of sleep disturbance that cannot be related to the physical aspects of pregnancy
  - Attempted suicide
  - Dropping out socially
  - Bland affect

- Did either parent formerly ever seriously consider an abortion?
  - Why didn't they go through with it?
  - Did they passively delay a decision until medically therapeutic abortion was not feasible?
- Did the parents ever seriously consider relinquishment?
  - Why did they change their minds?
  - The reality and quality expressed in the change of decision
- To whom does the mother turn for support?
  - How reliable and helpful are they to her?
  - Who accompanies the mother to the clinic?
  - Are any community agencies involved in a supportive way?
- Is the mother very alone and/or frightened?
  - Is this just because of the lack of education or understanding of pregnancy and delivery?
  - Is she overly concerned about the physical changes during pregnancy, labor, and delivery?
  - Do careful explanation, prenatal classes, and so on, dissipate these fears?
  - Does she tend to keep the focus of the interview on her fears and needs rather than any anticipation, excitement, or joy projected onto the new baby?
- The mother has many unscheduled visits to the prenatal clinic or the emergency room.
  - With exaggerated physical complaints that cannot be substantiated on physical examination or by laboratory tests
  - Multiple psychosomatic complaints
  - An overdependence on the doctor or nurse
- What are the patient's living arrangements?
  - Are the physical accommodations adequate?
  - Does she have a telephone? Is transportation available?
  - Are there friends or relatives nearby?
- The parents cannot talk freely on the above topics and avoid eye contact.
- What can you find out about the parents' backgrounds?
  - Did they grow up in a foster home?
  - Were they shuffled from one relative to another?
  - What type of discipline was used? (They may not see this as abusive.)
  - Do they plan to raise their children the way their parents raised them?

Source: Gray, Cutler, Dean, and Kempe, 1976. Reprinted with permission from Child Abuse and Neglect: The Family and the Community, copyright 1976, Ballinger Publishing Company.

Box 4.3
HIGH-RISK SIGNALS IN THE DELIVERY ROOM

Written form with baby's chart concerning parents' reactions at birth.
- How does the mother look?
- What does the mother say?
- What does the mother do?

The following phrases may help in the organization of information regarding observations for the above-mentioned form.

- Does the parent appear sad, happy, apathetic, disappointed, angry, exhausted, frightened, ambivalent?
- Does the parent talk to the baby, talk to spouse, use baby's name, establish eye contact, touch, cuddle, examine?
- Does the spouse, friend, relative offer support, criticism, rejection, ambivalence?

If this interaction seems dubious, further evaluation should be initiated. Concerning reactions at delivery include the following:

- Lack of interest in the baby, ambivalence, passive reaction
- Keeps the focus of attention on herself
- Unwillingness or refusal to hold the baby, even when offered
- Hostility directed toward father who put her "through all this"
  - Inappropriate verbalizations, glances directed at the baby, with definite hostility expressed
- Disparaging remarks about the baby's sex or physical characteristics
- Disappointment over sex or other physical characteristics of the child.

Source: Gray, Cutler, Dean, and Kempe, 1976. Reprinted with permission from Child Abuse and Neglect: The Family and the Community, copyright 1976, Ballinger Publishing Company.

and 28.5% of men report having experienced rape, physical violence, and or/or stalking by an intimate partner in their lifetime (Black, Basile, Breiding, et al., 2011). In a study carried out in Bangladesh, where more than 40% of Bangladeshi mothers and young children experienced IPV, it was found that the children suffered significantly more respiratory infection and diarrhea than children not exposed to IPV (Silverman, Decker, Gupta, et al., 2009).

Injuries in women resulting from family violence are often concealed or explained as accidental. The physician should be on guard for this. Marital discord is a common reason for chronic depression, especially in women. A wide variety of medical and psychological symptoms may have their roots in an

Box 4.4

HIGH-RISK SIGNALS IN THE POSTPARTUM PERIOD
(IN POSTPARTUM WARD AND IN WELL-BABY CLINIC)

- Does the family remain disappointed over the sex of the baby?
- What is the child's name?
  - Who is he or she named for/after?
  - Who picked the name?
  - When was the name picked?
  - Is the name used when talking to or about the baby?
- What was/is the husband's and/or family's reaction to the new baby?
  - Are they supportive?
  - Are they critical?
  - Do they attempt to take over and control the situation?
  - Is the husband jealous of the baby's drain on the mother's time and energy?
- What kind of support, other than family, is the mother receiving?
- Are there sibling rivalry problems? Does the mother expect any? How does she plan to handle them? Or does she deny that a new baby will change existing family relationships?
- Is the mother bothered by the baby's crying?
  - How does it make her feel? Angry? Inadequate? Like crying herself?
- Feedings
  - Does the mother view the baby as too demanding in his or her needs to eat?
  - Does she ignore the demands?
  - Is she repulsed by messiness, for example, spitting up?
  - Is she repulsed by sucking noises?
- How does the mother view changing diapers?
  - Is she repulsed by the messiness, smells, and so forth?
- Are the expectations of the child developmentally far beyond his or her capabilities?
- Mother's control or lack of control over the situation
  - Does she get involved and take control over the baby's needs and what's going to happen (waiting room and during the exam interaction)?
  - Does she relinquish control to the doctor, nurse, and so on (undressing, holding, allowing child to express fears, etc.)?
- Can the mother express that she is having fun with the baby?
  - Can she view him or her as a separate individual?
  - Can attention be focused on him or her and can she see something positive in that for herself?
- Can she establish and maintain eye-to-eye, direct contact with the baby?

- How does she talk with the baby?
- Are her verbalizations about the child usually negative?
- When the child cries, does she, or can she, comfort him or her?

Source: Gray, Cutler, Dean, and Kempe, 1976. Reprinted with permission from Child Abuse and Neglect: The Family and the Community, copyright 1976, Ballinger Publishing Company.

abusive relationship. Often, whether a woman reveals this to her physician depends on the perceived openness of the physician to what may be viewed by the patient as a shameful secret. The investigation of depression and symptoms arising from stress should always include inquiry about family relationships.

When a family physician confirms or strongly suspects that a woman or her children are at risk of domestic violence, the physician must assess the immediacy of the risk and help develop an escape plan if necessary. Most communities now have shelters and supports for abused women and their children. Having this information at hand and available in the family physician's office is an essential tool in family practice.

Another aspect of conflict is the stress induced by conflicting loyalties between different family members. This may be seen, for example, in a woman who is torn between her obligations to her children and to her elderly parents, or between commitments to job and family.

Divorce

Divorce is an experience analogous to bereavement in its capacity to cause grief. The same feelings of anger, bitterness, guilt, and self-doubt arise, without the comfort the bereaved can derive from memories of a loving relationship. Continuing conflict over the divorce settlement or over the children serve to intensify and prolong the pain.

Children are particularly vulnerable to the effects of divorce. About one-third of children are deeply distressed by divorce and continue to be distressed for many years. Very young children (up to age 5) show regression in development: feeding and toilet problems, enuresis, sleep disturbances, and separation anxiety. In early school-aged children, distress may be concealed by denial of difficulties. At this age, however, children may harbor strong feelings of guilt derived from their fantasy of having caused the separation. Distress may be expressed in the form of school problems, somatic symptoms, enuresis, and nightmares.

Older children are often shocked and incredulous. They may be directly involved in custody battles, and this is associated with later maladjustment. They suffer from conflicts of loyalty, which they may resolve by completely rejecting one parent. Adolescent children of divorced parents may have a particularly stormy adolescence and are likely to have a lower self-concept than their peers.

It is important for the family physician to identify and help the vulnerable children of divorced couples. The amount of distress in the children is proportional to the amount of conflict between parents. The Toronto Family Study (Homatidis, Johnson, Orlando, and Robson, 1986) found that vulnerable children had more school changes, fewer friends, more feelings of guilt, needed more help with schoolwork, and experienced the separation as very stressful. Other studies have shown that a good relationship with one parent, good peer relationship, academic success, and involvement in school counseling programs were associated with better adjustment.

Having identified vulnerable children, the physician can either provide counseling within the practice or ensure that the child and parents get help from an agency or school counseling service.

Younger children are often not told about an impending separation on the grounds that "they are too young to understand." This has the effect of increasing the child's anxiety and distress. The physician can help parents to understand the importance of explaining what is happening to the children.

Family physicians may in various ways become enmeshed themselves in divorce and custody proceedings. An attempt may be made by either party to enlist the physician's support in marital conflicts—a particularly difficult situation when husband and wife are both patients. On the other hand, if the physician can retain neutrality, he or she may be able to play a significant part in resolving the conflict. When divorce has become inevitable, the physician may be asked to give evidence in court, or to provide corroboration of abuse or of parenting failures. When disputes arise over visiting rights, the physician may be asked by the favored parent to certify that visits to the other parents make the child ill or anxious or that the child is being sexually abused.

Illness and Disability

Serious illness or disability has profound effects on the life of a family. The actual effect varies with the type of illness and the family member involved: a mentally or physically handicapped child; an adolescent with paraplegia, diabetes, or schizophrenia; a mother with multiple sclerosis; a father with cancer or alcoholism. The common factor in all these situations is the need for the other family members to adjust to the changed situation and to adopt new roles. With these adaptive changes come new risks to other members of the

---

CASE 4.5

An elderly woman with congestive heart failure was cared for during her long terminal illness by her husband. I saw him in the course of many home visits and although he always looked pale, I (IRMcW) never suspected anything amiss. Soon after the woman died, her husband came to see me complaining of severe fatigue. He had prostatic obstruction, renal failure, and uremia with secondary anemia, all of which had been present for the duration of his wife's illness.

---

family, which may in turn affect the member who is sick or disabled (Case 4.5). The harm caused by these changes is potentially preventable if members of the family can be helped to gain enough insight to avoid the risks. Glycemic control in adolescents with type one diabetes both affects and is affected by family stress (Tsiouli, Alexopoulos, Stefanaki, et al., 2013).

Counseling for families of patients with schizophrenia is a good example of what can be done to help families care for patients with chronic illness. Several studies have shown big reductions in relapse rates when families are either counseled in their own homes or invited to attend group sessions with other families (Leff, 1989). Themes running through the group sessions are education about schizophrenia, teaching about problem-solving, improving communication, and dealing with expressed emotion. Patients with schizophrenia are very vulnerable to criticism, hostility, and overinvolvement. Relatives may criticize patients for their apathy and lack of initiative, not realizing that these are manifestations of the illness. Family members can learn to control their negative emotions and to be more tolerant.

Although in the published studies therapy has been carried out by psychiatric teams, the methods could be adapted to family practice. The family physician or a counselor in the practice team could offer a series of sessions to a family in their home, or to members of several families at the practice center. In a less formal way, the physician could provide counseling during routine contacts with family members. The family doctor may be the only person who can reach those relatives who do not attend group sessions and who are likely to be in greatest need of help.

So much attention may be focused on a handicapped child or adolescent that the needs of a spouse or of siblings are not met. The strain of caring for a sick person may go unnoticed both by the physician and by other family members as they concentrate their attention on the sick member. Other members of the family may hide their illnesses or their despair until it becomes too late to help them. Medalie (1975) has stressed the need to be alert for the "hidden patient." Siblings of children with pervasive developmental disorder (PDD) are more likely to have more adjustment problems than siblings of children with Down syndrome or normal children. This appeared to be related to the parental distress that was highest in the PDD group (Fisman, Wolf, Ellsion, et al., 2000).

The question "And how are *you* doing?" can be sufficient to allow another family member to express his or her feelings. People from families with a member who is chronically sick have higher rates of illness themselves than people from families without chronic sickness.

Terminal illness is a particularly stressful time for families, whether the sick person is at home or in the hospital (Case 4.6). As well as grieving over the suffering, and physically exhausted by the demands on them, children or grandchildren may be disturbed by conflicts over sharing the burden of care, or by the resurgence of old conflicts that have remained dormant for years.

One could not imagine a clearer example of death from a broken heart. A "broken heart syndrome" (stress cardiomyopathy, myocardial stunning, takotsubo cardiomyopathy) has been described by Wittstein et al. (2005), and evidence for a physiological linkage through a strong neurohormonal surge has been found. This syndrome should be considered when patients present with symptoms of a myocardial infarction following strong emotional stress such as death of a loved one. In retrospect, her care might have been different if the palliative care team, coronary care team, and family doctor had recognized her as a highly vulnerable person. The risk of cardiac arrest might have been anticipated. Her intense suffering was inevitable, but an urgently convened family conference might have helped the family to respond by increasing their support.

CASE 4.6

The daughter of an elderly couple—a single woman—was dying of cancer in a palliative care unit. Despite vigorous efforts by the palliative care team, her pain remained uncontrolled and her suffering was intense. In the last few days of her life, her mother was admitted to the coronary care unit in another hospital with chest pain. After several days of observation, she was discharged home but continued to complain of pain and was very agitated. The family doctor, who was not involved in the care of the daughter, reassured her about the pain and prescribed a sedative. When her agitation continued, other members of the family became impatient with her, and one of her other children left and returned home. On the same day she died suddenly at home.

Communication problems are common, even in well-functioning families. According to Stedeford (1981), a psychiatrist who has done much work with the families of the dying, poor communication causes more suffering to dying patients and their families than any other problem except unrelieved pain. Married couples, even when very close to each other, may find it very difficult to talk to each other when one becomes terminally ill. Information may be withheld from key members of the family. A dependent child, for example, may not be told that his parent is dying. He may therefore feel, for the rest of his life, that he has been deprived of precious moments with his mother or father. A spouse may try to conceal the diagnosis from the patient, thus imposing intolerable strains on their relationship.

The adaptation of a family to a sick member may itself become a problem when it comes to rehabilitation. The spouses of alcoholics may become so used to their adaptive role that they find it difficult to relinquish control if their spouse recovers. A spouse may be drawn into facilitating alcohol abuse. Parents of a handicapped child may be so overprotective that the child is denied the opportunity to become independent. The sick role of an adult member may be reinforced so strongly by the family that rehabilitation becomes impossible.

Bereavement

The loss of a loved one is the greatest emotional trauma a person can experience. As we have seen, the loss has profound effects on both mind and body, making the bereaved person especially vulnerable to physical illness as well as to mental breakdown. However well prepared the person may be, the effect is one of devastation, isolation, and loss of purpose. Dr. Samuel Johnson described his own feelings after his wife's death in these words: "I have ever since seemed to myself broken off from mankind; a kind of solitary wanderer in the wild of life, without any direction or fixed point of view: a gloomy gazer on a world to which I have little relation" (Boswell, 1754).

Feelings of anger and guilt are common, and these are sometimes projected toward the physician ("If only he had diagnosed it sooner"). Friends can make the problem worse by trying to avoid discussion of feelings or even avoiding the bereaved person for fear of not knowing what to say.

Somatic symptoms are common: loss of appetite, loss of weight, diarrhea, and pain. The illness may be so severe as to suggest a life-threatening disease. There is a pitfall here for the unwary physician. If intensive investigations are set in motion without allowing the patient to express his or her grief, the result may be mental breakdown and suicide. It is sometimes forgotten, too, that other types of loss can cause grief—loss of a pregnancy, loss of health, of job, or of valued possessions, even the death of a family pet. For some, pets are their sole companion and may serve as surrogate children. Loss of a parent presents unique challenges, as it tends to bring to the forefront many, often previously repressed, issues in a person's life. The death of a child can widen any small cracks in a marital relationship, and without assistance, separation and divorce are common outcomes.

Family physicians encounter grief in many forms. In caring for a dying patient, they may be able to prevent some of the things that trouble the bereaved. They can reduce the dying person's pain and suffering to a minimum, protecting him or her from traumatic and disturbing investigations and therapies that cannot serve any useful purpose. They can ensure that the death is prepared for, so that there is no last-minute rush to the hospital by ambulance. They can assure the family that the patient is not suffering, tell them how well they are caring for the patient, and ensure that distant family members come in time to see the patient. They can be aware of family members who may find it difficult to express their needs, such as school-aged children.

After bereavement, family physicians can ensure that the family is offered support in bearing the grief, either from themselves or from another person. When bereaved persons become ill, they can remember that person's vulnerability and encourage the expression of feelings. Physicians, too, experience emotional reactions to the death of a patient, even if anticipated and planned for. These emotions may run the gamut from guilt to shame and personal loss. It behooves practitioners to be aware of these reactions and have in place a method of coping with them.

Poverty

Poverty is the strongest predictor of poor health in children, as indicated by mortality rates, activity limitations, and utilization of health care. The overwhelming majority of families who are failing to carry out their functions in childrearing are poor. In the United States, the Food Research and Action Center reported that more than 15.3 million children lived in households experiencing food insecurity (2014). Residential fires are among the leading causes of death due to injury in children aged 1 to 5 (Baker, O'Neill, Ginsburg, and Li, 1992). As of January 2014, there were 578,424 people experiencing homelessness in the United States, and 216,197 of that number were people in families. About 15% of this total are considered to be chronically homeless (National Alliance to End Homelessness, 2015).

The relationship between poverty and family function is a complex one. A strong family in a stable and supportive community can mitigate many of the adverse effects of poverty. On the other hand, poverty can weaken a family's ability to carry out its nurturing functions. Poverty is associated with pregnancy in poorly educated young single mothers, who have neither the earning capacity to provide for their children nor the parenting skills to care for them. Far from having supportive communities, they are condemned by their poverty to living in violent and socially disorganized neighborhoods.

Family physicians can do little to remedy these social ills in their relationships with families in their practice. Nevertheless, there is much they can do to mitigate their effects, in collaboration with nurses and social workers. Family doctors are often aware of vulnerable families whom they can support and put in touch with social agencies. They can be sensitive to the cues to family violence and competent in bringing it to notice and dealing with it. They can be especially attentive to the needs of children and adolescents from poor, unstable, or abusive families.

Even in the wealthiest countries, the poor have higher rates of illness and early death. The differences in death rates between social classes are not removed by having a national health service with free access to medical care. In Britain, for example, after more than 60 years of the National Health Service, there are still large differences between rich and poor. Some of these differences are no doubt due to environmental factors. Tudor Hart (1971) in Britain and Ford (1976) in the United States have shown that the poorest areas of the country also have the poorest health services.[2] Even though economic barriers may have been removed, there are other less visible barriers between the poor and the health services: difficulties with transport, long waits in clinics, lack of knowledge of services, communication problems, and the sheer weight of problems a family has to bear, of which illness is only one. Large income differentials between the wealthiest and the poorest in society have been found to be an independent factor in determining population health (Daniels, Kennedy, and Kawachi, 2000). Many of these problems can be eased by family physicians who help poorer families to use the health and social services and mobilize extra support for them. Shi, Starfield, and colleagues have found that access to primary care can mitigate the negative effect of large income differentials on health (Shi, Starfield, and Kawachi, 1999). Nevertheless, medical care has a limited role as a factor in social inequalities in health[3] (Marmot, Bobak, and Smith, 1995).

Thirty-six women staying in shelters or transitional housing were invited to form focus groups at five locations to discuss their health concerns. The groups, conducted by Susan Woolhouse, MD, explored the women's experiences and interactions with family physicians. Two dominant themes emerged. Power imbalances within patient–physician relationships could make women feel demeaned, marginalized, and unimportant, creating a reluctance to consult about their health. Women who described close and trusting relationships with their family physicians experienced support and collaboration, with continuity of care being of paramount importance (Woolhouse, Brown, and Lent, 2004).

A study in Scotland has compared affluent areas of the country with poor areas. More than 3,000 patients were surveyed and data collected on demographic and socioeconomic factors, health variables, and factors related to quality of care. Patients in the most deprived areas had more long-term illness, more multimorbidity, and more psychological problems. Patients in the more deprived areas had more problems to be discussed, but shorter time with their doctors than patients in affluent areas. General practitioners' stress was higher than in affluent areas (Mercer and Watt, 2007).

In poorer countries, poverty is a major reason for ill health through malnutrition, overcrowding, contaminated water, and ignorance of hygiene. Some of these problems may be so basic that the physician's most important task is to work with the community to raise standards of public health. In these conditions, however, a family approach to health is even more necessary. Teaching mothers about nutrition and about the management of infant diarrhea, for example, can improve child health and reduce infant mortality.

Uprooting

Migration of various kinds is one of the most traumatic experiences a family can undergo. The trauma varies with the type of migration, from the forced movement of refugees, to the "upwardly mobile" movement of a family on its way up the social scale. The trauma also varies with the cultural and language change involved in the move. Migration affects different members of a family in different ways. To an ambitious person, the move may be a challenge, to the spouse an alienating experience. A woman who moved to my (IRMcW) practice with her husband from another part of the country said she felt like "a snail without a shell." Younger children may be unaffected, older children disturbed by breaks in friendships and school careers. Migration is associated with an increase in illness rates and with an increase in utilization of health services.

Unemployment

Loss of job, with its resulting loss of income, loss of self-respect, and loss of social status is traumatic both for the individual and for the family. When the loss of job is associated with failure of a business or a family farm, the effect is even greater. Unemployment is reported to be associated with higher illness and death rates.

HOW FAMILY DOCTORS WORK WITH FAMILIES

We know very little about how family physicians work with families as groups. Very little research has addressed this question. Apart from Huygen's (1982) book and some case studies, the literature on the subject has been mainly concerned with theory development. One thing we know is that family physicians rarely function as family therapists. Almost certainly, family physicians do help families in their own way, by providing information and support at times of vulnerability, and by helping family members toward self-knowledge. Only long-term descriptive studies will tell us how this is done and how effective the help is.

Although a family physician may not be able to act as a family therapist in his or her own practice, he or she can help selected families by referring them for family therapy. Many families, however, are resistant to family therapy, lacking even the recognition that they have a problem. Family physicians still must work with these families as best they can.

Useful questions to include when discussing important health issues with a patient include the following: How has this problem affected you and your family? Who knows about this problem? What suggestions has your family made? These will naturally open up discussion about the family context of the issue.

THE FAMILY CONFERENCE

We do not know how often family physicians see entire family groups together. Encounters with parent–child and husband–wife pairs are probably frequent in most practices. Encounters with larger groups may occur naturally at times of crisis and during home visits, but these can rarely be as effective as a specially arranged family conference.

A family conference is especially helpful when a life-threatening or disabling disease has been diagnosed, when difficult treatment or placement choices have to be made, and when a family member is terminally ill (Schmidt, 1983). Who attends the conference will vary with circumstances. Usually it will include the patient and all close family members who are locally available. Besides the family physician, it may include other members of the healthcare team: a nurse, social worker, or consultant, who is involved in the patient's care.

The conference can deal with both cognitive and affective issues. Providing information to the whole family together can minimize the risk of misinformation, especially if questions are invited and responded to with care.[4]

The conference can provide an opportunity for family members to express feelings that they have found difficult to express before (Case 4.7). With good listening skills, the physician may pick up cues regarding family conflicts or a family member who is especially vulnerable. This may, for example, be a member who sits silent throughout the conference, or one who does not attend at all, even though he or she is readily available.

CASE 4.7

An elderly woman who was dying of liver cancer was being cared for at home by her widowed daughter, who was also working full-time as a librarian. Two teenaged granddaughters also lived in the home. The patient also had another daughter living nearby. The patient wanted to die at home and the whole family supported her in this. The burden of care, however, was falling mainly on the daughter, who was beginning to show signs of exhaustion. The rest of the family seemed unaware of this, and she had been unable to express her feelings to them.

At a family conference held in the home, the patient, her two daughters, and two granddaughters were present. The family physician, attending nurse, and a volunteer from a hospice organization were also present. The patient's daughter was able to express her feelings of exhaustion and despair, and the other members of the family understood for the first time how close to breakdown she was. Arrangements were made to provide her with relief and support. The physician and nurse answered questions about the patient's symptoms and clarified the arrangements for getting help in case of crises. The patient was able to remain at home until her death.

PRECEPTS OF FAMILY CARE

The following precepts summarize the content of this chapter. We regard them as the basic responsibilities of a family physician to the families of his or her patients.

1. Look out for vulnerable families and give them extra support.
2. Provide good information at times of serious illness. Ask, "Do you have any questions?"
3. "Be there" at times of crisis: serious illness, terminal illness, and bereavement.
4. Take the initiative at times when you may be needed—on discharge from the hospital, for example. Do not assume that people will know when to call you for advice or assistance.
5. Look out for vulnerable family members, the "hidden patient."
6. Look out for patients who are family scapegoats or are presenting symptoms of a family problem.
7. Avoid being drawn into taking sides in family conflicts.
8. Offer a family conference at critical times.

THE UNIVERSAL IMPORTANCE OF THE FAMILY

The family is important in all parts of the world. The principles set out in this chapter are as important—if not more important—in poverty-stricken parts of the world as they are in affluent countries. Dr. Cicely Williams, a pediatrician who spent her life working in Africa, and who was the first person to describe kwashiorkor, was emphatic about the need to involve the family if child health was to be improved. In her Blackfan Lecture (1973) at Boston Children's Hospital, she said, "the conditions that mostly damage children are gastroenteritis, respiratory diseases, dyspepsia, worms and maternal inadequacy. . . . Malnutrition and 'failure to thrive' are of course due to numerous causes, not only to insufficient food."

The public health services can improve the macroenvironment by instituting water supply, refuse disposal, pest control, food hygiene, and so forth. But it is the microenvironment in the home and its surroundings that are most important to the child. These are controlled by the parents and depend on their values and their diligence.

Given the literature that has evolved in the past few decades making clear the link between prenatal and childhood environment and health later in life, it is important for family physicians to dedicate their moral authority and energy toward community efforts and national policies to address the inequalities and violence that are part of too many childrens' lives (Boyce, 2009).

Whether in rich or poor countries, "developed" or "developing," the health of individuals is influenced by family life, and families are affected by the illnesses and misfortunes of their members.

NOTES

1. We are indebted to Dr. Michael Brennan for these observations.
2. The Inverse Square Law, published by Tudor Hart in 1971, states that areas with greatest need for medical care tend to be provided with fewer resources. For a first-hand account of practice among the inner-city poor, see David Hilfiker's *Not All of Us Are Saints: A Doctor's Journey with the Poor* (New York: Ballantine Books, 1994).
3. For a discussion of social inequalities in health, see Marmot, Bobak, and Smith (1995). Poverty does not account for the social class gradient in mortality and morbidity rates. These decrease with every step upward in social status from lowest to highest. The difference between the two highest levels clearly cannot be attributed to poverty. Moreover, the differences are found in most of the major causes of illness and death. There is no simple explanation for the relationship between social class and health. Social class is related to many factors with known relationships to health: early life experience, education, material conditions, health behavior, negative emotions arising from lack of control over one's life, and amount of social support. In this regard, it seems significant that differences between countries in the

social class gradient are related more to differences in the distribution of wealth than differences in overall wealth.

4. For an excellent guide, see Conducting a Family Conference, chapter 6 in *Family-Oriented Primary Care* by Susan McDaniel, Thomas Campbell, and David Seaburn (New York: Springer-Verlag, 1990).

REFERENCES

American Academy of Pediatrics. 2003. Report of the Task Force on the Family. *Pediatrics* 111(6):1541–1571.

Baker SP, O'Neill B, Ginsburg MJ, Li G. 1992. *The Injury Fact Book*, 2nd ed. New York: Oxford University Press.

Batty GD, Morton SMR, Campbell D, Clark H, et al. 2004. The Aberdeen Children of the 1950's cohort study: Background, methods and follow-up information on a new resource for the study of life course and intergenerational influences on health. *Paediatric and Perinatal Epidemiology* 18:221–239.

Black MC, Basile KC, Breiding MJ, Smith SG, Walters ML, Merrick MT, Chen J, Stevens MR. 2010. The National Intimate Partner and Sexual Violence Survey: 2010 Summary Report. Centers for Disease Control and Prevention. http://www.cdc.gov/violenceprevention/pdf/nisvs_executive_summary-a.pdf

Boswell J. 1754. Boswell's Life of Samuel Johnson. Vol II. John Murray. London.

Boyce WT. 2009. The family is (still) the patient. *Archives of Pediatrics & Adolescent Medicine* 163:768–770.

Brennan M. 1974. Personal communication.

Centers for Disease Control and Preventions; Injury Prevention & Control: Division of Violence Prevention. *The ACE Study.* http://www.cdc.gov/violenceprevention/acestudy/index.html

Daniels N, Kennedy B, Kawachi I. 2000. *Is Inequality Bad For Our Health?* Boston, MA: Beacon Press.

Day T. 1995. *The Health Related Costs of Violence Against Women in Canada, The Tip of the Iceberg.* London, ON: Centre for Research on Violence against Women and Children.

Dingle JH, Badger GF, Jordan WS. 1964. *Illness in the Home: A Study of 25,000 Illnesses in a Group of Cleveland Families.* Cleveland, OH: Western Reserve University Press.

Doherty WJ, Baird MA, eds. 1987. *Family Centered Medical Care: A Clinical Casebook.* New York: Guilford Press.

Duvall EM. 1977. *Marriage and Family Development*, 5th ed. Philadelphia, PA: Lippincott.

Feldman R, Rosenthal Z, Eidelman AI. 2014. Maternal-preterm skin-on-skin contact enhances child physiologic organization and cognitive control across the first 10 years of life. *Biological Psychiatry* 75(1):56–64.

Fisman S, Wolf L, Ellison D, Freeman T. 2000. A longitudinal study of siblings of children with chronic disabilities. *Canadian Journal of Psychiatry* 45(4):369–375.

Food Action and Research Center. 2014. *Hunger and Poverty in the U.S.* http://frac.org/reports-and-resources/hunger-and-poverty/

Ford AB. 1976. *Urban Health in America.* New York: Oxford University Press.

Gray JD, Cutler C, Dean J, Kempe CH. 1976. Perinatal assessment of a mother–baby interaction. In: Kempe CH, Helfer RE, eds., *Child Abuse and Neglect: The Family in the Community.* Cambridge: Ballinger.

Haggerty RJ, Roghmann KH, Pless IB. 1975. *Child Health and the Community.* New York: John Wiley.

Hart JT. 1971. The inverse care law. *Lancet* 696:405.

Heise L, Pitanguy J, Germain A. 1994. *Violence against women: The hidden health burden.* World Bank Discussion Papers. Washington, DC.

Hinkle LE. 1974. The effect of exposure to culture change and changes in interpersonal relationships in health. In: Dohrenwerd BP, Dohrenwerd BS, eds. *Stressful Life Events: Their Nature and Effects.* New York: John Wiley.

Homatidis G, Johnson L. Orlando F, Robson B. 1986. *The Toronto Family Study.* Toronto: Toronto Board of Education Publications.

Huygen FJA. 1982. *Family Medicine: The Medical Life History of Families.* New York: Brunner/Mazel.

Klaus AS, Kennell JH. 1976. *Maternal–infant Bonding.* St. Louis, MO: C. V. Mosby.

Kraus AS, Lilienfeld AM. 1959. Some epidemiologic aspects of the high mortality rate in the young widowed group. *Journal of Chronic Disease* 10:296.

Laughlin L, 2014. *A Child's Day: Living Arrangements, Nativity, and Family Transitions: 2011 (Selected Indicators of Child Well-Being).* http://www.census.gov/content/dam/Census/library/publications/2014/demo/p70-139.pdf.

Leff J. 1989. Family factors in schizophrenia. *Psychiatric Annals* 19(10):542.

Marmot M, Bobak M, Smith GD. 1995. Explanations for social inequalities in health. In: Amick BC III, Levine S, Tarlow AR, Walsh DC, eds., *Society & Health.* New York: Oxford University Press.

Maughan B, McCarthy G. 1997. Childhood adversities and psychosocial disorders. *British Medical Bulletin* 53:156.

McCain M, Mustard F. 1999. *The Early Years Study: Reversing the Real Brain Drain.* Ontario, The Canadian Institute for Advanced Research, and The Founders' Network.

McEwen BS, Seeman T. 1999. Protective and damaging effects of mediators of stress: Elaborating and testing the oncepts of allostasis and allostatic load. *Annals of New York Academy of Sciences* 896(1):30–47.

Medalie JH. 1975. The hidden patient. Lecture at Quail Hollow Conference. November. Case Western Reserve School of Medicine.

Medalie JH, Goldbourt U. 1976. Angina pectoris among 10,000 men: Psychosocial and other risk factors as evidenced by a multivariate analysis of a 5-year medicine study. *American Journal of Medicine* 60(6):910–921.

Mercer SW, Watt GC. 2007. The inverse care law: Clinical primary care encounters in deprived and affluent areas of Scotland. *Annals of Family Medicine* 5(6):503–510.

Meyer RJ, Haggerty RH. 1962. Streptococcal infections in families, factors altering individual susceptibility. *Pediatrics* 29:539.

Miller FJW, Court WKM, Walton WS, Knox EG. 1960. *Growing up in Newcastle upon Tyne.* London: Oxford University Press.

Mistry R. 2002. *Family Matters.* Toronto: McClelland and Stewart.

National Alliance to End Homelessness. *Snapshot of Homelessness.* http://www.end-homelessness.org/pages/snapshot_of_homelessness.

Nesser WB. 1975. Fragmentation of black families and stroke susceptibility. In: Kaplan BH, Cassel JC, eds., *Family and Health: An Epidemiological Approach.* Chapel Hill: University of North Carolina Press.

Pless IB, Satterwhite BB. 1973. A measure of family functioning and its application. *Social Science and Medicine* 7:613.

Ramsey CN, Abell TD, Baker LC. 1986. The relationship between family functioning, life events, family structure, and the outcome of pregnancy. *Journal of Family Practice* 22:521.

Ransom DC, Vandervoort HC. 1973. The development of family medicine: Problematic trends. *Journal of the American Medical Association* 225:1098.

Roland A. 1988. *In Search of the Self in India and Japan*. Princeton, NJ: Princeton University Press.

Sarkadi A, Kristiansson R, Oberklaid F, Bremberg S. 2008. Fathers' involvement and children's developmental outcomes: A systematic review of longitudinal studies. *Acta Paediatrica* 97:153–158.

Schmidt DD. 1983. When is it helpful to convene the family? *Journal of Family Practice* 16:967.

Seeman TE, Crimmins E, Huag M-H, et al. 2004. Cumulative biological risk and socioeconomic differences in mortality: MacArthur studies of successful aging. *Social Science and Medicine* 58:1985–1997.

Segalen M. 1996. The Industrial Revolution: From proletariat to bourgeoisie. Chapter 6 in Burguiere A, Klapishc-Zuber C, Segalen M, Zonabend F. eds., *A History of the Family: Volume II: The Impact of Modernity*. Cambridge, MA: The Belknap Press of Harvard University Press. Cambridge, MA.

Shi L, Starfield, Kennedy B, Kawachi I. 1999. Income inequality, primary care, and health indicators. *Journal of Family Practice* 48(4):275–284.

Silverman JG, Decker MR, Gupta J, Kapur N, Raj A, Naved RT. 2009. Maternal experiences of intimate partner violence and child morbidity in Bangladesh: Evidence from a national Bangladeshi sample. *Archives of Pediatrics & Adolescent Medicine* 163(8):700–705.

Smith K, Joshi H. 2002. The Millennium Cohort Study. *Population Trends* (Spring):30–34.

Stedeford A. 1981. Couples facing death: Unsatisfactory communication. *British Medical Journal* 183:1098.

Tsiouli E, Alexopoulos EC, Stefanaki C, Darviri C, Chrousos GP. 2013. Effects of diabetes-related family stress on glycemic control in young patients with type 1 diabetes: Systematic review. *Canadian Family Physician* 59:143–149.

Vespa J, Lewis JM, Kreider RM. 2013. *America's Families and Living Arrangements: 2012*. http://www.mwcog.org/uploads/committee-documents/kV1YX19a20140512145731.pdf.

US Census Bureau, 2013. https://www.census.gov/hhes/www/poverty/about/overview/.

Walsh F. 2012. *Normal Family Processes: Growing Diversity and Complexity*. Fourth Edition. The Guildford Press. New York.

Williams CD. 1973. Health services in the home. *Pediatrics* 52:773.

Wittstein IS, Thiemann DR, Lima JAC, et al. 2005. Neurohormonal features of myocardial stunning due to emotional stress. *New England Journal of Medicine* 352:539–548.

Woolhouse S, Brown JB, Lent B. 2004. Women marginalized by poverty and violence: How patient–physician relationships can help. *Canadian Family Physician* 50:1388–1394.

CHAPTER 5

✿

A Profile of Family Practice

It is difficult to convey in statistical terms a true picture of the content of family practice. One approach is to record the diagnosis made at each patient–doctor encounter. By this means, it is possible to obtain an accurate picture of the family physician's experience with well-defined diseases such as diabetes. Many illness episodes seen by family physicians, however, are much more difficult to define and label. The reader will obtain some idea of the difficulty by reading Case 9.1 in Chapter 9. This patient's problems cannot be expressed by simple disease labels. There is no diagnosis in the usual sense of the term. Another approach is to record the patient's main symptom or complaint. Here again, however, the result may be a very partial picture of the illness because a statement of the symptoms says little or nothing about its origins. If we were classifying Case 9.1 by disease labels, we could call the illness anxiety state or insomnia. If we were classifying the case by symptoms, we could call it insomnia or gastrointestinal symptoms. Whichever route we take, we provide only a partial picture, because we are doing something equivalent to taking a two-dimensional slice through a three-dimensional object. Another difficulty is that we have no assurance that any two physicians will classify the same illness in the same way. If one physician classifies the illness as anxiety state, it will appear in the statistics under the rubric of mental illness. If another classifies it as gastrointestinal symptoms (not yet diagnosed), it will appear under the rubric of gastrointestinal diseases. Given these difficulties of nomenclature and standardization, it is small wonder that there are wide variations in such estimates as the amount of psychiatric illness in family practice.

Nevertheless, there are some important areas of agreement regarding the content of family practice in countries with high general standards of living. The collection of reliable data has been enhanced by the development of standardized coding systems for primary care (e.g., ICHPPC-2, and ICPC-2-R), by the training of recorders, and by the validation of data. Morbidity studies, some of them national in scope, have been carried out in the United States, Britain, Canada, the Netherlands, Australia, Norway, West Germany, Austria, and Barbados. In this chapter we have used several of these studies to create a profile of the work of the family physician, emphasizing especially those features common to all these parts of the world.

CLASSIFICATION OF PRIMARY CARE

Difficult as it may be, some way of classifying and recording the experience of family practice is necessary if we are to make comparisons between practices or countries, to relate process of care to outcome, or to follow trends in illness over time. It is also necessary if we are to learn from our experience by retrospectively reviewing our cases in different disease categories. Accurate classification is required for studies of the natural history of disease and for clinical trials.

Before the development of the International Classification of Primary Care (ICPC), only the ICD (International Classification of Disease) was available. The ICD was based on well-defined disease categories and therefore was more suitable for classifying hospital discharges and causes of death than for the earlier manifestations of illness seen in primary care. The ICD classified illness at a high level of abstraction; family physicians operate for much of the time at lower levels of abstraction. Moreover, the ICD, lacking organizing principles, had "become an unstructured amalgam of chapters based variously on anatomy, clinical manifestations, changing views of 'causation,' clinical specialties, and age groups" (White, 1985). The ICPC was first published in 1987 by the World Organization of National Colleges, Academies, and Academic Associations of General Practitioners/Family Physicians (WONCA). Since publication, it has received widespread acceptance and use, especially in Europe and Australia. Originally designed for paper records, ICPC-2-R was released in 2005 for use in electronic databases.

The ICPC broke new ground by classifying three elements of an encounter between patient and doctor: the reason for encounter (RFE), the diagnosis or problem, and the process of care. Rather than being organized around endpoints of illness (definitive diagnoses or causes of death), the ICPC is based on episodes of care, defined as "a problem or illness in a patient over the entire period of time from its onset to its resolution" (Lamberts and Wood, 1987). One episode therefore, may last over many encounters, and a single encounter often includes several different illness episodes in various states of evolution. An episode of care is different from an episode of illness, which is the period during which a patient has symptoms, and from an episode of disease, which is a health problem from onset to resolution or death. A person may have an illness or disease without coming under care, and may have care (e.g., prenatal) without having an illness or disease. The duration of care for a disease may be different from the duration of the disease.

Classifying the RFE is especially important in family practice, where it has much stronger influence in determining costs than it has in specialty care, where diagnostic labels tend to drive investigations (Bernstein, Hollingworth, and Viner, 1994).

The structure of the ICPC is biaxial, with 17 chapters on the horizontal axis and 7 components on the vertical (Figure 5.1). In the chapters, body systems take precedence over etiology. The patient's reason for encounter is the patient's given reason as interpreted by the doctor. Most are symptoms and complaints, which are recorded under the appropriate chapter heading. Each chapter has rubrics for fear or disability associated with a symptom. If the RFE is a preventive procedure, prescription, test result, or medical certificate, this is recorded under the appropriate chapter heading under components 2, 3, 4, or 5. The process of care and the diagnosis are encoded and recorded under the appropriate chapter heading. With this structure, the ICPC can provide a profile of family practice that represents its complexity (see Figure 5.1).

As in all classification systems, the accuracy of the ICPC depends on the skill of the recording physician. The RFE is not necessarily the same as the

COMPONENTS \ CHAPTERS	A—General	B—Blood, blood forming	D—Digestive	F—Eye	H—Ear	K—Circulatory	L—Musculoskeletal	N—Neurological	P—Psychological	R—Respiratory	S—Skin	T—Metabolic, Endocrine, Nutr.	U—Urinary	W—Pregnancy, Child bearing, Family planning	X—Female genital	Y—Male gential	Z—Social
1. Symptoms and complaints																	
2. Diagnostic, screening, prevention																	
3. Treatment, procedures, medication																	
4. Test results																	
5. Administrative																	
6. Other																	
7. Diagnoses, disease																	

Figure 5.1:
The biaxial structure of ICPC.

presenting complaint, and underlying reasons may not emerge at the first encounter. Much depends on the physician's knowledge of the patient and consulting skills. Consistency in assigning diagnostic labels is difficult to attain in the many illnesses that cannot be differentiated to more than low levels of abstraction. All classification systems are simplifications of complex processes. We cannot expect them to fully represent the complexity of family practice. Case 5.1 outlines a case consisting of two episodes of care: cancer of the uterus (an intercurrent illness) and diabetes (a chronic one).

Symptoms

Table 5.1 gives the ranking order of the 30 most common problems, complaints, or symptoms presented to family physicians in the Netherlands, Japan, Poland, and the United States (Okkes et al., 2002).

CASE 5.1 AN EPISODE OF CARE

First visit: Mrs. C is an 80-year-old woman who lives alone since her husband died 8 years ago. She is active in her local church and is locally well known for continuing to regularly attend classes at a local fitness club. She has been diagnosed with diabetes for the past 10 years and takes an active interest in the management of it. Her glycosylated hemoglobin has consistently indicated good control. She attends her physician's office today, however, outside of her usual time for checkup. She relates that she has now come up with the courage to tell her physician that she had an episode of vaginal bleeding 3 months ago. This settled down over 2 days but then recurred only 3 days ago and that prompted her to make this appointment. She freely admits that she is afraid of cancer. "I have a lot more things that I want to do." Her physician arranges for a repeat appointment to undertake an endometrial biopsy.

RFE X12 (postmenopausal bleeding), X 25 (fear of cancer); Diagnosis X12, X 25

Second visit: the bleeding has settled down and no new symptoms are elicited. An endometrial biopsy is completed in the office without problems.

RFE X37 (diagnostic procedure, histological)

Third visit: The results of the biopsy confirm endometrial carcinoma. When this information is conveyed to her, she became understandably upset and had many questions about what treatments were available. She can't understand how she could have cancer when she feels so well. Her physician spends time discussing next steps and arrangements are made for her to see a gynecologist.

RFE X60 (attending to receive test results), X45 (health advice/ information)

Diagnosis X 77 (malignant neoplasm genital female other) X60 (test results), X 67 (referral to specialist)

Fourth visit: After seeing the gynecologist and being told that she would have surgery "as soon as possible," she wishes to discuss her concerns with her family physician. Will she need to have chemotherapy? She feels well now, should she go through with treatment that she feels will make her feel sick?

RFE X45 (health advice/information) Diagnosis X77 (malignant neoplasm genital female other), X 58 (therapeutic counseling)

Fifth visit: Six weeks after complete hysterectomy, she is feeling reasonably well, though still a bit weak. She has been told by the gynecologist that they were able to "get everything" and there appears to be no cancer remaining. Nevertheless, she is to see an oncologist in the next week for consultation. Her blood sugars indicate that control has not been as good as in the past, even though she has lost some weight after the surgery. Her family physician reviews the need for more regularity in her diet and adjusts her medication. Her daughters have become more solicitous and interfering (in her opinion), and she expresses discomfort about this.

RFE X45 (health advice re: test results), Z20 (relationship problem parent/children), Diagnoses X 77 (malignant neoplasm genital female other), T90 (diabetes non-insulin dependent), T45 (health counseling/advice)

Sixth visit: She returns to see her family physician after seeing the oncologist, who has not recommended any further treatment at this time, but will see her regularly in follow-up. She asks if her family physician can do the follow up: "That cancer clinic makes me nervous." Her blood sugars are once again in good control and she is feeling generally better. She wants to discuss living wills with her family physician.

RFE X45 (health advice), P01 (feeling anxious/nervous), Diagnosis X 77 (malignant neoplasm genital female other), T90 (diabetes non insulin dependent), P74 (anxiety state).

Only 35 groups of symptoms/complaints covered the top 30 in all databases, and this list represented 45%–60% of all reasons for encounter. Further, the top 30 represented 70%–75% of all encounters per 1,000 patients per year. Limitations to this study are that the data are derived from research practices and may not be representative of all family practices in the represented countries, and that the US data did not include reasons for encounter. Differences exist between the countries in the degree to which family practice contributes to psychological and gynecological care.

Table 5.1. MOST FREQUENT (GROUPS OF) REASONS FOR ENCOUNTER IN THE FORM OF A SYMPTOM/COMPLAINT PER 1000 PATIENTS PER YEAR, STANDARDIZED FOR THE 1996 SEX/AGE DISTRIBUTION OF THE US POPULATION

ICPC Codes	Symptom/Complaint	Netherlands	Japan	Poland	United States (% Family Physician)
R05/R07	Cough/sneezing/nasal congestion	163	292	684	295 (41)
R21/R22/R23	Throat/voice/tonsil symptom/complaint	66	81	250	102 (33)
A02/A03	Fever/chills	71	158	155	99 (29)
L02/L03/L05	Low back/back/flank symptom/complaint	88	28	64	135 (51)
D01/D06	Abdominal pain	77	34	76	42 (34)
A04	Tiredness	76	21	35	60 (26)
R02/R03	Shortness of breath/wheezing	73	9	14	59 (27)
S06/S07	Redness of skin	72	52	42	64 (31)
N01	Headache	48	49	39	68 (40)
H01	Earache	47	12	24	59 (33)
L15	Knee symptom/complaint	45	20	28	55 (12)
P03	Feeling depressed	16	–	8	53 (16)
S04	Localized swelling skin	53	14	19	28 (56)
L14	Leg/thigh symptom/complaint	38	11	14	51 (25)
K01/K02/L04	Heart/chest pain/tightness	48	15	49	42 (34)
D09/D10	Nausea/vomiting	34	49	24	42 (37)
F05/F07	Vision problems	8	2	38	48 (8)
P01	Feeling anxious/nervous/tense	26	1	14	47 (17)
U01/U02/U03	Urination symptom/complaint	22	3	47	37 (25)

(continued)

Table 5.1. CONTINUED

ICPC Codes	Symptom/Complaint	Netherlands	Japan	Poland	United States (% Family Physician)
L01	Neck symptom/complaint	36	16	18	44 (48)
L08	Shoulder symptom/complaint	42	12	16	40 (52)
S03	Warts	40	1	4	12 (27)
D11	Diarrhea	20	38	21	28 (36)
S02	Pruritis	37	19	25	25 (29)
L12	Hand/finger symptom/complaint	27	12	14	36 (21)
D02/03	Stomach pain/heartburn	28	25	33	34 (33)
L17	Foot/toe symptom/complaint	34	10	19	22 (17)
N17	Vertigo	29	14	17	32 (34)
H02	Hearing complaint	29	2	15	12 (15)
R09	Sinus symptom/complaint	24	2	14	29 (37)
H13	Plugged feeling in ear	22	1	10	12 (36)
P06	Sleeping disturbance	18	6	9	20 (25)
S18	Laceration	18	17	14	10 (46)
D19/D20	Mouth/tongue/teeth symptom/complaint	15	15	12	2 (51)
S12	Insect bite	3	11	2	3 (42)
	Total top 30s	1491	1052	1867	1747
	All symptoms/complaint reasons for encounter per	3362	1923	3375	2598 (31)
	1000 patients per year				

Based on top 30 of the reasons from the Netherlands, Japan, Poland, and United States (from NAMCS data). Okkes IM, Polderman GO, Fryer GE, et al. 2002. The role of family practice in different health care systems: A comparison of reasons for encounter, diagnoses, and interventions in primary care populations in the Netherlands, Japan, Poland, and the United States. *Journal of Family Practice* 51(1):72.

In a comparison of problems dealt with by family physicians in Australia and New Zealand and pediatricians, internists, and family physicians in the United States, the frequency of health problems managed showed considerable overlap (Figure 5.2). There is remarkable similarity in the clinical problems dealt with in primary care, even when there are difference in healthcare systems (Bindman, Forrest, Britt, et al., 2007).

Diagnoses

Table 5.2 shows the number and proportion of visits for the top 20 diagnoses broken out by sex. The Direct Observation in Primary Care (DOPC) study provides important insight into the content of the practices of 138 family physicians in the state of Ohio. In this multi-method study, 4454 patient visits were observed by trained research nurses.

The nurses gathered information on the content of each visit, using validated instruments (Davis Observation Code), direct observation of services offered, a patient exit questionnaire, medical record review, a practice environment checklist, billing data and ICD-9-CM diagnoses, a physician questionnaire, and field notes. The most common diagnostic clusters were hypertension, upper respiratory infection, and general medical examination. The top 25 diagnoses represented 61% of visits. The fact that nearly 40% of

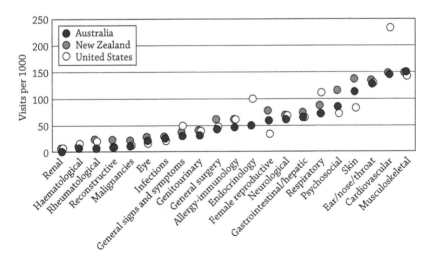

Figure 5.2:
Age-standardized frequency of health problems managed in primary care in Australia, New Zealand, and the United States: 2001–2002.
Reprinted with permission from Bindman AB, Forrest CB, Britt H, et al. 2007. Diagnostic scope and exposure to primary care physicians in Australia, New Zealand, and the United States: Cross sectional analysis of results from three national surveys. *BMJ* 334:1261–1264.

Table 5.2. TWENTY LEADING PRIMARY DIAGNOSIS GROUPS FOR OFFICE VISITS: UNITED STATES, 2015

Primary Diagnosis Group and ICD-9-CM Code(s)[1]		Number of Visits in Thousands	(standard error in thousands)	Percent Distribution	(standard error of percent)	Female[2] Percent Distribution	(standard error of percent)	Male[3] Percent Distribution	(standard error of percent)
All visits		1,008,802	(46,471)	100.0	...	100.0	...	100.0	...
Routine infant or child health check	V20.0–V20.2	44,634	(4,724)	4.4	(0.4)	3.7	(0.4)	5.4	(0.6)
Essential hypertension	401	38,916	(3,845)	3.9	(0.3)	3.5	(0.4)	4.4	(0.4)
Arthropathies and related disorders	710–719	36,130	(3,999)	3.6	(0.4)	3.7	(0.4)	3.4	(0.3)
Acute upper respiratory infections, excluding pharyngitis	460–461, 463–466	32,207	(3,102)	3.2	(0.3)	3.2	(0.3)	3.3	(0.3)
Spinal disorders	720–724	31,593	(4,165)	3.1	(0.4)	2.9	(0.4)	3.5	(0.4)
Diabetes mellitus	249–250	30,560	(4,369)	3.0	(0.4)	2.5	(0.4)	3.8	(0.5)
Malignant neoplasms	140–208, 209–209.36, 209.7–209.79, 230–234	29,155	(4,310)	2.9	(0.4)	2.5	(0.4)	3.4	(0.4)
Rheumatism, excluding back	725–729	21,835	(2,282)	2.2	(0.2)	2.4	(0.3)	1.9	(0.2)
Normal pregnancy	V22	20,879	(2,595)	2.1	(0.2)	3.6	(0.4)	...	...
General medical examination	V70	19,705	(1,968)	2.0	(0.2)	1.5	(0.2)	2.5	(0.3)
Gynecological examination	V72.3	16,345	(2,402)	1.6	(0.2)	2.8	(0.4)	...	...
Follow-up examination	V67	15,603	(2,132)	1.5	(0.2)	1.6	(0.2)	1.4	(0.2)
Otitis media and eustachian tube disorders	381–382	14,650	(1,545)	1.5	(0.1)	1.1	(0.1)	1.9	(0.2)
Specific procedures and aftercare	V50–V59.9	14,286	(1,836)	1.4	(0.2)	1.3	(0.3)	1.6	(0.2)
Asthma	493	14,232	(2,195)	1.4	(0.2)	1.4	(0.3)	1.5	(0.2)

Diagnosis	ICD-9-CM code	Number (SE)			
Heart disease, excluding ischemic	391–392.0, 393–398, 402, 404, 415–416, 420–429	12,405 (1,156)	1.2 (0.1)	1.2 (0.1)	1.3 (0.1)
Disorders of lipoid metabolism	272	12,350 (1,777)	1.2 (0.2)	0.9 (0.2)	1.6 (0.2)
Cataract	366	11,266 (1,990)	1.1 (0.2)	1.2 (0.2)	1.0 (0.2)
Allergic rhinitis	477	11,057 (2,252)	1.1 (0.2)	1.0 (0.2)	1.2 (0.3)
Benign neoplasms	210–229, 209.4–209.69, 235–239	10,663 (1,131)	1.1 (0.1)	1.1 (0.1)	1.0 (0.1)
All other diagnoses[4]		570,331 (27,399)	56.5 (0.9)	56.5 (1.0)	56.5 (1.1)

. . . Category not applicable.
[1]Based on the International Classification of Diseases. Ninth Revision, Clinical Modification (ICD-9-CM) (US Department of Health and Human Services, Centers for Disease Control and Prevention, Centers for Medicare and Medicaid Services. Official version: International Classification of Diseases, Ninth Revision, Clinical Modification, Sixth Edition. DHHS Pub No.(PHS) 06-1260). However, certain codes have been combined in this table to form larger categories that better describe the utilization of ambulatory care services.
[2]Based on 586,671,000 visits made by females.
[3]Based on 422,131,000 visits made by males.
[4]Includes all other diagnoses not listed above, as well as unknown and blank diagnoses.
Reprinted with permission from the National Ambulatory Medical Care Survey, 2010.

visits were not classifiable in one of these clusters again emphasizes the great variety of problems addressed in family practice (Stange, Zyzanski, Jaén, et al., 1998). These tables illustrate some of the key features of morbidity in family practice: the great variety of problems encountered; the high incidence of infectious disease, especially of the respiratory tract; the high prevalence of chronic disease, especially hypertension, diabetes, ischemic heart disease, and arthritis; the high frequency of depression and anxiety; and the low frequency of diseases such as cancer, which are so common in hospital practice.

The Bettering Evaluation and Care of Health (BEACH) initiative in Australia is the only continuous, randomized study of general practice activity in the world and includes management activity such as prescriptions, referrals, and investigations. It was started in 1998, and each year 1000 randomly selected general practitioners record standardized data on 100 consecutive patients. As of 2013 this database consists of 1.5 million encounters from 14,793 participants in 9630 practices (Britt, Miller, Henderson, et al., 2013). There were on average 1.55 problems dealt with in each encounter. Sixty-two percent of encounters had one problem recorded; 35% had two to three problems, and 3% had four recorded problems. Of all problems, chronic ones represented 36% and new problems 38%. Table 5.3 lists the most commonly encountered problems and Table 5.4 the most common chronic problems. The top seven in this category represented 51.7% of all chronic problems. Due to the continuous nature of this database, it is possible to look at long-term trends in reasons for encounters. Over the decade from 2005–2006 to 2013–2014, there was an increase in encounter time (from 14.1–14.8 minutes), an increase in the number of problems managed (from 1.46–1.58 per encounter), and an increase in the rate of chronic conditions managed (from 5.2–5.6 per encounter). Among the chronic conditions, there was a significant increase in nongestational diabetes, depression, esophageal disease, atrial fibrillation/atrial flutter, hypothyroidism, shoulder syndrome, and unspecified chronic pain (Britt, Miller, Henderson, et al., 2014). Some of these changes are likely attributable to the aging of the general population over this time period.

Multimorbidity

One characteristic of family practice that is not captured in tables of this kind is multimorbidity, which is defined as the simultaneous occurrence of several medical conditions in the same person. Because family physicians explicitly take responsibility for a comprehensive approach to their patients, multimorbidity represents a greater proportion of the workload in this discipline than in many specialties. Starfield, Lemke, Bernhardt, et al. (2003) found that, for both index conditions and their comorbidities, visits to primary

Table 5.3. MOST FREQUENTLY MANAGED PROBLEMS

Problem Managed	Number	Percent of Total Problems (n = 152,517)	Rate per 100 Encounters (n = 98,564)	95% LCL	95% UCL	New as Percent of all Problems[a]
Hypertension*	8482	5.6	8.6	8.1	9.1	5.0
Check-up (air)*	6304	4.1	6.4	6.0	6.8	45.1
Upper respiratory tract infection	5716	3.7	5.8	5.3	6.3	77.4
Immunization/vaccination (all)*	4922	3.2	5.0	4.5	5.5	61.3
Diabetes (all)*	4186	2.7	4.2	4.0	4.5	5.3
Depression*	4084	2.7	4.1	3.9	4.4	14.6
Arthritis (all)*	3743	2.5	3.8	3.6	4.0	18.2
Lipid disorder	3292	2.2	3.3	3.1	3.6	10.9
Back complaint*	2906	1.9	2.9	2.8	3.1	23.3
Prescription (all)*	2677	1.8	2.7	2.4	3.0	5.8
Gastro-oesophageal reflux disease*	2538	1.7	2.6	2.4	2.8	15.8
Acute bronchitis/bronchiolitis	2306	1.5	2.3	2.1	2.5	70.9
Asthma	2124	1.4	2.2	2.0	2.3	17.1
Anxiety*	2085	1.4	2.1	1.9	2.3	16.3
Test results*	2019	1.3	2.0	1.8	2.2	29.4
Contact dermatitis	1764	1.2	1.8	1.7	1.9	48.0
Urinary tract infection*	1678	1.1	1.7	1.6	1.8	63.7
Sleep disturbance	1534	1.0	1.6	1.4	1.7	18.8
Vitamin/nutritional deficiency	1466	1.0	1.5	1.3	1.6	32.5
Administrative procedure (all)*	1414	0.9	1.4	1.3	1.6	42.2

Reprinted with permission from Britt H, Miller GC, Henderson J, et al. *General Practice Activity in Australia; 2012–13. BEACH: Bettering the Evaluation and Care of Health.* Sydney: Sydney University Press, University of Sydney Library. 2013.

Table 5.4. MOST FREQUENTLY MANAGED CHRONIC PROBLEMS

Chronic Problem Managed	Number	Percent of Total Chronic Problems (n = 54,944)	Rate per 100 Encounters (n = 98,564)	95% LCL	95% UCL
Hypertension (non-gestational)"	8474	15.4	8.6	8.1	9.1
Diabetes (non-gestational)"	4157	7.6	4.2	3.9	4.5
Depressive disorder"	4038	7.3	4.1	3.9	4.3
Chronic arthritis"	3728	6.8	3.8	3.5	4.0
Lipid disorder	3292	6.0	3.3	3.1	3.6
Oesophageal disease	2568	47	2.6	2.4	2.8
Asthma	2124	3.9	2.2	2,0	2.3

Reprinted with permission from Britt H, Miller GC, Henderson J, et al. *General Practice Activity in Australia; 2012–13. BEACH: Bettering the Evaluation and Care of Health.* Sydney: Sydney University Press, University of Sydney Library. 2013.

care physicians greatly exceeded visits to specialists, the only exception being some uncommon chronic conditions. In a cross-sectional study using video recordings of 229 patient encounters to 30 general practitioners in the United Kingdom, it was found that there was an average of 2.5 problems per encounter and that 41% had three or more problems. Mean consultation time was 11.9 minutes and increased by 2 minutes for each additional problem. In family practice, both patients and physicians come to the encounter with unique agendas, and Table 5.5 illustrates the types of problems raised and who raised them (patient or physician) (Salisbury, Procter, Stewart, et al., 2013).

Multimorbidity impacts family practice in a number of ways:

1. Healthcare delivery is complicated and individual patient encounters more complex. Family physicians address more than three problems more than one-third of the time (Beasley et al., 2004).
2. Clinical practice guidelines (CPGs) generally focus on one disease at a time and do not take into consideration that most patients who are meant to be targeted by them have more diseases than the one covered by them; randomized control trials (many of which underpin the CPGs) usually exclude participants with multimorbidity, casting doubt on their applicability or transferability to family practice (Fortin et al., 2006).
3. There is a major impact on time management (Ostbye et al., 2005).
4. Multimorbidity affects the cognitive strategies of family physicians (Christensen, Fetters, and Green, 2005) (for more on multimorbidity, see Chapter 16).

Table 5.5. TYPES AND FREQUENCIES OF PROBLEMS

Problem ICPC Heading	Problem Type	Frequency	%	Who Raised the Problem?[a]			
				Patient	%	GP	%
W	Pregnancy, childbearing, family planning	16	2.8	15	93.8	1	6.3
S	Skin	46	8.2	42	93.3	3	6.7
N	Neurological	24	4.3	21	91.3	2	8.7
L	Musculoskeletal	107	19.0	95	88.8	12	11.2
D	Digestive	46	8.2	39	88.6	5	11.4
U	Urological	19	3.4	16	84.2	3	15.8
R	Respiratory	44	7.8	37	84.1	7	15.9
H	Ear	9	1.6	7	77.8	2	22.2
X	Female genital	12	2.1	9	75.0	3	25.0
P	Psychological	43	7.6	32	74.4	11	25.6
F	Eye	11	2.0	8	72.7	3	27.3
T	Endocrine/metabolic and nutritional	36	6.4	24	66.7	12	33.3
Z	Social problems	12	2.1	7	63.6	4	36.4
K	Cardiovascular	34	6.0	21	61.8	13	38.2
Y	Male genital	11	2.0	6	60.0	4	40.0
A	General and unspecified	86	15.2	48	57.1	36	42.9
B	Blood and immune mechanism	8	1.4	3	37.5	5	62.5
Total		564	100	430	77.3	126	22.7

[a]Problems raised by third parties (n = 8) are omitted for ease of presentation. ICPC = International Classification of Primary Care.

Reprinted with permission from Salisbury C, Procter S, Stewart K, et al. 2013. The content of general practice consultations: Cross-sectional study based on video recordings. *British Journal of General Practice* 63(616):e751–e759.

SOURCES OF VARIATION IN FAMILY PRACTICE

Although the average morbidity and utilization patterns in family practice are remarkably similar in all parts of the world with a similar standard of living, there are some major differences between practices. The following are the main sources of variation:

1. *Local conditions.* The strongest influence on family practice is the local context, including the population structure, economic conditions, the physician–population ratio, availability of other primary care services, and administrative constraints. In poor communities with a low doctor–population ratio, family physicians see more patients per hour. When the ratio becomes extremely low, physicians have to delegate much of the patient care to other personnel and act as resources, teachers, and administrators for a primary care organization. The use of diagnostic tests is related to local resources.The services provided by family physicians are influenced by the availability of other primary care services in the area. Where there are specialized emergency services, family physicians are less involved with trauma. The same applies with such services as family-planning clinics, sexually transmitted disease clinics, well-baby clinics, and so on. The availability of other physicians providing primary care (pediatricians, obstetricians, internists) has a strong influence on the content of family practice. Increasingly, some family physicians are taking on tasks that are often considered part of secondary care, and provide a service to their colleagues (see Chapter 22, "Consultation and Referral"). Because alternative primary care services are more readily available in urban areas, rural family physicians usually provide a wider range of services. Scope of practice is understood to be the range of services, both office-based and non-office-based, provided by family physicians. Utilizing data from the National Family Physician Workforce Survey, Wong and Stewart (2010) found that geographic factors, such as province of practice and whether it was rural, explained most of the differences.
2. *The age of the physician.* As doctors grow older, so do their patients. A family practice is like an organism, developing, changing, and adapting over the years as the physician also grows older and changes. Demographic differences between practices result in differences in morbidity patterns and therefore in utilization. For these reasons, older doctors see more chronic illness and do less obstetrics.
3. *The gender of the physician.* Female physicians see a higher proportion of female patients than male physicians. In the National Ambulatory Medical Care Survey (NAMCS) studies, 75% of the patients seen by women physicians were female, compared with 58% seen by male physicians. This appears to be a common finding in countries where women have only

recently begun to enter family practice in large numbers. Whether it will change as the number of women family physicians begins to equal or exceed the number of male family physicians remains to be seen.

4. *Distribution of diagnoses.* Some diagnoses are associated with high—or low—utilization patterns (Lamberts, 1984). Chronic disease, for example, is associated with a high encounter rate, but few new episodes of illness or new problems, and few out-of-hours calls. Childhood illness is associated with many new problems, many out-of-hours calls, and a low encounter rate per episode. Psychological and social problems (problem behavior) are associated with both a large number of episodes of illness and a large number of encounters per episode.

5. *Vocational training.* Family physicians who are graduates of vocational or residency training programs show differences from those who did not receive such training. One study showed that residency-trained physicians were more likely to have practices organized for prevention, with such tools as age–sex registers, prevention flow charts, and recall systems (Audunsson, 1986). In a Canadian study, Borgiel et al. (1989) found that vocational training in family medicine was significantly and positively related to criteria for quality in charting, periodic health maintenance, medical care, and use of indicator drugs. Since those studies, residency and vocational training has become the norm in many countries. More recently, preventive services in Canadian family practices have been found to be more likely to be associated with female physicians and those whose practices were organized into family health teams or networks, or in community health centers (Thind, Feightner, Stewart, et al., 2008). Physicians practicing solo or international medical graduates were relatively less likely to deliver recommended preventive services. In an attempt to answer the question of whether family physicians who received vocational training deliver better quality care, a review of the literature consisting of 25 studies found that graduates of such programs provide better quality patient care, and have increased knowledge, improved general practice skills, increased confidence, and better adherence to practice guidelines (Harre Hindmarsh, Coster, et al., 1998).

In some jurisdictions there is a separation between general practice and hospital inpatient care. If this applies to obstetrics, then obstetrics may be completely excluded from general practice, or the general practitioner's role may be limited to antenatal and postnatal care.

The service profile of general practitioners in Europe was found to vary according to whether or not they performed a gatekeeping role in the healthcare system as well as remuneration methods. "[T]he concept of comprehensive and family care is included in the usual definitions of general practice, but, in some countries, separate provision is made for gynecology and pediatrics"

(Boerma, Van Der Zee, and Fleming, 1997). Remuneration variables, such as incentives, also have an effect on the workflow of family practitioners.

In economically advanced countries, family physicians can usually take it for granted that basic public health services like clean water, sanitation, and food inspection are provided. In other countries this is not so, and family practice will be correspondingly different. Even in developed countries, there are often communities where standards of public health are poor enough to make an impact on the content of practice. Because these are unusual, family physicians in developed countries are not usually well trained in the environmental aspects of family practice.

REFERENCES

Audunsson GG. 1986. Preventive infrastructure in family practice. Master of Clinical Science thesis, University of Western Ontario.

Beasley JW, Hankey TH, Erickson R, et al. 2004. How many problems do family physicians manage at each encounter? A WReN Study. *Annals of Family Medicine* 2(5):405–410.

Bernstein RM, Hollingworth GR, Viner GS. 1994. Something old, something new, something borrowed: A review of standardized data collection in primary care. *Journal of the American Informatics Association*: Proceedings from the 18th Annual Symposium on Computer Applications in Medical Care.

Bindman AB, Forrest CB, Britt H, et al. 2007. Diagnostic scope and exposure to primary care physicians in Australia, New Zealand, and the United States: Cross sectional analysis of results from three national surveys. *BMJ* 334:1261–1264.

Boerma WGW, Van Der Zee J, Fleming DM. 1997. Service profiles of general practitioners in Europe. *British Journal of General Practice* 47:481–486.

Borgiel AEM, Williams JI, Bass MJ, et al. 1989. Quality of care in family practice: Does residency training make a difference? *Canadian Medical Association Journal* 40:1035.

Britt H, Miller GC, Henderson J, et al. 2013. *General Practice Activity in Australia; 2012–13. BEACH: Bettering the Evaluation and Care of Health*. Sydney: Sydney University Press, University of Sydney Library.

Britt H, Miller GC, Henderson J, et al. 2014. *A Decade of Australian General Practice Activity 2004–05 to 2013–14: BEACH Bettering the Evaluation and Care of Health*. Sydney: Sydney University Press, University of Sydney Library.

Christensen RE, Fetters MD, Green LA. 2005. Opening the black box: Cognitive strategies in family practice. *Annals of Family Medicine* 3:144–150.

Fortin M, Dionne J, Pinho G, et al. 2006. Randomized controlled trials: Do they have external validity for patients with mulitple comorbidities? *Annals of Family Medicine* 4(2):104–108.

Harre Hindmarsh J, Coster GD, Gilbert C. 1998. Are vocationally trained general practitioners better GPs? A review of research designs and outcomes. *Medical Education* 32(3):244–254.

Lamberts H. 1984. *Morbidity in General Practice: Diagnosis Related Information from the Monitoring Project*. Utrecht: Huisartsenpers.

Lamberts H, Wood M, eds. 1987. *ICPC: International Classification of Primary Care.* Oxford; New York: Oxford University Press.

National Ambulatory Care Medical Survey. 2010. http://www.cdc.gov/nchs/data/ahcd/namcs_summary/2010_namcs_web_tables.pdf.

Okkes IM, Polderman GO, Fryer GE, et al. 2002. The role of family practice in different health care systems: A comparison of reasons for encounter, diagnoses, and interventions in primary care populations in the Netherlands, Japan, Poland, and the United States. *Journal of Family Practice* 51(1):72.

Ostbye T, Yarnall YSH, Krause KM, et al. 2005. Is there time for management of patients with chronic diseases in primary care? *Annals of Family Medicine* 3:209–214.

Salisbury C, Procter S, Stewart K, et al. 2013. The content of general practice consultations: Cross-sectional study based on video recordings. *British Journal of General Practice* 63(616):e751–e759.

Stange KC, Zyzanski SJ, Jaén CR, et al. 1998. Illuminating the "black box": A description of 4454 patient visits to 138 family physicians. *Journal of Family Practice* 46(5):377.

Starfield B, Lemke KW, Bernhardt T, et al. 2003. Comorbidity: Implications for the importance of primary care in "case" management. *Annals of Family Medicine* 1(1):8–14.

Thind A, Feightner J, Stewart M, et al. 2008. Who delivers preventive care as recommended? Analysis of physician and practice characteristics. *Canadian Family Physician* 54(11):1574–1575.

White KL. 1985. Restructuring the International Classification of Diseases: Need for a new paradigm. *Journal of Family Practice* 21(1):17–18, 20.

Wong E, Stewart M. 2010. Predicting the scope of practice of family physicians. *Canadian Family Physician* 56(6):e219–e225.

ᴄᴧ☊

Philosophical and Scientific Foundations of Family Medicine

L ike any other branch of science or technology, medicine is based on theory. It is, of course, quite possible to practice for an entire lifetime without being aware of the theory, let alone questioning it. Remarkable as it may seem, the curriculum in most medical schools devotes very little time to examining the ideas on which medicine is based. Small wonder, then, that for many physicians the ideas are a given and discussions about them are considered unprofitable. For some periods of medical history, this does not matter very much: physicians can practice quite confidently and successfully without examining their assumptions, even if it means ignoring for the time being some problems that do not seem to fit. There are other times, however, when problems we have conveniently set aside become more difficult to ignore. At these times, medicine is driven back to an examination of its fundamentals.

Academic family medicine has emerged during one of these periods of reassessment: in a sense, it is itself the product of a ferment of ideas. To understand family medicine, therefore, it is necessary to have a grasp of the ideas on which medicine is based. Moreover, it is important for a newly emergent discipline to be based on firm theoretical foundations. Thomas Kuhn's theory of paradigm change provides a useful frame of reference for a discussion of medical theory.

PARADIGM CHANGE IN SCIENCE

In his influential book, *The Structure of Scientific Revolutions*, Thomas Kuhn (1967) has challenged the conventional view of how science progresses. Kuhn begins by challenging the view that science develops by the accumulation of individual discoveries and inventions. It is true, he says, that for certain periods of time, science may appear to develop cumulatively, but this can be misleading. Such a progression only takes place after a scientific community has agreed on a set of shared assumptions about the phenomena that form the subject matter of the science. Once the assumptions have been made, they are no longer questioned. They become embedded in the education of scientists in such a way that they exert a deep hold on the scientific mind, all the deeper for the fact that they are not made explicit. Kuhn refers to this set of received beliefs in a science as a *paradigm*.[1] He calls the cumulative research that follows the acceptance of a paradigm *normal science*. He describes research in normal science as "a strenuous and devoted attempt to force nature into the conceptual boxes supplied by professional education" (Kuhn, 1967, p. 5).

To take an example from medicine, we might say that one of the assumptions of the existing medical paradigm is that there are such entities as diseases. Once this assumption was made, it became the agenda of normal medical science to describe and establish causes for these entities. But the justification for the assumption was not discussed in the education of physicians. The entities became our conceptual boxes, into which we attempted to force the natural phenomenon of illness.

The formation of a scientific discipline begins with the acceptance of its first paradigm. The earlier stages in the history of a science are marked by many competing schools of thought. During this phase, observations are made and facts are gathered, but in the absence of a paradigm there is no organizing principle to indicate to the observer how the facts relate to each other. Kuhn calls this the *preparadigm phase*. Although this early fact-gathering has been essential to the origin of many sciences, the result is usually, in Kuhn's words, "a morass." "No natural history," says Kuhn, "can be interpreted in the absence of at least some implicit body of intertwined theoretical and methodological belief that permits selection, evaluations, and criticism" (Kuhn, 1967, p. 17).

The preparadigm phase is succeeded by a phase in which one of the competing schools of thought is accepted as a paradigm. To be accepted, a theory must seem better than its competitors in tying together and explaining the facts, but it need not, and never does, explain all the facts. The acceptance of a paradigm is the occasion for the formation of a professional discipline, with its own journals, scientific societies, and textbooks. Once a paradigm is accepted, the individual scientist can take it for granted. He need no longer "attempt to build his field anew, starting from first principles and justifying the use of each concept introduced." The process of normal science is referred to by Kuhn as "mopping up." The acceptance of a paradigm provides a research agenda that can keep workers in the field busy for generations.

The process of change begins when normal science encounters anomalies. Because no paradigm is a complete fit with nature, anomalies are always present. At first, however, these may be ignored, or not even perceived, for perceptions are influenced by expectations. Eventually, the anomalies are increasingly recognized. They attain both observational and conceptual recognition, and then, often after a period of resistance, are accommodated within a new paradigm. Sometimes, the anomalies are related to the use of a scientific instrument. Scientists' expectations are influenced not only by their theories but by their instruments. Instruments are designed with particular observations and results in mind. When the observations are different from those expected, the anomaly puts an entirely new perspective on the instrumental procedure. The discovery of X-rays by Roentgen, for example, violated deeply entrenched expectations. At the time of the discovery, cathode-ray equipment of the kind used by Roentgen was in use in many laboratories. Other workers must have produced X-rays without observing them. The anomaly was presumably blocked out of their awareness because to have acknowledged it would have been tantamount to rethinking all the previous work done in this field.

In some cases, the emergence of anomalies leads to a state of crisis. Failure of normal science to solve the problems created by the anomalies produces a sense of insecurity. From this state of crisis a new paradigm emerges, claimed by its proponents to be more successful in accounting for the anomalies. A period of conflict ensues, with one of three outcomes: success of the old paradigm in handling the crisis; failure of either paradigm to deal with it; or the triumph of the new paradigm.

The change from an old to a new paradigm is revolutionary rather than cumulative. It has been likened to a change of visual Gestalt: a fundamental shift in worldview. In Kuhn's words, it is "a reconstruction of the field from new fundamentals, a reconstruction that changes some of the field's most elementary theoretical generalizations" (Kuhn, 1967, p. 85). The change, however, does not necessarily add any new facts. Just as in a change of visual Gestalt, the picture itself does not change; the paradigm shift is an altered perception of how the facts are related. The fundamental nature of paradigm shift explains some of the features of the conflict. Because it is ultimately about matters that have never been made explicit, it may become extremely bitter and irrational. Adherents of the old paradigm may be incapable of understanding the new one. Proponents of a new paradigm often arise from the periphery of the discipline or from outside it altogether, or they may be young members of the discipline who are able to see it with fresh eyes.

If anomalies are always present, what produces the heightened awareness of them that leads to a state of crisis? There appears to be no single answer. Sometimes, the anomaly calls into question a fundamental generalization of the paradigm; or the anomaly may have practical implications; or a minor anomaly may become a major one when a new experimental technique is developed. Kuhn also mentions social influences in the precipitation of a crisis. At the time of the Copernican revolution, there were strong social pressures for change. The Ptolemaic system developed between 200 BC and 200 AD was very successful in predicting the changing positions of both stars and planets. Ptolemaic astronomy is still in use today as a practical approximation. The minor anomalies in the Ptolemaic system became the subject of normal astronomical science in the succeeding centuries. Discrepancies were eliminated by making minor adjustments to the theory, but the cumulative effect was a theory of enormous complexity, which, by the sixteenth century, was widely recognized as having failed to solve the traditional problems. In addition to this, there was social pressure for calendar reform, making a solution to the problem of precession of the equinoxes particularly urgent.

Kuhn has not been alone in questioning our assumptions about scientific progress.[2] In *Science and the Modern World*, Whitehead (1926, p. 48) wrote,

> When you are criticizing the philosophy of an epoch, do not chiefly direct your attention to those intellectual positions which its exponents feel it necessary explicitly to defend. There will be some fundamental assumptions which adherents of all the variant systems within the epoch unconsciously presuppose. Such assumptions appear so obvious that people do not know what they are assuming because no other way of putting things has ever occurred to them.

In her book *Philosophy in a New Key*, Susanne Langer (1979) observes that when an epoch changes, it is not the answers to questions that change, it is the questions themselves. The way a question is framed limits the possible answers. When an epoch changes, questions asked in the previous epoch are not answered differently: the questions themselves are rejected, along with the assumptions behind them. For example, we might respond to the question "Is disease X organic or psychogenic?" by saying, "Diseases aren't organic or psychogenic."

The unquestioned assumptions behind a paradigm become embodied in language. The very words we use express our assumptions as if they were given, so when a paradigm changes, it is often necessary to find new words to replace the old. Only in this way can we break free from the shackles that words impose on us. For example, the conventional language of medicine expresses our culture's assumptions about the separation of mind and body in words like psychosomatic and somatization.[3]

PARADIGM CHANGE IN MEDICINE

Opinion is divided on whether or not Kuhn's theory applies to medicine. Kuhn himself maintains that paradigm change occurs in applied disciplines, and even in subdisciplines. Our own view is that the theory fits well with the changes occurring in medicine. The old paradigm, also known as the biomedical model,

can be described as follows. Patients suffer from diseases that can be categorized in the same way as other natural phenomena. A disease can be viewed
independently from the person who is suffering from it and from his or her
social context. Mental and physical diseases can be considered separately, with
provision for a group of psychosomatic diseases in which the mind appears to
act on the body. Each disease has a specific causal agent, and it is a major
objective of research to discover them. Given a certain level of host resistance,
the occurrence of disease can be explained as a result of exposure to a pathogenic agent. The physician's main task is to diagnose the patient's disease and
to prescribe a specific remedy aimed at removing the cause or relieving the
symptoms. To achieve this, the clinician is provided with an intellectual tool,
the clinical method known as differential diagnosis. The physician is usually a
detached observer and the patient a passive recipient in this process.

This paradigm provides a good fit with certain categories of illness, especially those that dominated medical practice in the nineteenth century. With
the major exogenous infections such as cholera and typhoid, and with diseases resulting from nutritional deficiencies, the idea of specific causal agents
is a useful one. Causal agents are understood to be rooted in biochemical processes that are determined by genetic makeup and altered by environmental
influences. Under certain conditions, the paradigm is still successful today. In
other settings, notably in family practice, it is encountering anomalies that
are increasingly difficult to ignore. Because family physicians are among the
first to encounter changes in morbidity, they have also been among the first to
encounter the anomalies in the old paradigm. In fact, they have been encountering them for many years. The old paradigm has never had a very good fit
with family practice, and we believe it probable that many family physicians
have only partially accepted it.

ANOMALIES ENCOUNTERED BY THE OLD PARADIGM
The Illness/Disease Anomaly

A large proportion of the symptoms presented by ill people seen in family practice cannot be assigned to a disease category based on a physiological or anatomical abnormality. These symptoms are referred to as medically
unexplained symptoms (MUS). Some examples are given in Table 6.1. In the
first, Blacklock (1977) examined the records of successive patients presenting with chest pain in a general practice. Only half received a specific diagnosis based on pathology. In the second, the Headache Study Group (1986)
followed up 265 patients for a year after they presented in general practice
with new headaches. Only 27% received a diagnosis based on demonstrable
physical changes, such as classical migraine or sinusitis. In the third, Wasson
and his colleagues (1981) followed up adult males for 3 months after they

Table 6.1. PERCENTAGE OF SYMPTOMS PRESENTED TO PRIMARY PHYSICIANS
RECEIVING A SPECIFIC DIAGNOSIS

	Symptom	Study Method	Percentage Receiving Specific Diagnosis
Blacklock (1977)	Chest pain	Chart review	50
Wasson et al. (1981)	Abdominal pain in adult males	Chart review Questionnaire	21
Headache Study Group (1986)	Headache	Physician questionnaire Patient interview	27

presented with abdominal pain to primary care clinics at veterans' hospitals. Only 30% received pathology-based diagnoses. Of course, the remaining patients in all these examples could be given labels such as intercostal myalgia, tension headache, or irritable colon, but these categories are devoid of predictive or inferential power. These early research results in family medicine have been supported by recent results. At least one-third of those presenting to a general medicine outpatient clinic are classified as idiopathic, meaning "symptom-only" in etiology, and at least a quarter will have such symptoms persist at 1 year follow-up (Khan, Khan, Harezlak, et al., 2003). Even after 5-year follow-up of patients presenting with physical symptoms 35% remained unexplained and, importantly, contrary to common belief, most patients with MUS did not have a mental disorder (Jackson and Passamonti, 2005).

The Specific Etiology Anomaly

If the occurrence of disease depended mainly on the presence of specific causal agents, we would expect that, in a homogeneous population sharing the same environment, different diseases would be distributed evenly across the population. Hinkle (1974) showed that this is not the case. In a 20-year study of a group of women, similar in age, occupation, background, and environment, they found that 25% had 52% of the illness, and another quartile had only 6% of the illness. They conjectured that the women with high illness rates were susceptible to particular recurring complaints such as headaches, or had a defect in one organ system. This proved not to be the case. The more illnesses a woman had, the more different types of illness she had, and the more organ systems were involved. They then conjectured that these women were susceptible to diseases of a particular etiology, some to infections, some to allergies, and so on. Again, they found this not to be so. Those with the greatest number of illnesses had illnesses of many different causes, more major illness, and more disturbances of mood, thought, and behavior. The main determinant of health and disease in this population was not the presence of specific agents, but the general susceptibility of the individual women.

Even with infectious diseases, the doctrine of specific etiology is not very useful in technologically advanced societies, where the citizens are protected against most highly virulent agents. As Dubos (1965) has observed, most of the agents associated with current diseases are ubiquitous in the environment, exist in the body without causing harm under ordinary circumstances, and have pathological effects only when the infected person is under physiological stress. An understanding of health and disease, therefore, requires not only a knowledge of disease agents, but of those factors that protect the host from these agents, or make them more vulnerable to them. Even *Streptococcus and Helicobacter pylori* can be present in the throats and stomachs of healthy people without causing harm.

The Mind/Body Anomaly

Under the old paradigm, mind and body were separated, except in certain "psychosomatic" diseases in which psychological factors were thought to be causal. The concept of causation was strongly influenced by the prevailing doctrine of specific etiology. Psychological and social factors were thought to act directly to produce pathological change. Different factors, moreover, were thought to be specific for each psychosomatic disease. This view has now become untenable in the light of recent discoveries. Factors such as social isolation and stressful life events are associated with higher mortality from all causes, not only from certain psychosomatic diseases. Eight prospective, population-based studies have shown an association between social integration and mortality rates from all causes (Berkman, 1995). In the Alameda County Study, men and women with the fewest social ties were 1.9 to 3.1 times more likely to die in the 9-year follow-up period than those with the most social ties. This was after correcting for other determinants of health (Berkman and Breslow, 1983). Five studies have shown that patients who lack support, live alone, or have not been married have an increased risk of death after a myocardial infarction (Berkman, 1995). In one study, men who were socially isolated were twice as likely to die over a 3-year period after the infarct as those who were not isolated. When this was combined with a general measure of life stressors, the risk increased to four to five times that of men in the low-risk categories (Ruberman et al., 1984). Close and supportive relationships have been found to be associated with lower morbidity and mortality (Fagundes, Bennett, Derry, et al., 2011).

Studies of different populations have shown consistently that recent stressful life events are associated with an increased risk of illness of many kinds. People who have experienced recent stressful life events, or who are psychologically vulnerable, have greater deterioration of overall health, more diseases of the upper respiratory tract, more allergies, more hypertension, and a greater risk of coronary disease and sudden death (Dohrenwend and Dohrenwend, 1974; Jemmott and Locke, 1984). Coker, Tyrell, and Smith (1991) inoculated healthy volunteers aged between 20 and 55 with either a cold virus or placebo. The rates of respiratory infection and colds increased with the level of psychological stress in a dose–response manner.

Short-term stressors such as student exam stress can delay wound repair and modulate the immune response to a vaccine (Kiecolt-Glaser, McGuire, Robles, and Glaser, 2002a). Chronic stress, such as caring for a spouse or parent with dementia, has been associated with prolonged endocrine and immune dysregulation, as well as changes in health, vaccine response, and wound healing. Burnout, imprisonment, job stress, and unemployment have also been associated with immune modulations (Kiecolt-Glaser, McGuire, Robles, and Glaser, 2002b).

Kiecolt-Glaser, McGuire, Robles, and Glaser (2002c) regard the link between personal relationships and immune function as one of the most robust findings in psychoneuroimmunology: for example, higher natural killer (NK) cell activity was associated with higher level of support in women whose husbands were being treated for cancer. A low sense of coherence in healthy adults was associated with the poorest level of NK cell lysis (sense of coherence is a construct formulated by Antonovsky, 1979). High hostility individuals exhibited greater increases in NK cell cytotoxicity following self-disclosure than those with low hostility (Kiecolt-Glaser, McGuire, Robles, and Glaser, 2002b).

Events involving a loss of important personal relationships appear to have the greatest potential for harm (Kiecolt-Glaser and Glaser, 1995). This emerges strongly in studies of the mortality of bereavement. One prospective study of conjugal bereavement, for example, found increased mortality among widowers, especially between the ages of 55 and 74, for 10 years after the deaths of their wives (Helsing, Szklo, and Comstock, 1981). Divorce and marital separation are also associated with increased risks of illness that are even greater, on an actuarial basis, than those associated with bereavement (Kiecolt-Glaser and Glaser, 1995). Close, supportive relationships have been linked to lower levels of inflammation, whose presence has been linked to many age-related diseases (Fagundes, Bennett, Derry, et al., 2011). Disruption of relationships is a possible explanation for the association between unemployment and an increase in rates of illness and death (Jin, Shah, and Svoboda, 1995).

In addition to the evidence on the effects of social integration and stress, a large body of research supports the influence of personality traits and emotions on the outcome of some disease states. The strongest associations are those between anger, hostility, and depression and poor outcomes in coronary heart disease (CHD) (Siegler, Costa, Brummett, et al., 2003). There is some evidence linking emotional suppression with breast cancer incidence and the occurrence of CHD. There is evidence to suggest that pessimism and fatalism may be associated with poorer outcomes in AIDS, cancer, and CHD (Scheier and Bridges, 1995).

Scheier and Bridges (1995) contend that age and stage of disease seem to modulate the strength of the relationship between emotional variables and health. These variables appear to have a stronger effect in younger than in older people and in the earlier rather than the later stages of disease.

The lack of specificity of illness after stressful life events has focused attention on the neuroendocrine and immune systems as the possible pathways through which the emotions can alter susceptibility to illness. Depression of immune function has been found in widowers and widows, divorced men and women, family caregivers of patients with Alzheimer's disease, and students under academic stress (Kiecolt-Glaser, Dura, Speicher, et al. (1991)). Discussing psychological factors on immune function, Kiecolt-Glaser and Glaser, (1995) write, "However, only a few studies have so far shown a correlation between stressors, immunodepression, and illnesses" (Keicolt-Glaser and Glaser, 1995, p. 269).We do not know how far immune function must be suppressed to make a person more vulnerable to disease."(. Kiecolt-Glaser and Glaser (1995) suggest that stress-related immunosuppression may have its most serious consequences in people whose immune function is already impaired, such as the aged. As noted earlier, however, a number of studies have shown stronger relationships between emotional factors and health status in younger than in older people, and no studies have reported the opposite (Scheier and Bridges, 1995). The answers to these questions have therapeutic implications, for the same questions could be asked about the therapeutic effect of supportive therapies.

The strongest refutation to dividing the mind and the body has been the discovery that receptors for neuropeptides are found throughout the body, not only in nervous tissue. Our entire body is capable of responding to our cognitions and our emotions. We can no longer think of the mind as being located in the brain alone. It is not accurate even to think in terms of a *connection* between the mind and body. Rather it is best to conceive of a mind/body unity (Dreher, 2003).

THERAPEUTIC IMPLICATIONS OF THE MIND/BODY UNITY

Because of the strong evidence for the health consequences of emotions, relationships, and social integration, we must ask whether supportive therapies can affect the duration or outcome of illness. Several studies have shown that assurance given to patients prior to surgery can reduce the length of postoperative recovery. Patients who reported that their doctors had ascertained the patient's meaning of the illness recovered more quickly from a variety of minor illnesses than patients whose doctors did not ascertain the meaning (Bass, Buck, Turner, et al., 1986).

Several randomized controlled trials have compared groups of cancer patients receiving psychosocial supportive treatment with groups of cancer patients receiving no supportive therapies. No significant difference in life span was found (Goodwin, Leszcz, Ennis, et al., 2001; Kissane, Love, Hatton, et al., 2004).

It seems clear, therefore, that supportive group therapy does not prolong the life span in breast cancer patients under the conditions tested. However, this does not prove that the mind has no effect on survival in cancer. Cunningham makes it clear that these studies show "that certain types of short-term group psychological interventions fail to prolong the *mean* or *median* life span of *groups* of cancer patients. ... What should not be dismissed, however, is the possibility that some therapies may have the potential to extend life in certain patients under some conditions. To rule this out risks making a type II error that could inhibit further research on an issue that is of great importance to many cancer patients" (Cunningham and Edmonds, 2005, p. 5263).

Cunningham cites evidence from his own studies that patients who have gone through a significant life change after psychotherapy, which includes spiritual aspects of healing, survive much longer than their expected prognosis (according to a panel of oncologists). Patients in the same study who did not go through a life change did not have prolonged survival.

A randomized controlled trial cannot resolve this question. Research on the effects of psychotherapy is not the same as research on a new drug. There are ways of assessing whether a patient has responded to the drug. The only way of knowing whether a patient has gone through a life change is to examine patients one by one.

In addition to the evidence for the therapeutic benefits of social support, many studies have shown that adults and children can learn to voluntarily control autonomic physiological responses and to alter their cellular and humoral immune responses by relaxation/imagery, self-hypnosis, and/or biofeedback (Hall, Minnes, and Olness, 1993). Children can reduce the frequency of migraine headaches by self-hypnosis (Olness, MacDonald, and Uden, 1987). Studies in cancer patients suggest that self-hypnosis can lessen pain in patients with breast cancer, and that relaxation and imagery can reduce the nausea and vomiting associated with chemotherapy. Other studies suggest that both individual and group therapies enhance coping skills and reduce anxiety and depression in cancer patients (Classen, Hermanson, and Spiegel, 1994).

There are important implications for family physicians. The support provided by the family doctor, like other supportive therapies, can help improve patients' health and enhance their general resistance; it can combine cognitive approaches with emotional expression and support, and the family doctor is well placed to mobilize support from the patient's family. Other members of the primary care team are also important sources of support. All these therapeutic interventions act not on specific disease states, or on causal agents, but on the patient's resistance, helping patients to become agents of their own healing.

Reviewing the subject of social environment and host resistance, Cassel (1976) made three postulates:

1. Social factors enhance or lower susceptibility to disease generally, not to specific diseases.
2. The mechanisms involved are general in nature.
3. Social supports act by buffering the effects of environmental stressors.

The experimental evidence accumulated has supported these postulates.

Much of the discussion of the role of the social environment in disease has been concerned with the concept of *stress*, a term that is often used rather loosely. In his pioneering work on stress, Selye (1956) used the term to indicate a bodily state resulting from the interaction of the organism with noxious stimuli. The stress state described included adrenal hypertrophy and elevated corticosteroid levels. Since this time, the term *stress* has been used to denote both the stimulus and the response. The response is mediated through the hypothalamic-pituitary-adrenal (HPA) axis. Confusion can be avoided by using *stressor* for the former and *stress state* for the latter. With social stressors, the issue is complicated by the fact that there is no constant relationship between stressor and stress state. Whether or not a social stimulus is stressful depends very much on its meaning for the individual and on his or her psychological vulnerability. Hinkle and his colleagues (1974), for example, observed that women with high illness rates were of a different personality type from women with low illness rates.

The relationship of stressors to mental health has been controversial. In the past the prevailing view was that stress is of little significance in accounting for variations in mental health. Using a new method of assessing traumatic events, however, Turner, Wheaton, and Lloyd (1995) reported significant associations between traumatic events in childhood and adult life, and subsequent mental illnesses such as major depression and substance abuse. The lifetime risk of illness increased with the number of traumas prior to the age of 18, and the risk of a recurrence of the illness was strongly associated with the number of additional traumas experienced since the first episode. The childhood traumas included physical abuse, separation from home, substance abuse in a parent, parental unemployment or divorce, serious injury, and sexual abuse (in females). Adult traumas included divorce, substance abuse in spouse, physical abuse by spouse, and infidelity by spouse. The authors noted that the average age at the first episode of illness was 21 and suggested that preventive efforts should be targeted to children and adolescents. Although many of these traumas are unavoidable, their effects on the young can be mitigated. All types of child abuse (physical abuse, sexual abuse, and exposure to intimate partner violence) has been found to be associated with mental conditions in adulthood. The number of abuse types demonstrates a dose–response relationship with increasing odds of mental conditions later in life (Afifi, MacMillan, Boyle, et al., 2014).

Because social stimuli act by virtue of their symbolic meaning for the individual, their pathogenicity is of a different order from that of physicochemical stimuli. The latter tend to damage the organism directly; the former act indirectly by modifying the host's response to disease agents.

As family physicians, interested in health as well as disease, we should also think in terms of factors that increase host resistance and strengthen resistance against noxious stimuli. Psychological factors such as coping ability may increase resistance. Social factors can be not only stressful, but supportive. Antonovsky (1979) has called these factors *general resistance resources* (GRR). There is evidence that social supports can modify the harmful effects of stressful life events. In a prospective study of pregnant women, Nuckolls, Cassel, and Kaplan (1972) studied the relationship of life events and social supports to complications of pregnancy. Life changes were recorded at the 32nd week of pregnancy, using Holmes and Rahe's cumulative life change index (1967). At the same time, social supports were measured by an instrument designed to record the woman's feelings about her pregnancy, her relationship with her husband, and her perception of support from her family and community. After delivery, the records were reviewed blindly for complications of pregnancy or delivery. Ninety percent of women with high life change scores and low social supports had one or more complications. Among women with equally high life change scores, but high social supports, only 33% had one or more complications. In a large prospective study in Israel, Medalie and Goldbourt (1976) found that men with severe family problems were three times more likely to develop angina than those with few family problems. In men with high anxiety levels, the risk of developing angina was significantly lower in those who received much support and love from their wives than in those who did not. Social support protects men from the health consequences of loss of employment, including the physical indicators of arthritis (Cobb and Kasl, 1977; Gore, 1978). A number of studies also indicate that social support influences the course and outcome of illness and injury (Turner, 1983).

There is evidence for the influence of social support on mental health, especially on depression (Turner, 1983). Much of this evidence points to the protective or buffering effects of social supports in individuals experiencing stressful events. Other studies, however, have suggested that social support has a main and independent relationship with mental health, in addition to moderating the effect of stressful life events. Education of families in coping and providing support reduces the relapse rate in patients with schizophrenia (McFarlane, 1992). After an extensive review of the evidence, Turner (1983) draws three tentative conclusions:

1. Social support tends to matter for psychological well-being independent of stressor level.
2. Support tends to matter more where stressor level is relatively high.
3. The extent to which conclusions 1 and 2 are true varies across subgroups of the population (e.g., by social class).

Evidence is accumulating linking social support and personal relationships to gene expression, intracellular signaling mechanisms, and inflammatory biomarkers (Kiecolt-Glaser, Gouin, and Hantsoo, 2010).

Another issue raised by social support research is the one of causal inference. It is well recognized that social support is not simply a matter of a network of relationships. What matters to a person is his or her subjective feeling of being "loved, wanted, valued, esteemed, and able to count on others should the need arise" (Cobb, 1976, p. 300). The perception of being loved and esteemed may be strongly influenced by the person's own self-esteem: his or her social supports may be as much a reflection of the individual's mental health as the cause of it. How then can we be sure that the association between low social support and poor mental health is causal in one direction? In human behavior, cause and effect rarely act in a linear unidirectional manner. Causation in complex systems is circular or spiral, each effect having reciprocal effects on the cause by feedback loop, as well as more distant effects on other parts of the system. A person's early life experience may make him or her vulnerable to depression. Frequent depressions may lead to a withdrawal from social contacts. The lack of social contacts may then act to reinforce the depression and delay recovery. Given the complexity of causation in human affairs, we cannot assume that cause and effect are all in one direction. Nevertheless, after an extensive review of the evidence, Turner (1983) concludes that an important part of the causation goes from support to psychological distress. The fact that we cannot isolate simple causal chains does not mean that we cannot act on our knowledge about the importance of life experience and social supports. We know enough to give close attention to a patient's supporting relationships in all types of illness, and especially to the support we ourselves can provide.

Thinking of the mind/body as a unity makes the notion that there is a group of psychosomatic diseases untenable. Social and psychological factors may be influential in any disease state, either as a cause of the disease itself or as a factor determining its severity and course.

THE PLACEBO EFFECT

In some respects, *placebo effect* is an unfortunate name for the phenomenon, because it focuses attention on the placebo as a substance administered to the patient. In fact, the placebo effect does not depend on the administration of a substance. It may follow any therapeutic modality, including those where no physical treatment of any kind is given. The placebo effect occurs when a patient responds to the form but not the content of therapy. The patient exhibits a biological response to the symbolic significance of the treatment. Moerman (1983) prefers to call this "general medical effectiveness," rather than placebo effectiveness.

The placebo effect occurs if a patient in a healing context is administered an intervention as part of that context, if the patient's condition is changed, and if the change is attributable to the intervention, but not to any specific therapeutic effect or to any known pharmacologic or physiologic property of the intervention (Brody, 1980). By using the term *changed* rather than *improved*, this definition allows for the fact that the placebo effect can be harmful as well as therapeutic. It also excludes general effects of the intervention that may not be symbolically mediated, such as diet and exercise.

A recent experiment exemplifies the power of the placebo effect in patients with severe coronary disease. Patients with end-stage coronary disease had long-term beneficial effects of placebo therapy in a study of angiogenesis and laser myocardial revascularization trials. Patients were randomly assigned to therapy or placebo. Improvements in mean angina class, exercise treadmill time, and quality of life were mostly maintained at 90 days from baseline. The benefits of placebo therapy were maintained at 2-year follow-up (Rana et al., 2005). In a systematic review of the use of a placebo arm in the evaluation of surgical interventions, it was found that in 51% of such trials the effect of placebo did not differ from that of surgery (Wartolowska, Judge, Hopewell, et al., 2014).

It is important to correct some misconceptions about the placebo effect. Some of these are not so much misconceptions as attempts to explain it away as a matter of little significance. The first is that placebo effectiveness is only found in subjective conditions such as pain and anxiety. In fact, placebos affect objectively measurable processes as well as subjective reports. The second is that placebos are harmless. In fact, placebos can produce undesirable effects and addiction like pharmacologically active drugs. The third misconception is that only highly suggestible or neurotic personality types respond to placebos. People responding to placebos are of very varied personality types (Brody, 1980). The fourth is that the placebo effect is constant at about 35% of patients. Placebo effectiveness has been found to vary between 10% and 90% (Moerman, 1983), 35% being the generally accepted mean figure.

The explanation of the placebo effect that fits best with the evidence is provided by the meaning model (Brody, 1980). This may be stated as follows. The placebo effect is most likely to occur when the following conditions are met:

1. The patient is provided with an explanation of his or her illness that is consistent with his or her worldview.
2. Individuals in socially sanctioned caring roles provide support for the patient.
3. The healing intervention leads to the patient acquiring a sense of mastery and control over the illness.

The placebo response can be learned by association, as in classical conditioning. Pavlov was the first to report a conditioned placebo effect in dogs who showed morphine-like effects, whenever they were placed in the experimental chamber where they had previously received morphine. Several studies have shown that the placebo response can be conditioned in humans (Peck and Coleman, 1991). Olness and Ader (1992) have reported on the case of a child with lupus erythematosus who needed only half the usual dose of cyclophosphamide after conditioning with cod liver oil. Because classical conditioning depends on a response to something that symbolizes the unconditioned stimulus, the symbolism of our therapeutic acts assumes practical importance. The continuing patient–doctor relationship and the familiar surroundings of the practice are fertile ground for symbols of healing. Conditioning is maintained and enhanced by every new experience of effective treatment. On the other hand, the effect can be reduced or extinguished by negative experiences. The familiar doctor's face, in a familiar place, associated with healing on many past occasions, is a strong foundation for the working of the placebo effect.

Slow progress continues to be made in our understanding of the placebo effect. Setting an interdisciplinary research agenda is an important step in this direction (Guess, Kleinman, Kusek, and Engel, 2002). There is much still to be learned about the patient–doctor relationship in family medicine.

PHYSIOLOGICAL PATHWAYS

Research points to the nervous, endocrine, and immune systems as the main pathway by which nonmaterial phenomena influence bodily health. The cardinal manifestations of the general adaptation syndrome (GAS) described by Selye (1956) are adrenal hypertrophy, thymic involution, and elevated corticosteroid levels. High levels of corticosteroids are immunosuppressive, and high physiological levels are required for several normal immune functions. In the GAS, noxious stimuli cause the hypothalamus to release a corticotropin-releasing factor, which in turn causes the pituitary to release adrenocorticotropic hormone (ACTH). This stimulates the adrenal cortex to secrete corticosteroids. Thyroid, growth and sex hormones, and insulin are also required for the normal development and function of the immune system.

Walter Cannon (1932), the American physiologist who gave us the concept of homeostasis, also described the fight-or-flight response—a sympathetic outflow leading to the secretion of norepinephrine in target organs and epinephrine in the adrenal medulla. Lymphocytes have receptors for catecholamines, and stimulation of the beta-adrenergic (epinephrine) fibers decreases cellular immune response. Beta-adrenergic drugs have been shown to be immunosuppressive. Studies in animals have shown relationships between social environment, changes in the endocrine system, and morbidity and mortality. Abrupt change in the social environment in mice, either from isolation to group or vice versa, results in adrenal hypertrophy and increased growth of an implanted tumor. Male mice housed one or two per cage had a lesser ability to reject lymphosarcoma than those in larger groups. Anxiety stress in mice increases the risk of malignancy, and this increased risk is associated with elevated plasma corticosterone. Benign virus infections can also produce an elevated corticosterone level and increase the risk of malignancy. Some of the evidence from animal experiments is conflicting. Stressful stimuli have been found in some experiments to reduce the risk of malignancy. The contradictions may be explained by the finding that chronic stress can produce immunosuppression, followed by immunoenhancement (Riley, Fitzmaurice, and Spackman, 1981). Activation of T lymphocytes releases lymphokines that control lymphoid cell activation, transformation, and clonal expansion. The experimental evidence suggests two regulatory mechanisms for the immune system: homeostatic autoregulation depending on internal immunologic signals, and an external system mediated by the central nervous and endocrine systems (Besedovsky and Sorkin, 1981). The way in which these control systems interact is extremely complex, making inferences about cause and effect very uncertain.

Our ability to maintain homeostasis is essential to survival, and chronic states of hyperarousal add to the allostatic load, which represents the strain on the organism and can lead to dysregulation of various systems (McEwen and Norton, 2002).

THE IMMUNE SYSTEM

Until recent years, the immune system was regarded as isolated from other body systems. Research in the field of psychoneuroimmunology (PNI) has now shown close reciprocal relationships between the immune and neuroendocrine systems. The autonomic nervous system, through its innervation of lymphoid organs, provides a pathway for communication between both systems. Cells of the immune system have receptors for neuropeptides and the latter have been shown to modulate immune response. Every hormone secreted or regulated by the pituitary gland has some effect on the immune system (Bellinger, Madden, Felten, and Felten, 1994). The cells of the immune system can produce substances previously identified as neurotransmitters, suggesting that there is a commonality of signal molecules that can act on the nervous system, the immune system, or both.

Felten and Felten (1991) describe the implications of recent research in these terms:

> The unequivocal demonstration of direct neural innervation between the nervous and immune system and the demonstration of functional consequences of signaling in both directions suggest that these two great memory and communication systems, poised to respond to internal and external challenges for the protection and preservation of the organism, are interdependent. No longer can we think of the immune system as autonomous, and no longer can we think of behavior and neural responsiveness as unaffected by the immune status of the organism (Felten and Felten, 1991, p. 52).

One of the most striking examples of the relationships between behavior and the immune system is the fact that the immune response can be altered by conditioning. In other words, the immune system can learn from experience. In the same way as Pavlov's dogs learned to salivate at the sound of a bell, animals learn to alter their immune response when given an inert substance previously paired with a suppressor or enhancer of immune response. In a key experiment by Ader and Cohen (1991), saccharin paired with the immunosuppressant cyclophosphamide was administered to rats, which were immunized 3 days later with sheep red blood cells (SRBC). On the day of immunization, the animals were divided into three groups. One group received a second dose of saccharin; one received a second dose of cyclophosphamide; and the third were not re-exposed to either substance. Antibodies to SRBC were measured 6 days later. The animals given a second dose of saccharin and those given a second dose of cyclophosphamide showed reduced anti-SRBC response compared with those who did not receive a second dose, and with unconditioned animals injected with SRBC. As already indicated, we also know that humans can be conditioned in the same way to respond to an inert substance (placebo).

The significance of this finding is the response of the immune system to a symbol of the active agent. The organism responded to the stimulus because it had meaning for it. This process is difficult to describe in the ordinary mechanistic language of medical science. To capture it, we have to use words like *meaning, message,* and *symbol.* If we insist on eschewing such terms, we miss the point that organisms in health and disease respond at multiple levels, and that each level poses its own questions for us, as well as its own therapeutic possibilities. As well as asking the lower level question, "What are the neuronal and chemical pathways?" we should ask the upper level question, "Can humans help to heal themselves by altering their immune response by their own volition?"

A NEW PARADIGM

In spite of its many critics, the biomedical model reigned supreme for most of the twentieth century; the model is exemplified by the clinicopathological conference, a procedure that has shown generations of students how to approach a patient's clinical problem. An invited clinician would be presented with a patient's history, physical signs, and test results, after which he or she would present a differential diagnosis and a probable diagnosis, giving his or her reasons. The pathologist would then present the definitive diagnosis. Within its limits, it was an excellent teaching tool, but patients' personal aspects were rarely mentioned, and the patient's own story was not included.

The biomedical model was very successful and continued to be so within the walls of the teaching hospital. Outside the walls, however, it was very different. Until very recently, general practitioners were trained in teaching hospitals according to the biomedical model. In practice, they found that many of their patients had illnesses that did not fit with any diagnosis, or had problems that were a complex of illness, problems of living, and emotional turmoil.

It is not surprising, therefore, that one of the earliest attempts to change the medical model came from a group of general practitioners working with Michael Balint, a psychoanalyst and physician, who sat with the group while they discussed patients who troubled them. The result was Balint's book, *The Doctor, His Patient, and the Illness*.(1957). The book and the seminars that followed had a profound effect on general practice and "marked the beginning of a shift away from the purely biomedical model of medical practice which was the prevailing one at the time" (Gillies, 2005, p. 2). Although influential in general practice, Balint's teaching made no impact on the medical schools.

Twenty years later, another psychoanalyst, George Engel, published a seminal paper on the shortcomings of the biomedical model, advocating a biopsychosocial model based on general system theory. Engel, himself, was not satisfied with the name *biopsychosocial* and welcomed the term *infomedical* coined by Foss and Rothenberg, whose book had a foreword by Engel (Foss and Rothenberg, 1987). A term for a new paradigm should convey its essence, and while *infomedical* made a step forward by focusing on the crucial role of information at all levels of the human body, it fails to include a holistic approach, which is so central to family medicine.

We have called this the Goldstein paradigm in honor of Kurt Goldstein (1878–1965) (Goldstein, 1995), scientist, neurologist, psychologist, and above all a pioneer of the holistic approach to medicine. Although his major work was in neurology, we in family medicine share with him the conviction that it is impossible to consider any illness without reference to the patient's self. The essence of the Goldstein paradigm is to see the patient as a whole, an integrated being with a history, a present, and a future that is ensconced in myriad psychological realities, social relationships, and environmental challenges, against a background of genetic propensities. Within this ontological framework, symptoms are seen as a manifestation of the organism attempting to achieve a new adaptation to circumstances brought about by an illness or accident. At times, these adaptations can have consequences that are more far reaching than the original deficit or illness. To fully understand a symptom complex, therefore, you must take a holistic view. Meticulous observation and understanding of the patient's self are necessary for the physician to assist the patient through a period of chaos to a new equilibrium.

The new paradigm is especially applicable to family medicine. We define ourselves in terms of relationships, not by diseases or technologies. We form relationships with patients before we know what their illnesses will be. Our commitment to them, therefore, is unconditional. We are available to them for any problem they bring to us. Our special skill is the assessment of undifferentiated clinical problems. Our long-term relationships with patients and their families give us privileged knowledge about their lives, gathered often by listening to their stories. We tend, therefore, to think in terms of individuals: of patients, rather than abstractions. General practice is the only major field of medicine that transcends the dualistic division between mind and body. Note, however, that this does not mean bringing mind and body together—a much more difficult task. In a relation-based discipline, says Gillies (2005), decision-making must include both emotional and intellectual aspects.

To bring about paradigm change in medical practice, however, it is necessary to describe in detail a new clinical method, as is done in Chapter 9.

As the consultation begins, the patient is seen as a whole, before any attention to detail. The encounter is an emotional engagement between doctor and patient. The doctor's attention should be outward toward the patient, and his feeling with, or his compassion for, the patient should be an imaginative grasp of the patient's whole situation (Macnaughton, 2002). The capacity of bodily empathy is central to the general clinical competence of the family practitioner. Bodily empathy is a route to the understanding of the emotions and bodily experience (Rudebeck, 1992).

Whatever the outcome of the consultation, the doctor may reflect on the knowledge he or she has gathered of the patient's life history and family relationships—knowledge that may have relevance for the present illness, being careful not to make unfounded assumptions.

Almost any illness has reverberations among the patient's relationships. A new illness may have an impact on existing chronic illnesses or disabilities. The patient's reason for coming may be a problem of living, or a problem of living affecting a chronic illness.

> Medicine is, at the very deepest level concerned with loss, or the possibility of loss. In many illnesses and consultations, general practitioners deal with patients who are afraid of loss: loss of function due to illnesses or ageing, loss associated with the stigma of a disease, loss of employment, friends or family, or even their own lives . . . a consultation that seems to be about a minor symptom may have been interpreted by the patient as an indicator of serious, perhaps fatal disease. At the very heart of meaning, is this knowledge of the possibility, and in the end, the inevitability of loss. (Gillies, 2005, p. 34)

Facing this suffering, week in, week out, makes great demands on us. Avoidance is a great temptation. Yet it is so important that we give ourselves to these suffering patients. At the same time, we must be quite clear that what we are doing is not self-serving. This is why self-knowledge, and an understanding of our own countertransference, is so important for physicians, and especially for general practitioners (see Chapter 24, "Continuing Self-Education").

The patient-centered clinical method is described in detail in Chapter 9. Its essence is to ascertain the meaning of the illness to the patient. A proper use of the method requires that we carefully listen to the patient's needs, be sensitive to his or her cues and body language, and explore the circumstances surrounding the onset of the patient's symptoms. The patient's illness is not separate from the patient's life. That ideas and events in the patient's life can trigger or cause the illness is one of the differences between the Goldstein paradigm and the biomedical paradigm. It follows, also, that bringing this knowledge to the patient can be therapeutic (Broom, 2007).

According to the emerging paradigm—designed to take into account the anomalies referred to earlier—disease is not separated conceptually from the person, nor is the person separated from his or her environment. Conventional disease categories are still used as a frame of reference, but always in context. All illnesses affect the patient at multiple levels. All have multiple causes, although it may be useful to focus therapy on a single causal chain. Causation acts not only in a linear, but also in a reciprocal fashion. The relationship between doctor and patient has a profound effect on the illness and its course. The task of the physician is to understand the nature of the illness on all its levels. For practical purposes, attention may be focused on only one level, at least for a time. In all serious illness, however, attention should be paid at multiple levels. Our *clinical method* should be adequate to this task. To understand the illness at the higher psychological and social levels, the physician has to identify with the patient and his or her loved ones through qualities of empathy and compassion. This is necessary both for humanitarian reasons and for the scientific practice of medicine. It is through these relationships that new qualities emerge in all the participants.

The new paradigm has important implications for clinical method and for how the physician treats the patient. The contrast between the old and the new paradigms is illustrated very vividly by the clinicopathological conference (Clinicopathological Conference, 1968).

The subject of the conference was a 50-year-old man with adult celiac disease, resistant to treatment. Initially, the patient had responded well to a gluten-free diet, but he had later gone downhill very rapidly and died. In opening the discussion, the professor of medicine asked, "Why did this patient's intestine suddenly become wrecked and remain so wrecked that he died from his disease?"

After a discussion about the pathology of the patient's intestine, the professor commented:

> So it appears that we are completely at sea over the cause of the gut lesion in this man. This is not like the ordinary coeliac disease with a response to a gluten-free diet. This is an exception which in Dr._____'s experience affects about 30% of the patients he sees. . . . But of some 30% of adult patients who will not respond to a gluten-free diet only a few will be like this, running almost a malignant course resulting in death; and the question we have to ask is what would cause it. Dr._____ "you were this patient's family physician, would you like to comment . . . ?" (Clinicopathological Conference, 1968, p. 681)

To this, the patient's family physician replied:

> I would like to suggest that the main reason for this [failure to account for the course of the illness] is the inadequacy of the concepts which they [the discussants] are using in their attempted explanations. If we treat the patient as a biochemical machine and exclude any concepts which refer to him as a person, then it seems to me that explanations of his illness must be extremely limited. If we turn our attention to this man's life pattern and what little we know of his inner feelings, this illness becomes much more understandable. Perhaps we should be using more relevant concepts as the basis for our explanations.
>
> In this case, I know there were major emotional conflicts in all the main areas of his life.
>
> The onset of the illness followed the death of his father, an event with which a lot of family feeling was associated. The exacerbation of his illness coincided with rising tension between himself and his adopted daughter within the context of a sterile marriage. The final stage of his illness coincided with the collapse of his work relationship after a long period of devoted service. . . . I feel that he died because all that he had lived for had somehow come to nothing.

To this the professor of medicine responded,

> Thank you very much. The possibility of a psychogenic influence in coeliac disease has been suggested by Pauley, and clearly if the basic abnormality of coeliac disease is due to a genetically determined enzyme defect, I would find it difficult to believe that psychogenic influences could play much part. It is more likely to be a sensitivity. Do you think that the mucosal lesion was due to an enzyme factor, Dr.——?

This encounter between a professor of medicine and a family physician is full of interest, for it brings into sharp focus the two contrasting views of disease we have been discussing. Note that the family physician answered the professor's question very precisely. He had not asked "Why did the patient get celiac disease?" but "Why did the patient die?" The family physician shifted the focus of the discussion from the organ and the disease to the whole person and his response to his environment. In his reply, however, the professor showed himself to be the prisoner of his concepts. First, he was unable to transcend disease categories and think in terms of the patient as an organism rather than a case of celiac disease. Second, he was unable to think about cause in any other way than as a specific etiology. The likelihood of a genetically determined enzyme deficiency was thought to rule out any possibility of environmental factors acting concurrently.

This exchange took place in 1968, before the scientific evidence for the influence of relationships and emotions on health had begun to accumulate. The professor's reluctance to discuss this aspect of the case is therefore understandable. He was also constrained by a model of disease that is unable to account for it. This has not changed.

Although we have been thinking of recent changes in medical thought in terms of old and new paradigms, a more historical perspective indicates that the new paradigm is not without precedent. Crookshank (1926) has traced two theories of medicine back to the schools of Cos and Cnidus in ancient Greece. To the school of Cos, understanding a disease included understanding the patient in his or her environment. Therapy consisted of prescribing a regimen that would help the patient to overcome his or her disease. To the Cnidians, diseases were entities in their own right. The task of the physician was to categorize the disease and to prescribe the specific remedy. For a more extensive discussion of the Coan and Cnidian schools, see Chapter 9.

These two philosophies have vied with each other over the centuries, one or other being dominant at different times. The wisest physicians have been those who have taken something from each. What I have described as the new paradigm is the heir of the Hippocratic tradition. Of course, historical events and movements never recur in exactly the same way. The new paradigm is new in the sense that, although it has roots in tradition, it also embodies all that we have learned from the experience of the past 100 years. The patient-centered clinical method is a way of implementing these principles in current practice (see Chapter 9).

THE BIOLOGICAL BASIS OF FAMILY MEDICINE

Medical science is based on a mechanistic metaphor of biology. Its ideal goal, as expressed by the geneticist Arthur Zucker (1981, p. 145), is "diagnostics accomplished by a biochemical–biophysical survey of the body. Ideally, psychological problems could be captured by this technique. It is part of the assumption of reductionist medicine that, at the very least, mental states have clinically useful physical correlates."

Reduction undoubtedly confers benefits by reducing the number of explanatory principles for otherwise disparate phenomena (Foss, 1994). As Foss points out, however, reduction can become generalized into reductionism: "a belief in the universal applicability of *upward* causation: the universe is composed of fundamental entities—organs, cells, organelles, genes, ultimately perhaps elementary particles—whose intricate interactions account for complex behaviour" (Foss, 1994, p. 33). The difference between reduction and reductionism is illustrated by the development of sumatriptan for migraine. Reducing migraine to its biochemical correlate produced a clinically useful drug. But to suggest that the syndrome is now fully explained, or that pharmacotherapy is a complete solution to the problem of migraine, is reductionism.

The biologist F. E. Yates (1993) writes:

> . . . biological sciences now suffer from permeation by a mechanistic reductionism in the guise of two limiting and inappropriate metaphors: (1) the dynamic metaphor of organisms as machines, and (2) the information metaphor, of life as a text written in DNA . . . both metaphors are false and destructive of conceptual advances in the fundamental understanding of complex living systems that self-organize, grow, develop, adapt, reproduce, repair, and maintain form and function, age and die. The rise of the sciences of complexity offers a fresh, non-reductionist avenue toward the nature, origin, and fabrication of life (Yates, 1993, p. 189).

Even though the body has machine-like features, everything we do for the health of the body depends on the healing powers of nature. At its most successful, medicine works in supporting these natural processes. Surgeons drain abscesses, set fractures, repair wounds, and relieve obstructions. Immunization strengthens the organism's defenses. The most effective drugs are those that support natural defenses and maintain balance in the milieu interieur. The traditional regimens of balanced nutrition, rest, sound sleep, exercise, relief of pain and anxiety, and personal support are all measures that support the organism's healing powers.

Family medicine is based on an organismic metaphor of biology. It is natural for family physicians to think organismically. "In contrast with physics, biology presents diversity and specialness of form and function, and sometimes a striking localness of distribution of its objects. Biological systems are complex by any definition of the term" (Yates, 1993, p. 189).

What does it mean to think organismically? An organism is a particular, that is, "it occupies a region of space, persists through time, has boundaries, and has an environment" (Gorovitz and MacIntyre, 1976, p. 56). The point about particulars is that their behavior cannot be explained or predicted solely by applying the general laws of science. The degree to which a law will apply to a particular organism will depend on its history and its context or environment. There is an inherent uncertainty about all particular applications of general scientific principles. The more complex the particular organism, the greater the uncertainty, and a sick patient is a very complex organism. Family medicine operates at a high level of complexity.

Organismic thinking is multilevel and nonlinear. Organisms maintain themselves in a state of dynamic equilibrium by a reciprocal or circular flow of information at all levels, and between organism and environment. Through these multilevel channels, change in any part can reverberate through the whole organism and to its surroundings. The necessity of constant information flow can be seen in the destabilizing effects on humans of sensory deprivation. Information is carried in the form of symbols conveying messages that are decoded at the appropriate level of the organism. At lower levels, information is carried by hormones and neurotransmitters. At the level of the whole organism, it is carried by stimuli reaching the special senses, such as the words and other symbols by which meaning is expressed in human relationships. This provides the background for our accumulating knowledge of the effect of relationships on health and disease.

The transition from mechanistic to organismic thinking requires a radical change in our notion of disease causation. We have learned to think of a causal agent as a force acting in linear fashion on a passive object, as when a moving billiard ball hits a stationary one. In self-organizing systems such as living organisms, causation is nonlinear. The multiple feedback loops between organism and environment, and between all levels of the organism, require us to think in causal networks, not straight lines. The organism, moreover, is not a passive object. The "specific cause" of an illness may only be the trigger that releases a process that is already a potential of the organism. The causes that maintain an illness and inhibit healing may be different from the causes that initiated it, and they may include the organism's own maladaptive behavior. Therapeutic measures may act not on a causal agent but on the body's defenses, as appears to be the case with the therapeutic benefits of human relationships. In a complex system, cause and effect are not usually close to each other in time and space (Briggs and Peat, 1989); and because organic processes are maintained or changed by multiple influences, it is difficult to predict the consequences of an intervention. It is true that we can still isolate one link in the causal network as our point of intervention, as when we prescribe an antibiotic, but even in these instances we should be aware of the whole context in which we are operating, and of the reciprocal effects of our intervention. The complexity of the illnesses we encounter in family medicine makes it natural for us to think in this way. Does isolation from social supports cause depression, or does depression cause the isolation? Did this life event cause the depression, or was it only the trigger, releasing a depression in a susceptible individual? In human science we can establish relationships between events, but it is often difficult to establish cause. Does this imply therapeutic impotence? No, but it does require a change from simplistic causal thinking to thinking about how change can be facilitated in complex systems.

SELF-ORGANIZING SYSTEMS

General system theory is a response to the limitations of nineteenth-century science. The mechanistic worldview and reductive methods of nineteenth-century science were not able to deal adequately with organic phenomena such as organization and growth. The reductive method dealt with problems by cutting them down to size, separating them from their surroundings, and reducing them as far as possible to simple, linear, causal chains. System theory seeks to do the opposite: to approach problems by including all their significant relationships. A system is defined by Von Bertallanfy (1968, p. xx) as "a dynamic order of parts and processes standing in mutual interaction with each other." Some of the basic concepts of system theory are as follows.

Nature is ordered as a hierarchy of systems, both living and nonliving. Living systems go from organelle to cell, to tissue, to organ, to organism, to family, to community, to society. Each level in the hierarchy is both a whole in itself and part of a greater whole: in Koestler's (1979) words, it is Janus-faced, having one face toward a higher order system and another toward a lower order subsystem (see Figure 6.1). Systems are related to each other, not only hierarchically and vertically, but also horizontally. The immune system "talks" to the nervous system on the same level of the vertical hierarchy. Social systems—family, community, culture—relate to each other on the same level, and a person can be a component of all three.

If we think in terms of human systems, a person is at the highest level of the organismic hierarchy and at the lowest level of the social hierarchy. Each system has features that are unique to that level and can only be explained by criteria that are appropriate to that level. A social system like the family, for example, cannot be explained in biological terms, and a living system cannot be explained in terms of physics and chemistry. Nor can a system be understood by studying each part individually. Understanding the whole requires a

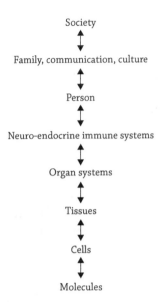

Figure 6.1:
Systems hierarchy (level of organization).
Based on Engel CL. 1980. The clinical application of the biopsychosocial model. *American Journal of Psychiatry* 137:535.

knowledge of the purpose of the system and how its parts interact to attain that purpose. This feature of systems is known as emergence. A system has properties that are not present in the individual parts: they arise from the relationship between the parts—the organization. When a system is broken down into its component parts, the emergent properties are lost.

All living systems are open systems, in that they exchange both energy and information across the system interfaces or boundaries. Each system exists in a state of dynamic internal equilibrium between its parts and in a state of external equilibrium with the systems that form its environment. If the equilibrium is disturbed by changes inside or outside a system, corrective forces come into play, which may restore the equilibrium or return the system to a new steady state. Mutual interdependence of a system's parts is a basic concept of system theory. Any change in a part produces changes in the whole and, because nature is a continuum, the change reverberates up and down the system hierarchy.

These changes cannot be broken down into simple causal chains without grossly oversimplifying the process. To do so is to think in the closed-system way typical of nineteenth-century science. The limitations of this mode of thought have been illustrated by the effects on whole ecosystems of technological innovations like pesticides. In a complex system, cause does not operate in a linear fashion. A chronic illness may cause depression, which may in turn lead to neglect of treatment, resulting in a worsening of the illness, which then exacerbates the depression, and so on.

Living systems have regulatory mechanisms to maintain their equilibrium. One of these is cybernetic regulation, which involves three steps: the return of information by feedback loop from the system's output; matching of this information to the system's rules; and adjusting the output to correct any mismatch. In system theory, the terms *positive* and *negative feedback* are used in a different sense from those we are accustomed to in education. In teaching, negative feedback implies criticism of a student's performance; positive implies praise. In systems language, negative feedback stabilizes a system by reducing deviation from its normal range, as when a thermostat adjusts a heating or cooling system. Positive feedback amplifies a deviation and drives the system into excess. If a doctor confronted by an angry patient responds with anger (positive feedback), the patient is likely to become angrier, then the doctor angrier still, in an escalation of emotion that threatens the relationship. If the doctor makes a conciliatory response (negative feedback), the patient's anger is likely to be reduced, with a stabilizing effect on the relationship.

A living system is constantly adjusting itself to feedback from its own body—engaging in a monologue with itself. In proprioception, for example, the motor impulses of muscles are fed back to the central nervous system through a sensory loop via receptors in tendons and joints. The term *umwelt* was introduced by the ethologist von Uexküll to express the idea that an organism's environment is not simply a neutral piece of space "out there," but rather a subjective universe constructed of features that have a meaning for it (von Uexküll, Geigges, and Herrmann, 1993). The *umwelt* of a bat is a subjective world of sonar impulses; a dog inhabits a world of smells. A blind person, deprived of one mode of perception, has to construct a new *umwelt* based on the remaining senses. The blind person's stick becomes a probe, transmitting vibrations from the environment. As Kay Toombs (1995) has observed, serious disabilities, whether motor or sensory, always require a change in our subjective universe—a reconstruction of our world in synchrony with our altered activities and perceptions. Because our sense of self comes from the sense of coherence generated by the internal monologue, and by the interaction with our environment, any serious disturbance of the interactions is a crisis for our "self." This can be seen in the effects of sensory deprivation and social ostracism, as well as in the onset of blindness, deafness, and other disabilities.

Living systems also experience growth, development and adaptation, all of which require change in response to new conditions. A family changes as its children grow through adolescence to adulthood. The healthcare system changes in response to new health problems. If a system cannot adapt to a changing environment, it may disintegrate and collapse.

One of the most important contributions of system theory has been the conceptual separation of the regulating from the dynamic processes of systems. Because information is the key to regulation, this is equivalent to the separation of information from energy. This distinction between information and energy helps us to see how very large dynamic effects can be set in motion or released by the very small amounts of energy required to process information. An electronic signal can explode a bomb. Breaking an electric circuit can open a large metal door. The ingestion of a minute amount of antigen can lead to fatal anaphylaxis in a sensitized individual. A minor annoyance may trigger a depression in a person predisposed by heredity and life experience. In all these cases, the information acts by releasing energy that is already present in the system. The distinction between the regulating and dynamic processes of systems has implications for our thinking about the causes of events. The cause of anaphylactic shock is both the hypersensitivity of the individual and the antigen that releases the anaphylactic response.

The flow of information is essential to the function of medical systems: the doctor–patient system, the doctor–family system, and the different teams that make up the healthcare system. Failure of communication is the most common reason for medical error. Yet we still pay much more attention to the technical aspects of care than to communication.

THE QUESTION OF MEDICAL KNOWLEDGE

This brings us to a discussion of the knowledge required of the physician working in the new paradigm—the question of the epistemology of medicine. Epistemology (from the Greek *episteme*, "knowledge") is the theory of knowledge. The epistemology of medicine is concerned with questions such as "What is medical knowledge, what should we know about our patients, and how can this knowledge be acquired?"

Since the nineteenth century, medicine has been dominated by the positivist view of knowledge—the belief that the only valid knowledge is that obtained by the empirical method: the verification of hypotheses by recourse to data accessible to our five senses. In the English-speaking tradition, empiricism is indissolubly associated with the experimental method. In the Continental tradition, other rigorous routes to scientific knowledge are recognized: in German, *natur wissenschaften* and *geistenwissenschaften*; in French, *la science de la nature* and *la science de l'humanité*. In medicine, we have recognized only one of these routes to valid knowledge, and this route has, to us, become synonymous with science. Medical scientists sometimes make a distinction between hard and soft data, usually implying a judgment about their relative value. To do this is to compare two categories of data that are not comparable. Data from natural science are about the world of the senses; data from human science are about meaning. Both types of data can be verified, but the means of verification are different.

The physical phenomena of the illness of a patient are all empirically verifiable. The mental phenomena, however—the thoughts and feelings, and personal perceptions—require a different form of inquiry. In European philosophy this is known as hermeneutic (*hermeneutike*, the art of interpretation) or phenomenological inquiry. In empirical inquiry, as it is commonly understood, the observer collects data with his or her five senses from an object, in this case a patient. Hermeneutic inquiry is intersubjective. One person, in this case a physician, reaches an understanding of another's thoughts, feelings, and sensations by entering into a dialogue in which the meaning of words and other symbols is progressively clarified. In an intersubjective inquiry, neither party is unchanged by the process. In this case, the patient may gain a deeper level of self-knowledge as well as a resolution of her existential crisis; the physician also may learn something about the human condition, and perhaps about herelf.

Knowledge attained by hermeneutics is intersubjective and is, therefore, not scientific in the conventional sense of the term. Yet it has its own canons of verification. In this case, verification depended on intersubjective agreement between doctor and patient. In other cases, verification may include more than two people. Another physician, for example, may verify a colleague's understanding of a patient's pain. The whole process of taking a history is hermeneutic, in that it seeks to understand a patient's sensations, perceptions, and feelings. Although in medicine we have followed the trend toward positivism, we have all the time, without acknowledging the fact, been relying on knowledge that can be obtained only by intersubjective agreement.

In the historical perspective, positivism can be viewed as a modern heresy. All the great religions and schools of philosophy are remarkably consistent about many things, including their teaching about levels of being. This distilled wisdom of the ages, called the *perennial philosophy* by Leibniz and others, recognizes a hierarchy of levels of existence. The simplest has three levels: the transcendental, the mental, and the physical. Whitehead (1926) maintained that if we wish to know the general principles of existence, we must start at the top and work down. Each higher level has capacities not found at lower levels. The higher cannot be derived from the lower. The characteristics of water cannot be predicted from the properties of hydrogen and oxygen. Biology cannot be fully explained in terms of physics, or psychology in terms of biology. Each higher level includes the lower levels, but transcends them.

Each level of being has its own level of knowing. To have knowledge at any of the levels, the understanding must be adequate to the thing known. "When the level of the knower is not adequate to the level of the object of knowledge," wrote Schumacher (1977, p. 42), "the result is not a factual error, but something much more serious: an inadequate and impoverished view of reality."

For the physical level, the way of knowing is sensory. As we well know, the simple use of the senses is not usually enough. Our perceptions have to be trained. In this way, the radiologist "sees" more in an X-ray film than a clinician; an ophthalmologist "sees" more in a retina than an internist. For the mental level, the way of knowing is symbolic. We understand another person's thoughts and feelings by interpreting symbols: words, gestures, movements, and expressions. Again, simple listening is not enough. Our inward ear has to be trained so that we can listen in the way described later in this chapter. And even this is not enough. How can we understand the inner life of another person? The perennial philosophy is clear on this: we can understand others only to the extent that we know ourselves. How could we understand what a patient means by pain unless we had experienced pain ourselves? Schumacher (1977, p. 83) wrote:

> A person who had never consciously experienced bodily pain, could not possibly know anything about the pain suffered by others. The outward signs of pain—sounds, movements, a flow of tears—would of course be noticed by him, but he would be totally inadequate to the task of understanding them correctly. No doubt he would attempt some kind of interpretation; he might find them funny or menacing or simply incomprehensible. The invisibilia of the other being—in this case his experience of pain—would remain invisible to him. . . . The example of bodily pain is instructive precisely because there is no subtlety about it. . . . Few people doubt the reality of pain, and the realization that here is a thing we all recognize as real, true, one of the great "stubborn facts" of our human existence, which nonetheless is unobservable by our outer senses, may come as a shock. If only that which can be observed by our outer senses is deemed to be real, "objective," scientifically respectable, pain must be dismissed as unreal, "subjective," unscientific. And the same applies to everything else which moves us internally: love and hatred, joy and sorrow, hope, fear, anguish and so on.

It is at the mental level that we understand the meaning of a person's experience and the values he lives by. It is at this level that we encounter the spiritual aspects of medicine, the things that give significance to a person's life.

For the transcendental, the way of knowing is contemplative and intuitive. Knowledge at this level is difficult to express in words and cannot be attained by the intellect alone. We know a person has attained it because it transforms the whole personality. This level of knowing also requires an understanding adequate to the level of being.

The kind of preparation that can give us both self-awareness and an insight into the inner lives of others cannot be a matter for the intellect alone. This kind of understanding comes from the heart. The first prerequisite is faith that there is a level of meaning beyond the reach of our senses. Without such faith, we are not likely to have the commitment to undertake the search for this understanding. The intellect and the heart are not—or should not be—in conflict. The understanding that comes from the heart can enrich the intellect, and the intellect can act on the heart's insights. Each form of understanding reflects a different kind of truth. For the intellect, truth is the truth of a proposition, to be established by logical argument. For the heart, truth is something that penetrates one's whole being and transforms one's life. The truth of a proposition can be accepted without having the slightest impact on the way we live. Limiting our understanding to the intellect alone gives us a shallow and impoverished vision of reality. Samuel T. Coleridge saw this happening even in his own day: "I have known some men who have been rationally educated as it is styled. They were marked by a microscopic acuteness, but when they looked at great things, all became blank and they saw nothing" Coleridge (1853, p. 609).

It follows, then, that medicine should include both knowledge derived from empirical science and knowledge derived from hermeneutics. Using Dr. Stetten's case as an example (see Chapter 7), it should include both a knowledge of vision and a knowledge of the experience of blindness. These two fields of knowledge are of a very different order. One is a knowledge of abstractions; the other is a knowledge of concrete experience as it is lived. Whitehead (1926, p. 197) criticized professional education for its concentration on abstractions, the result of which is people with minds in a groove:

> to be mentally in a groove is to live in contemplating a given set of abstractions. The groove prevents straying across country and the abstraction, abstracts from something to which no further attention is paid. But there is no groove of abstraction which is adequate for the comprehension of human life. Thus, in the modern world, the celibacy of the medieval learned class has been replaced by a celibacy of the intellect, which is divorced from the concrete contemplation of complete facts.

THE PLACE OF THE OBSERVER

One of the assumptions of positivism has been the separation of the observer from the observed and the subjective from the objective. Medicine has followed science in its view of the physician as a detached and uninvolved observer. In our clinical records, the history is often written under the heading of subjective and the physical examination under objective. What this implies is that the knowledge gained from these two modes of inquiry is of a different order: in the physical examination, knowledge of the bodily state comes from the physician's five senses without interpretation by the patient; in the history, knowledge comes from the patient's interpretation of his or her bodily sensations and feelings. These differences dissolve on analysis. The physical signs are not raw data; they are the physician's interpretations of his or her own sensations. Physicians do not feel the liver or hear pleural friction: they feel a resistance as they palpate the abdominal wall, or hear a sound in the chest that they interpret as pleural friction. Clinicians often disagree about physical signs, and postmortem findings often contradict the physical examination. The examination is also not without the patient's interpretation. The decision to remove the appendix may depend on the patient's "Yes, that hurts." The knowledge gained from the history is interpreted not only by the patient, but by the physician. The result is some sense of order that the clinician has given to the patient's story, an order that has a meaning in the context of a disease taxonomy.

The distinction between subjective and objective data is artificial because perception and interpretation always go together. Learning to be a skilled observer is a training in interpretation. Well-trained and experienced clinicians can achieve close agreements on their observations, so we call their findings objective. But the criterion of objectivity is intersubjective agreement by different observers: reproducible findings require observers who are skilled in the use of their senses and their instruments.

The separation of observation from interpretation was expressed by Newton's dictum: "hypotheses non fingo." Phenomena, he believed, should be described without prior hypotheses, by an observer who is neutral and detached. Newton's viewpoint has dominated Western thought, with a few dissenting voices, notably that of Johann Wolfgang von Goethe, who maintained that the observer, as part of nature, stood within the phenomena observed. Not until our own century, however, has there been a revolutionary change of view. The change has come in physics: according to quantum theory, the consciousness of the observer is essential to the observation; moreover, it is the act of observation that collapses the probability functions of quantum mechanics into actualities (Harman, 1994). So far, other fields of science have not followed physics in making this change. But when we look closely at the conduct of science, or think about our own experience in research, we find the person of the observer involved at every stage.

In his searching inquiry into the nature of scientific knowledge, Michael Polanyi (1962) rejects as false the ideal of scientific detachment. Scientific knowledge comes from the exercise of the knower's intellectual powers and his passionate participation in the act of knowing. "Personal Knowledge [is] manifested in the appreciation of probability and of order in the exact sciences ... and in the way the descriptive sciences rely on skills and connoisseurship. At all these points, the act of knowing includes an appraisal; and this personal co-efficient, which shapes all factual knowledge, bridges in doing so the disjunction between subjectivity and objectivity. It implies the claim that man can transcend his own subjectivity by striving passionately to fulfil his personal obligations to universal standards" (Polanyi 1962, p. 17).

Establishing contact with the reality hidden in nature involves the recognition of order. This comes, not from a study of separate parts, but from an intuition of how the parts are organized together in the whole. The observer does this by identifying with the phenomena. Piaget (1973) described this as a process by which the subject assimilates the object and accommodates to it. The higher the whole is in the systems hierarchy, and the greater its degree of complexity, the more involvement by the observer is required. It is this kind of involvement that is required by the Goldstein model. To attend to a patient's illness at all its levels, the physician must identify with the patient as a whole person with memories, emotions, interpretations, values, and intentions. To do this accurately, avoiding the many pitfalls, we have to attend to our own emotions, interpretations, and intentions. The physician is not only an observer of the patient, but a meta-observer of self and patient altogether.

The training of an observer in medicine or any other branch of science or technology is a training in the skills of attention, observation, and interpretation. What the new paradigm requires is that the physician becomes aware of himself or herself as an agent with the patient in bringing forth order and meaning from the patient's experience of illness: " . . . the individual in search of knowledge is locked in an embrace with the world. Out of this knowledge emerges a generated reality that bears the imprint of both natures involved in the process" (Goodwin, 1994, p. 215).

Although we should be prepared by self-reflection, in actual practice the self/other distinction between doctor and patient may almost disappear. The craftsman feeling at one with his material, the surgeon absorbed in an operation, the inhabitant's sense of connectedness with her own landscape, the intimacy between doctor and patient: all are familiar to us. By "dwelling in" an experience with our whole being, we gain what Polanyi (1962) calls "tacit knowledge": the embodied knowledge that cannot be fully articulated in words and concepts. The difference between theoretical and embodied knowledge—"knowing about" and "knowing"—can be appreciated by reflecting on the experience of using a new drug. Even though we have full information about the drug—its absorption, excretion, half-life, dosage range, and so on—we feel awkward in using it at first. It is not until we have experienced it in action with many patients—learned its nuances, its different effects on different people, the variations in its actions—do we then begin to use the drug as an extension of ourselves.

Broom invokes Husserl's concept of the life-world. "If we want to see the world more the way it is we need a radical change of attitude, when we turn from the objectified meaning of the sciences to meaning as immediately experienced in the *leberswelt* or 'life-world" (Kockelmans, 1999)" (Broom, 2007, p. 100)).

The notion of the life-world is very relevant to the "seeing" of meaningful disease. The life-world is the real, experienced, lived in world—a much richer world than that of mere objects, or that defined by the objective existence of things. The life-world *gives rise* to the scientific world, but it is much more than the world described by science (Broom, 2007).

The trouble is that we are so often blind to the patient's life-world: a world which, if we knew it, can explain the meaning of the disease that we have diagnosed—a meaning which perhaps reached far into the past, and which may hold the prospect of a therapy. We are blind because the paradigm that rules our medical schools does not believe such things exist.

Broom wrote:

> When I work with patients, with disease, I employ a phenomenological method continuously. Typically, I start with my attention on the "thing" of illness, the disease manifestation, and then I slide my attention seamlessly towards, the "meaning" of the same illness, whilst still holding them together in the same clinical time/space. Throughout the consultation I am moving seamlessly backwards and forwards, backwards and forwards, attending to the physical "object," disease aspect in one moment, and then attending to the subjective "meaning" aspect in another moment; in a zig zag way I am gradually building a picture of multifactorial, multidimensional emergence and perpetration of disease in this person in front of me. (Broom, 2007, p. 120)

The nature of this weaving back and forth has been described as well in the patient-centered method (Stewart, Brown, Weston, et al., 2014).

Broom's method is reminiscent of Balint's teaching, especially Balint's way of listening with total attention. There is, however, one big difference. Balint makes a clear distinction between patients with clear-cut diseases, and with neurotic illnesses; Broom seeks for meaning in all diseases.

Family physicians have the great advantage of knowing the life stories of many of their patients. When new illnesses make their appearance, our store of knowledge can be a starting point, with cues as to the meaning of the "new" illness. But we must not be too complacent: we may not know our patient as well as we think we do (Case 6.1).

ABSTRACTION AND EXPERIENCE (MAP AND TERRITORY)

The importance of abstraction in human understanding is illuminated by Alfred Korzybski's (1958) vivid metaphor of the map and the territory. We make a map by abstracting certain features from a territory and ignoring others. The features we abstract will depend on the purpose of the map: topographical, geological, ethnographic, and so on. To be useful, the map should have the same structure as the territory but, in the words of Korzybski's aphorism, "the map is not the territory." Knowing the map is not the same as knowing the territory. A native of the territory knows it by living in it and

---

CASE 6.1

I (IRMcW) had cared for an elderly couple for a number of years. The husband was disabled by a neurological illness that had progressed until he had great difficulty in walking. Intensive investigation had not resulted in a diagnosis. Also in the home was an elderly woman whom I used to see when making home visits. I understood that she was the wife's aunt.

   I used to see the husband and the aunt quite frequently, but the wife was in good health until one day she came to the surgery (office) complaining of persistent watery stools. Suspecting ulcerative colitis, I referred her to a surgeon who confirmed the diagnosis and his report came with a cryptic remark about the patient's aunt. When the patient came back to see me, she told me that she had suddenly discovered that the "aunt" was actually her mother. I already knew that the aunt owned the house and used this power to make their lives difficult, but of course I did not know her true relationship. Feeling somewhat humiliated, I asked her why she had told the specialist, but not me, her family doctor. "Well" she said, "when I was going to see the specialist my husband said: tell him everything." Is it not possible that the meaning of her illness was the life change she had undergone? At this stage of my career I did not give it a thought. Nor did I ask her how the news came to her, or how it had affected her.

---

identifying with it. The native is immersed in his landscape: his experience of it is sensuous, affective. Korzybski calls this experience a "first order abstraction." It does not distinguish between body and mind: the experience is one of immediate feelings and is ultimately indescribable—in Polanyi's (1962) terms, it is tacit knowledge. A word may be found for it, but "the word is not the thing." Once we have used a word, it becomes a second-order abstraction.

   The maps and schemas we have constructed have added enormously to our knowledge of the world. In medicine, we take people with similar illnesses and identify features that they have in common, while ignoring the many things they do not share. These collections of abstractions we call diseases, and our classification system is a map of the territory of illness experienced by our patients. The system greatly increases our knowledge by the power of generalization. Once we have correctly classified (diagnosed) the patient's illness (found our place on the map), we can make inferences about its course and outcome, its relationship to other illnesses, its response to treatment, and so on.

   The power of generalization increases with each degree of abstraction, the ultimate degree being a scientific law or mathematical formula. In medicine, some of our categories are low-level abstractions, such as the clusters of clinical observations we call syndromes. At the next level, other ways of describing the illness are added—pathological, biochemical, radiological— each one increasing the power of generalization. Names are given to each level of abstraction, and the language is also a map of the territory. The words in Table 6.2 stand for increasing degrees of abstraction from patients' original experience to the highest levels arising from "translation" of the illness into the languages of physical pathology and, finally, a diagnostic code.

The power of the abstraction depends on its having the same structure as the illness it represents—a feature exemplified by the case of multiple sclerosis. However, no abstraction is ever a complete picture of what it represents: it becomes less and less complete as the levels of abstraction and power of generalization increase. Every patient's illness is different in some way. As we increase the levels of abstraction, the differences are ironed out in the interests of increasing our power of generalization. And something very important is lost in the process. As we increase the levels of abstraction, the affective contribution to our understanding of the original experience becomes less and less. Abstraction distances us from experience. We cannot experience the beauty or the terror of a landscape by reading the map. Of course, one can get passionate about maps. There is a thrill in making a good diagnosis (finding our place on the map), and there can be beauty in a radiograph. But this is not the same as a feeling for the patient's experience of illness.

"The map is not the territory" seems like a statement of the obvious, yet we repeatedly fall into the trap of mistaking the abstraction for the experience it represents. We ask whether such and such a disease is an "entity," when what we really mean is, "Does the map have the same structure as reality?" Patients may be told, "the disease you think you have doesn't exist," and, by many subtle cues, they may feel that they are not believed. The doctor, perhaps unconsciously, feels that because the illness is not on his map, the patient is not ill.

Table 6.2. LEVELS OF ABSTRACTION IN A PATIENT WITH MULTIPLE,
FLUCTUATING, NEUROLOGICAL SYMPTOMS AND SIGNS

Level 1	Level 2	Level 3	Level 4	Level 5
Patient's sensation and emotions	Patient's expressed complaints, feelings, interpretations	Doctor's analysis of illness: clinical assessment	MRI scan	EMR
Preverbal	Second-order abstraction	Third-order abstraction	Fourth-order abstraction	Fifth-order abstraction
Illness	"Illness" (doctor's understanding)	"Disease" (clinical diagnosis: multiple sclerosis)	"Disease" (definitive diagnosis: MS)	ICD code-G35

It is often taught that a "disease" is the cause of a "syndrome," when these really are different levels of abstraction.[4] Western medicine often reverses the status of abstraction and experience: a patient's illness is not considered "real" until it has been put on the map. The opposite is true; diseases, like maps, are not "real"—they are mental constructs having the same structure as reality. Sometimes we find that our maps are wrong. Mitral valve prolapse, for example, should not have been on any map; the relationship we had mapped between symptoms and valve prolapse turned out not to correspond to relationships in the real world. Sometimes the map is correct, but we misread it. A patient's backache may be called osteoarthritis on the strength of X-ray changes that are normal for his age. Such spurious diagnoses can have serious consequences in delayed recovery and inappropriate management.

One of the features of family practice is intimacy arising from long-term patient–doctor relationships, so much so that family physicians often tend to think more in terms of individual patients than in terms of abstractions. Describing a series of interviews with general practitioners, Reid (1982, p. 325) noted that some "could not talk about general practice except in terms of their specific patients." Our experience does not allow us to forget the limitations of abstractions, even when we use them. Korzybski maintained that we should constantly remind ourselves of the uniqueness of each object. We need to remind ourselves that knowing the map is not the same thing as understanding the patient's illness experience—the first order, preverbal experience. Patients are very sensitive to the difference. The path to this understanding is not abstraction, but identification. This nonverbal identification with the patient may be the most important factor in healing. Identification engages all our cognitive powers, especially our feelings. Undifferentiated illness is illness that has not been through a process of abstraction by clinical assessment. The process of differentiation is one of increasing abstraction, and the level of abstraction reached depends on the extent to which the illness can be reduced to markers at the level of cells, molecules, and images. Much of the illness seen in family practice cannot be reduced in this way, and so, for much of the time, family physicians operate at lower levels of abstraction.

Because Western medicine and the modern paradigm of knowledge are heavily biased toward abstraction, we all tend to feel drawn away from the attempt to identify with the patient's experience. The biopsychosocial model is itself an abstraction; so is the system theory on which it is based. The model could be misconstrued simply as a call to interpret the patient's illness in terms of biological, psychological, and social science theory. When it comes to healing, abstractions can only get in the way. There comes a time when we have to set aside our maps and walk hand in hand with the patient through the territory.

NOTES

1. The word *paradigm* is now commonly used in many different contexts—so much so that it has lost much of its original meaning. Both molecular medicine and evidence-based medicine have been described as new paradigms (Robert Wood Johnson Commission, 1992; Glass, 1996), when, in Kuhn's terms, they are no more than developments within an existing paradigm.
2. Kuhn had a precursor in Ludwig Fleck, a Polish physician and scientist, who, in 1935 published a book in German, later to be translated into English as *The Genesis and Development of a Scientific Fact* (1979). At the time when the book was written, the idea that facts could have a natural history, and could go through a process of social conditioning, was so unfamiliar as to pass unnoticed. Fleck's book is of particular interest to us because he uses the discovery of the Wassermann reaction to illustrate his thesis.
3. For a fuller discussion of these implications, see McWhinney, IR. The importance of being different, *British Journal of General Practice* (1996), 46:433–436; McWhinney IR, Epstein RM, Freeman T, Rethinking somatization, *Annals of Internal Medicine* (1997), 126(9):747; and McWhinney IR, Epstein RM, Feeman T, Rethinking somatization, *Advances in Mind-Body Medicine* (2001), 17(4):232.
4. When a condition previously described as a syndrome is redefined as a disease by the inclusion of a specific pathology, the symptoms and signs that defined the syndrome become part of the new definition. The new category is symptoms and signs plus the pathology. Without the clinical features, the pathology would have no clinical significance. To say that the disease is the cause of the syndrome is tantamount to saying that the category is the cause of itself—the equivalent of saying that lions are the cause of quadripeds.

REFERENCES

Ader R, Cohen N. 1991. The influence of conditioning on immune responses. In: Ader R, Felton DL, Cohen N, eds., *Psychoneuroimmunology*. San Diego, CA: Academic Press.

Afifi TO, MacMillan HL, Boyule M, et al. 2014. Child abuse and mental disorders in Canada. *Canadian Medical Association Journal* 186: e675.

Antonovsky A. 1979. *Health, Stress and Coping*. San Francisco, CA: Jossey-Bass.

Bass MJ, Buck C, Turner L, et al. 1986. The physician's actions and the outcome of illness in family practice. *Journal of Family Practice* 23:43–47.

Bellinger DL, Madden KS, Felten SY, Felten DL. 1994. Neural and endocrine links between the brain and the immune system. In: Lewis CE, O'Sullivan C, Barroclough J, eds., *The Psychoimmunology of Cancer: Mind and Body in the Fight for Survival*. New York: Oxford University Press.

Berkman LF. 1995. The role of social relations in health promotion. *Psychosomatic Medicine* 57:245.

Berkman LF, Breslow L. 1983. *Health and Ways of Living: The Alameda County Study*. New York: Oxford University Press.

Besedovsky HO, Sorkin E. 1981. Immunologic-neuroendocrine circuits: Physiological approaches. In: Ader R, ed., *Psychoneuroimmunology*. New York: Academic Press.

Blacklock SM. 1977. The symptom of chest pain in family practice. *Journal of Family Practice* 4:429.

Briggs J, Peat DF. 1989. *Turbulent Mirror: An Illustrated Guide to Chaos Theory and the Science of Wholeness*. New York: Harper & Row.

Brody H. 1980. *Placebos and the Philosophy of Medicine*. Chicago: Chicago University Press.

Broom B. 2007. *MEANING-full DISEASE. How personal experience and meanings cause and maintain physical illness*. London: Karnac Books.

Cannon WB. 1932. *The Wisdom of the Body*. New York: W. W. Norton.

Cassel J. 1976. The contribution of the social environment to host resistance. *American Journal of Epidemiology* 104:107.

Classen C, Hermanson KS, Spiegel D. 1994. Psychotherapy, stress, and survival in breast cancer. In: Lewis CE, O'Sullivan C, Barroclough J, eds., *The Psychoimmunology of Cancer: Mind and Body in the Fight for Survival*. New York: Oxford University Press.

Clinicopathological Conference. 1968. A case of adult coeliac disease resistant to treatment. *British Medical Journal* 1:678.

Cobb S. 1976. Social support as a moderator of life stress. *Psychosomatic Medicine* 38:300.

Cobb S, Kasl SV. 1977. *Termination: The Consequence of Job Loss*. Washington, DC: US Department of Health Education and Welfare.

Coker S, Tyrell DAJ, Smith AP. 1991. Psychological stress and susceptibility to the common cold. *New England Journal of Medicine* 32:606.

Coleridge ST. 1853. *Biographia Literaria; or, Biographical Sketches of My Literary Life and Opinions*. New York: Harper.

Crookshank FG. 1926. The theory of diagnosis. *Lancet* 1:939.

Cunningham A, Edmonds C. 2005. Possible effects of psychological therapy on survival duration in cancer patients. *Journal of Clinical Oncology* 23(22):5263.

Dohrenwend BS, Dohrenwend BP (eds.). 1974. *Stressful Life Events: Their Nature and Effects*. New York: John Wiley.

Dreher H. 2003. *Mind-Body Unity: A New Vision for Mind-Body Science and Medicine*. Baltimore, MD; London: The Johns Hopkins University Press.

Dubos R. 1965. *Man Adapting*. New Haven, CT: Yale University Press.

Engel CL. 1980. The clinical application of the biopsychosocial model. *American Journal of Psychiatry* 137:535.

Fagundes CP, Bennett JM, Derry HM, Kiecolt-Glaser JK. 2011. Relationships and inflammation across the lifespan: Social developmental pathways to disease. *Social and Personality Psychology Compass* 5(11):891–903.

Felten SY, Felten DL. 1991. Innervation of lymphoid tissue. In: Ader R, Felton DL, Cohen N, eds., *Psychoneuroimmunology*. San Diego, CA: Academic Press.

Fleck L. 1979. *The Genesis and Development of a Scientific Fact*. Chicago: University of Chicago Press.

Foss L, Rothenberg K. 1987. *The Second Medical Revolution: From Biomedicine to Infomedicine*. Boston, MA: New Science Library, Shambhala.

Foss L. 1994. The biomedical paradigm, psychoneuroimmunology, and the black four of hearts. *Advances* 10(1):32.

Gillies JCM 2005. Getting it right in the consultation: Hippocrates; problem; Aristotle's answer. Occasional Paper 86, Royal College of General Practitioners.

Glass RM. 1996. The patient–physician relationship: JAMA focuses on the center of medicine. *Journal of the American Medical Association* 275:147.

Goldstein K. 1995. *The Organism: A Holistic Approach to Biology Derived from Pathological Data in Man*. New York: Zone Books.

Goodwin BC. 1994. Toward a science of qualities. In: Harman W, Clark J, eds., *New Metaphysical Foundations of Modern Science*. Sausalito, CA: Institute of Noetic Sciences.

Goodwin PJ, Leszcz M, Ennis M, et al. 2001. The effect of group psychosocial support on survival in metastatic breast cancer. *New England Journal of Medicine* 345(24):1719.

Gore S. 1978. The effect of social support in moderating the health consequences of unemployment. *Journal of Health and Social Behavior* 19:157.

Gorovitz S, MacIntyre A. 1976. Toward a theory of medical fallibility. *Journal of Medical Philosophy* 1:51.

Guess HA, Kleinman A, Kusek JW, Engel LW (eds.). 2002. *The Science of the Placebo: Toward an Interdisciplinary Research Agenda*. London: BMJ Books.

Hall H, Minnes L, Olness K. 1993. The psychophysiology of voluntary immunomodulation. *International Journal of Neuroscience* 69:221.

Harman W. 1994. A re-examination of the metaphysical foundations of modern science: Why is it necessary? In: Harman W, Clark J, eds., *New Metaphysical Foundations of Modern Science*. Sausalito, CA: Institute of Noetic Sciences.

Headache Study Group of the University of Western Ontario. 1986. Predictors of outcome in headache patients presenting to family physicians: A one year prospective study. *Headache* 26:285.

Helsing KJ, Szklo M, Comstock GW. 1981. Factors associated with mortality after widowhood. *American Journal of Public Health* 71(8):802.

Hinkle LE. 1974. The effect of exposure to culture change and changes in interpersonal relationships in health. In: Dohrenwend BS, Dohrenwend BP, eds., *Stressful Life Events: Their Nature and Effects*. New York: John Wiley.

Holmes TH, Rahe RH. 1967. The social readjustment rating scale. *Journal of Psychosomatic Research* 11:213.

Jackson JL, Passamonti M. 2005. The outcomes among patients presenting in primary care with a physical symptom at 5 years. *Journal of General Internal Medicine* 20(11):1032–1037.

Jemmott JB, Locke SE. 1984. Psychological factors, immunologic mediation and human susceptibility to infectious diseases: How much do we know? *Psychological Bulletin* 95:78.

Jin RL, Shah CP, Svoboda TJ. 1995. The impact of unemployment on health: A review of the evidence. *Canadian Medical Association Journal* 153:529.

Khan AA, Khan A, Harezlak J, et al. 2003. Somatic symptoms in primary care: Etiology and outcome. *Psychosomatics* 44(6):471–478.

Kiecolt-Glaser JK, Dura JR, Speicher CE, et al. 1991. Spousal caregivers of dementia victims: Longitudinal changes in immunity and health. *Psychosomatic Medicine* 53(4):345.

Kiecolt-Glaser JK, Glaser R. 1995. Psychoneuroimmunology and health consequences: Data and shared mechanisms. *Psychosomatic Medicine* 57:269.

Kiecolt-Glaser JK., McGuire L, Robles TF, Glaser R. 2002a. Psychoneuroimmunology and psychosomatic medicine: Back to the future. *Psychosomatic Medicine* 64(1):15.

Kiecolt-Glaser JK, McGuire L, Robles TF, Glaser R. 2002b. Psychoneuroimmunology: Psychological influences on immune function and health. *Journal of Consulting and Clinical Psychology* 70(3):537–547.

Kiecolt-Glaser JK, McGuire L, Robles TF, Glaser R. 2002c. Emotions, morbidity, and mortality: New perspectives from psychoneuroimmunology. *Annual Review of Psychology* 53:83–107.

Kiecolt-Glaser JK, Gouin J-P, Hantsoo L. 2010. Close relationships, inflammation, and health. *Neuroscience and Biobehavioral Reviews* 35(1):33–38.

Kissane DW, Love A, Hatton A, et al. 2004. Effect of cognitive-existential group therapy on survival in early-stage breast cancer. *Journal of Clinical Oncology* 22(21):4255–4260.

Kockelmans JJ. 1999. Phenomenology. In: Audi, R. (ed.) *The Cambridge Dictionary of Philosophy*, 2nd ed. Cambridge: Cambridge University Press.

Koestler A. 1979. *Janus: A Summing Up*. London: Picador.

Korzybski A. 1958. *Science and Sanity: An Introduction to Non-Aristotelian Systems and General Semantics*, 4th ed. Lake Bille, CT: International Non-Aristotelian Library.

Kuhn TS. 1967. *The Structure of Scientific Revolutions*. Chicago: University of Chicago Press.

Langer SK. 1979. *Philosophy in a New Key*. Cambridge, MA: Harvard University Press.

McEwen BS, Norton E. 2002. *The End of Stress as We Know It*. Washington, DC: National Academies Press.

McFarlane WR. 1992. Psychoeducation: A potential model for intervention in family practice. In: Sawa RJ (ed.). *Family Health Care*. Newbury Park, CA: Sage.

Medalie JH, Goldbourt U. 1976. Some epidemiologic aspects of the high mortality rate in the young widowed group. *Journal of Chronic Disease* 10:207.

Moerman DE. 1983. General medical effectiveness and human biology: Placebo effects in the treatment of ulcer disease. *Medical Anthropology Quarterly* 14:3.

Nuckolls KB, Cassel JC, Kaplan BH. 1972. Psychosocial assets, life crisis and the prognosis of pregnancy. *American Journal of Epidemiology* 95:431.

Olness K, Ader R. 1992. Conditioning as an adjunct in the pharmacotherapy of lupus erythematosus. *Developmental and Behavioral Pediatrics* 13:124.

Olness K, MacDonald JT, Uden DL. 1987. Comparison of self-hypnosis and propranolol in the treatment of juvenile classical migraine. *Pediatrics* 79:593.

Peck C, Coleman G. 1991. Implications of placebo theory for clinical research and practice in pain management. *Theoretical Medicine* 12:247.

Piaget J. 1973. *The Child and Reality*. New York: Grossman.

Polanyi M. 1962. *Personal Knowledge: Towards a Post-critical Philosophy*. Chicago: University of Chicago Press.

Rana J, Mannam A, Donnel-Fink L, et al. 2005. Longevity of the placebo effect in the therapeutic angiogenesis and laser myocardial revasculatization trials in patients with coronary heart disease. *American Journal of Cardiology* 95:1456–1459.

Reid M. 1982. Marginal man: The identity dilemma of the academic general practitioner. *Symbolic Interaction* 5(2):325.

Riley V, Fitzmaurice MA, Spackman DA. 1981. Psychoneuroimmunologic factors in neoplasia: Studies in animals. In: Ader R, ed., *Psychoneuroimmunology*. New York: Academic Press.

Robert Wood Johnson Commission Report on Medical Education. 1992. *JAMA* 268(9):1144–1145.

Ruberman W, Weinblatt E, Goldberg JD, et al. 1984. Psychological influences on mortality after myocardial infarction. *New England Journal of Medicine* 311:552.

Rudebeck CE. 1992. General practice and the dialogue of clinical practice. *Scandinavian Journal of Primary Care* Supplement 1.

Scheier MF, Bridges MW. 1995. Person variables and health: Personality predispositions and acute psychological states as shared determinants for disease. *Psychosomatic Medicine* 57:255.

Schumacher EF. 1977. *A Guide for the Perplexed*. New York: Harper and Row.

Selye H. 1956. *The Stress of Life*. New York: McGraw-Hill.

Siegler IC, Costa PT, Brummett BH, et al. 2003. Patterns of change in hostility from college to midlife in the UNC alumni heart study predict high-risk status. *Psychosomatic Medicine* 65(5):738–745.

Stewart M, Brown JB, Weston WW, et al. 2014. *Patient-Centered Medicine: Transforming the Clinical Method*, 3rd ed. Oxford: Radcliffe Medical Press.

Toombs SK. 1995. *The Meaning of Illness: A Phenomenological Account of the Different Perspectives of Physician and Patient*. Dordrecht: Kluwer.

Turner RJ. 1983. Direct, indirect and moderating of social support on psychological distress and associated conditions. In: Kaplan HB, ed., *Psychological Stress*. New York: Academic Press.

Turner RJ, Wheaton B, Lloyd DA. 1995. The epidemiology of social stress. *American Sociological Review* 60:104.

Von Bertallanfy L. 1968. *General System Theory*. New York: George Braziller.

von Uexküll T, Geigges W, Herrmann JM. 1993. A fresh look at the immune system: The principle of teleological coherence and harmony of purpose exists at every level of integration in the hierarchy of living systems. *Advances* 9(3):50.

Wartolowska K, Judge A, Hopewell S, et al. 2014. Use of placebo controls in the evaluation of surgery: Systematic review. *BMJ* 2014;348:g3253. doi: 10.1136/bmj.g3253.

Wasson JH, Sox HC, Sox CH. 1981. The diagnosis of abdominal pain in ambulatory male patients. *Medical Decision Making* 1:215.

Whitehead AN. 1926. *Science and the Modern World*. Cambridge: Cambridge University Press.

Yates FE. 1993. Self-organizing systems. In: Boyd CAR, Noble D, eds., *The Logic of Life: The Challenge of Integrative Physiology*. New York: Oxford University Press.

Zucker A. 1981. Holism and reductionism: A view from genetics. *Journal of Medicine and Philosophy* 6:2.

CHAPTER 7

✧

Illness, Suffering, and Healing

The central tasks of a physician's life are understanding illness and understanding people. Because one cannot fully understand an illness without also understanding the person who is ill, these two tasks are indivisible. One approach to the understanding of illness is through the application of our knowledge of science and technology. This will give us an understanding of the illness on one level, but it will not enable us to understand the patient as a person, with unique life story, feelings, values, and relationships. Nor will it help us to understand the deeper meaning the illness may have for him or her. Science, as seen in Chapter 6, gives us a knowledge of abstractions. These abstractions are very powerful. They enable us to make the precise inferences and predictions on which the technology of medicine is based. But they do so by ignoring and excluding the concrete experience of illness as lived through by the patient. In Richard Baron's words (1985), "a great gulf now exists between the way we think about disease as physicians and the way we experience it as patients."

The grip that abstraction has on modern medicine is, we believe, at the root of one of the paradoxes of the patient–doctor relationship. At a time when medicine has never been more technologically successful, physicians have never been more criticized and attacked. In the past three decades there has been a remarkable increase in the number of books and articles describing personal experiences of illness. These writings, by patients themselves or by their relatives, are often bitterly critical of physicians. They are uncomfortable for us to read, and it is tempting to become defensive or to dismiss the writers as complainers. It is important, however, that we pay attention to what they say. They tell us something about the state of medicine and, if we do not regard the criticisms as applying only to others, they can teach us something about ourselves.

Arthur Frank (1991) developed testicular cancer at the age of 40. "I always assumed," writes Frank,

> that if I became seriously ill, physicians, no matter how overworked, would somehow recognize what I was living through. I did not know what form this recognition would take, but I assumed it would happen. What I experienced was the opposite. The more critical my diagnosis became, the more reluctant physicians were to talk to me. I had trouble getting them to make eye contact; most came only to see my disease. This "it" within the body was their field of investigation; "I" seemed to exist beyond the horizon of their interest (p. 54). . . . After five years of dealing with medical professionals in the context of critical illness, as opposed to the routine problems I had had before, I have accepted their limits, even if I have never become comfortable with them. Perhaps medicine should reform itself and learn to share illness talk with patients instead of imposing disease talk on them. Or perhaps physicians and nurses should simply do what they already do well—treat the breakdowns—and not claim to do more (Frank, 1991, p. 14).

The novelist Reynolds Price (1994), writing of his experience with a spinal cord tumor and subsequent paraplegia and chronic pain, has good words for his surgeon but says this about his encounters with other doctors:

> . . . surely a doctor should be expected to share—and to offer at all appropriate hours—the skill we expect of a teacher, a fireman, a priest, a cop, the neighborhood milkman or the dog-pound manager.
>
> These are merely the skills of human sympathy, the skills for letting another creature know that his or her concern is honored and valued and that, whether a cure is likely or not, all possible efforts will be expended to achieve that aim or to ease incurable agony toward its welcome end. Such skills are not rare in the natural world. What else but the urge to use and perfect such skills on other human beings in need could drive a man or woman into medicine? What but massive failure to recognize one's stunted emotions before they blunder against live tissue—that and an avid taste for money and power? And having blundered on other creatures, how can the blunderer not attempt to change? Is he or she legally blind as well? Maybe we have the right to demand that such a flawed practitioner display a warning on the office door or the starched lab coat, like those on other dangerous bets—*Expert technician. Expect no more. The quality of your life and death are your concern* (Price, 1994, p. 145).

When Price was referred to a pain clinic for his chronic neurologic pain, the physicians there did not even mention therapies for pain that were available on another floor of the same building. Eventually, 2 years later, Price found that two of these—biofeedback and hypnosis—helped more than anything else to make his pain tolerable.

Some of the most revealing accounts of illness have come from physicians who have become patients. Dr. DeWitt Stetten (1981) wrote of his experience with progressive loss of vision caused by macular degeneration:

> Through all these years and despite many encounters with skilled and experienced professionals, no ophthalmologist has at any time suggested any devices that might be of assistance to me. No ophthalmologist has mentioned any of the many ways in which I could stem the deterioration in the quality of my life. Fortunately, I have discovered a number of means whereby I have helped myself, and the purpose of this essay is to call the attention of the ophthalmological world to some of these devices and, courteously but firmly, to complain of what appears to be the ophthalmologist's attitude: "We are interested in vision but have little interest in blindness." (Stetten, 1981, p. 458)

What we see in Dr. Stetten's physicians, I think, is an extreme literal-mindedness: a poverty of feeling that renders them incapable of recognizing the suffering of a person going through this devastating disruption of his "life-world," and a lack of that imaginative power that might have given them some sense of it. To these ophthalmologists, it appears, macular degeneration is a condition of the retina, not a human experience. The fault, moreover, is not unique to ophthalmologists. We are all guilty, family physicians included. In his attempts to compensate for his disorientation in space and time, Stetten learned about a machine that projects enormously magnified printed material onto a television monitor, the Talking Books Program, the Talking Clock, and a reading machine that converts the printed word to synthesized speech. In no instance did his information come from ophthalmologists.

Modern physicians have not been trained to understand illness as a human experience. In our formal education, we live mainly in a world of abstractions. Medical knowledge is defined implicitly as a knowledge of diseases. Macular degeneration is part of medical knowledge, but the experience of going blind is not. The boundaries drawn between specialties reflect this tacit definition of medical knowledge. The patient's adaptation to illness and disability may be defined as "rehabilitation," and therefore the concern of a different specialist or another profession. Patients often find such rigid boundaries difficult to understand. Even though some differentiation of function is inevitable, we need to be alive to the ways in which too rigid a drawing of boundaries can impair our capacity as healers. Because family medicine is defined in terms of relationships, we have no need to feel restricted by the way medicine is subdivided. The resources of the specialties can be used without relinquishing our healing role.

How can we teach ourselves to understand the experience of our patients? We can learn, first of all, by paying attention to their experience, by practicing the very difficult art of listening, by reading the appropriate literature, and by reflecting on our own experience.

Autobiographies and biographies that describe experiences of illness—now known as pathographies (Hawkins, 1993)—provide us with rich opportunities for deepening our knowledge and understanding. Although—like the ones we have quoted—they are sometimes critical of physicians, they are often profound meditations on illness and healing. Some are works of literature in their own right. Book-length pathographies are a recent phenomenon. Before 1950 they were rare; now there are many. Besides the books, there have also been numerous articles in magazines and medical journals. Why this abrupt appearance of a new literary genre? Hawkins (1993) sees it as a possible reaction to a medicine "so dominated by a biophysical understanding of illness that its experiential aspects are virtually ignored." (Hawkins, 1993, p. 11). She describes three groups of pathographies: testimonial, angry, and those advocating alternative therapies. Testimonial pathographies, mostly from the 1960s and 1970s, are didactic in intent, "blending a personal account of illness with practical information." In the 1980s these mainly uncritical accounts give place to those expressing anger at "a medical system seen as out of control, dehumanized, and sometimes brutalizing." (Hawkins, 1993, p. 4). According to Hawkins, two themes recur in these stories: "the tendency in contemporary medical practice to focus primarily not on the needs of the individual who is sick but on the nomothetic condition we call the disease, and the sense that our medical technology has advanced beyond our capacity to use it wisely" (Hawkins, 1993, p. 6). The third group, also a feature of the 1980s, is less critical of physicians, but treats orthodox medicine as only one of a large number of therapies available to sufferers.

To these three groups we would add another: books written by philosophers, anthropologists, physicians, and literary critics, who bring a professional interest and expertise to bear on the subject of illness narratives. Hawkins's book is one of these.

Some of these writers bring their professional expertise to bear on their own illness. Kay Toombs (1992) writes on the meaning of illness as a philosopher and sufferer from multiple sclerosis. Oliver Sacks (1984) brings his knowledge as a neurologist and medical theorist to bear on his own experience of illness.

Hawkins views pathography as "a re-formulation of the experience of illness," using formulation in Robert Lifton's (1967) sense of a restorative process. Like the authors of pathographies, Lifton is writing about a devastating experience: survival of the atomic attack on Hiroshima. Hawkins remarks (Hawkins, 1993, p. 24):

> [T]he act of formulation . . . involves the discovery of patterns in experience, the imposition of order, the creation of meaning—all with the purpose of mastering

a traumatic experience and thereby re-establishing a sense of connectedness with objective reality and with other people.

Note that what these reformulations provide—the sense of coherence, the feeling of mastery, the creation of meaning—are also the elements of a healing relationship. A pathography can be healing for its author and for its readers; it can also help physicians to be healers for their patients, to act as their guides through terrifying and devastating experiences. The message to us from many pathographies is that we have almost forgotten what it is to be a healer.

Perhaps because the patients' voice has been denied for so long, there has occurred many more venues for them to be heard. Illness blogs are common on the Internet; the *New York Times* regularly publishes a section entitled *Patient Voices*, and there is now *Patient Experience Journal* (http://pxjournal. org/journal/). All of these can help, to some extent, inform physicians about how their patients' lives are affected by illness, but none is a substitute for simple inquiry and active listening.

It is not easy for us to attend to our patients' experience. To do so requires us to step out of our usual way of attending to a person's illness. We are trained to see illness as a set of signs and symptoms defining a disease state as a case of diabetes or peptic ulcer or schizophrenia. The patient, on the other hand, sees illness in terms of its effects on his or her life. The physician, therefore, must learn to see illness as it is lived through, before it has been categorized and interpreted in scientific terms. Although every illness is different in some way because everybody's life story is different, there are certain common features of illness as a lived experience (Toombs, 1992).

THE PATIENT'S EXPERIENCE OF ILLNESS

A healthy person takes his or her body for granted. It does, of course, impose limitations on what he or she can do, but the person does not have to bring into consciousness the everyday acts of living. Writing this, one is not conscious of the movement of the hands. The sick, however, become very much aware of the body and the limitations it imposes. They have to think about activities that previously were carried out below the level of awareness. Will I manage this flight of stairs? Will I be able to get on the bus to do my shopping? Bodily functions, which previously formed the background to one's world, become the foreground; the rest of world recedes into the background. In health, the body and the self are one: we are *our* bodies. In sickness, the body becomes something other than the self, something alien, over which the self has limited control. At times, there is a sense that the damaged body has betrayed the person and is no longer to be trusted.

Physicians see illness in terms of a disturbance of bodily function. Patients see it as a disruption of their "being in the world."

> Critical illness leaves no aspect of life untouched. The hospitals and other special places we have constructed for critically ill persons have created the illusion that by sealing off the ill person from those who are healthy, we can also seal off the illness in that ill person's life. This illusion is dangerous. Your relationships, your work, your sense of who you are and who you might become, your sense of what life is and ought to be—these all change, and the change is terrifying. (Frank, 1991, p. 6)

In Kay Toombs's words, "A patient does not so much have an illness as exist an illness." She takes to the physician a problem of existence but finds the physician's attention directed to her body rather than to her problems with existence. The patient feels "reduced to a malfunctioning biological organism" (Toombs, 1992).

Chronic disease, especially if it brings successive losses of independence and control, often engenders profound sensations of grief. With grief come the feelings associated with it: sadness and anger, guilt and remorse. If the illness is one that carries a stigma—such as schizophrenia, epilepsy, cancer, or AIDS—then feelings of rejection may add to the grief. Anger may be projected onto the physician, who may be viewed as responsible for delays in diagnosis or errors in management. Given the insidious nature of many chronic illnesses and the difficulties of early diagnosis, family physicians are especially liable to encounter this level of hostility. When the patient feels responsible for causing his or her own disease, the anger is turned inward. Those physicians who would like to convince people that they are responsible for their own healing should consider the consequences in guilt and remorse if their efforts do not improve their health or prevent deterioration.

Fear and anxiety are ever-present in illness, even in minor illness. Fears are many and varied, rational and irrational. Physicians cannot assume that they know what patients' fears are until they make an effort to discover them. A patient may have come to terms with the fact that she has progressive cancer but may still fear that her death will be painful and distressing. Or she may fear for the future of her family. Dying patients may have a fear that they will be abandoned by their doctor if they complain too much. They then become reluctant to ask for a visit when they need one, and tolerate pain that could be controlled. This is why regular visits, rather than "on request," are so important for dying patients.

A number of physicians, most recently Eric Cassell (1990, 2013), have observed that illness may impair the faculty of reason. The most rational of people may become irrational, and even superstitious. This impairment of judgment is rarely considered when we are enjoined to give patients responsibility for decisions about their treatment. As an ethical principle, this is no doubt correct. In real life the issue is rarely so clearly defined.

The threats to self that illness brings—the disruption, loss of autonomy, loss of control, and loss of confidence—make sick persons very vulnerable. They not only feel vulnerable, they *are* vulnerable. This vulnerability makes it impossible for the relationship between the doctor and the sick patient to be an equal one, however much we may wish it to be so. This puts a great responsibility on physicians to respect patients' vulnerability and to use their power responsibly and with compassion.

Kay Toombs has commented on the changed sense of time and space that illness induces. The natural rhythms of the body—the rhythms of eating, sleeping, working, resting—are disturbed. The patient loses the sense of the future as a time of possibilities. Simple tasks like dressing and tying shoelaces may occupy a large part of the day. Hull (1992, p. 60) says of his experience as a blind person:

> Sighted people can bend time. For sighted people, time is sometimes slow and sometimes rapid. They can make up for being lazy by rushing later on. . . . For me, as a blind person, time is simply the medium of my activities. It is the inexorable context within which I do what must be done. For example, the reason why I do not seem to be in a hurry as I go around the building is not that I have less to do than my colleagues, but I am simply unable to hurry.

"Perhaps all severe disabilities," says Hull, "lead to a decrease in space and an increase in time" (p. 60). Toombs (1992, p. 67) remarks on how illness changes the character of one's sense of space. " . . . [O]bjects or locations [the bathroom, for example] which were formerly regarded as 'near' are now experienced as 'far.' . . . Spaciality . . . constricts in the sense that the range of possible actions becomes severely circumscribed. Rather than representing the arena of possible action, space is encountered as the restriction of possibilities."

Toombs (1992) writes of the "profound effects of the loss of upright posture" (p. 65). A person in a wheelchair at a social gathering, being low on the ground, may be treated like a child, in that people talk to their spouse about them, as if they were not able to speak for themselves.

In mental illness, the threat to the self is terrifying. The experience of dementia, depression, schizophrenia, or anxiety may produce the most intense suffering. The experience is not limited to those with severe mental illness. It is often surprising to find that patients who are mildly depressed will express fears of insanity.

An account of the experience of illness would not be complete without mention of the response to illness. People do triumph over their disabilities. The body has remarkable powers of compensation and adaptation. A newly defined self can emerge from suffering. Suffering engenders the kind of introspection that can add a new depth to the personality. Although the patient may have little control over the course of the illness, he or she is free to choose how to respond to it.

So far, we have been considering the experience of illness and disability in a person who was previously healthy. The process is one of alienation of the body from the self. The situation is different in those who are born with a disability. In these, the disabled body is the lived body, from the very beginning. Rather than the body becoming alien to the self, the body, with its disabilities, is the self. With some disabilities such as deafness, the person enters a culture with a strong sense of its place in the world (Sacks, 1989). A child may resist a parent's attempts to correct some disability on the grounds that if they corrected it, "it wouldn't be me." Rejection of the disability may be interpreted as rejection of the child. On the other hand, for those with acquired hearing loss, the disability is seen as alien to the individual's identity and something to which one must adapt (Shea, 2013). Harm may be done by attempts to correct "disabilities" that are themselves harmless variants. At one time, left-handed children were forced to use their right hands. Attempts to change those with a sexual orientation that differs from the majority, or to force those experiencing gender dysphoria to not change, are fraught with danger and suffering. When a child has severe disability that can be corrected, the process of adaptation is the reverse of that in a person with an acquired disability. The child, whose body and self have grown within their limitations, has to develop a different way of "being in the world"—a world with wider horizons.

Although all sufferers from chronic disease and disability have something in common, each patient's story is an individual one. The experience of illness also varies with the course the illness takes: a sudden or gradual onset; a one-time disability like stroke or injury, which then remains static; a progressively downhill course; or a process of remissions and relapses. Loss of vision, for example, is often a very long process ending in the state of blindness—a new way of being in the world. John Hull (1992) a university professor, describes his own experience:

> First, there was a period of hope that lasted for a year or 18 months. It was brought to an end by the deterioration of sight during the summer of 1981, although even as late as the summer of 1982, when I was still seeing a few lights, colours and shapes, I could not resist occasional flickers of hope.

> Secondly, there was a period of busyness in overcoming the problems. This began about the summer of 1981, when visual work became impossible, and lasted until about the summer of 1984. It was not until Easter of 1985 that I began to have a feeling that I did not need any more equipment. A main drive to create a workable office system took place during 1982 and 1983. During this time, blindness was a challenge.

The third stage began some time in 1983, possibly late in the year, and lasted for about a year. This was the time when I passed through despair. These were the years during which my sleep was punctuated by terrible dreams, and my waking life was oppressed by awareness of being carried irresistibly deeper and deeper into blindness.

The fourth and current period has begun since the autumn of 1984, i.e., since the recovery from the visit to Australia, during which time blindness had engulfed me. I began writing my book on adult religious education in October of 1984 and concluded it in March of 1985.

For most of the time now my brain no longer hurts with the pain of blindness. There has been a strange change in the state or the kind of activity in my brain. It seems to have turned in upon itself to find inner resources. Being denied the stimulus of much of the outside world, it has had to sort out its own functions and priorities. I now feel clearer, more excited and more adventurous intellectually than ever before in my life. I find myself connecting more, remembering more, making more links in my mind between various things I have read and had to learn over the years. Sometimes I come home in the evening and feel that my mind is almost bursting with new ideas and new horizons.

I continue to find deep need for that kind of sustenance. Even a single day without study, away from the possibility of learning something new, can precipitate a new sense of urgency and suffering. I still feel like a person on a kidney machine, but increasingly like a person who has managed to survive.[1] (pp. 139–140).

Primacy of the person has been mentioned as one of the fundamental principles of family medicine. To give primacy to the personhood of the patient requires that we attend very carefully to the meaning the illness has for him or her, not as an "add-on" after clinical diagnosis but as a central obligation. This has implications for our clinical method, which is discussed in Chapter 9.

SUFFERING

Eric Cassell (2013, p. 61) recognizes three aspects of suffering. First, suffering involves the whole person and "requires a rejection of the historic dualism of mind and body." Second, people suffer when threatened by distress, which can cause them serious harm. Third, "suffering can occur in relation to any aspect of the person."

Arthur Kleinman (Kleinman and Kleinman, 1997) adds that a suffering person not only perceives a threat, but also must resist it. Also, that suffering has a social dimension "that undergoes great cultural elaboration in distinctive local worlds." Frank regards telling stories as a form of resistance: "people tell uniquely personal stories, but they neither make these stories by themselves, nor do they tell them only to themselves. Stories of suffering have two sides: one expresses the threat of disintegration, the other the emphasis on resistance" (1997, p. 171). What Frank calls the quest narrative "recognizes that the old intactness must be stripped away to prepare for something new. Quest stories reflect a confidence in what is waiting to emerge from suffering."

The suffering of the woman in Case 7.1 was inevitably of the first kind, that which involves the whole person. There was, however, an outcome that was of very great importance to her: the continuing relationship between her daughters.

Physicians tend to equate suffering with pain and disease. As Eric Cassell observes, suffering is a very personal matter. How much suffering is caused by a pain or disease depends on many individual factors. The suffering caused by pain is greater if pain is chronic, if the reason for the pain is not known, and if the patient feels that it cannot be controlled. It is a common experience that patients with chronic cancer pain feel a great release from suffering when it has been demonstrated to them that their pain can be controlled by narcotics. Patients suffer more if their pain has not been validated by a physical diagnosis and if, as a result, their relatives or their physician convey disbelief in its reality.

The suffering produced by disruption of the sense of self depends on how a person defines his or her sense of self. A middle-aged laborer may be devastated by a physical disability that would cause little suffering to a sedentary worker. Loss of sexual function may be devastating to one person but of little importance to another. To a young woman without children, loss of her uterus may be the loss of her hope for the future; to a middle-aged woman, loss of her uterus may be a relief.

Suffering is increased if it is associated with guilt, if the pain and disability are caused by some foolish and avoidable error—an accident or some form of self-abuse, for example. The most intense form of suffering is vicarious suffering, the anguish of a relative who sees a loved one suffering, especially if the relative feels that he or she may be to blame. Parents suffer greatly through the misfortunes of their children and usually feel that they are to blame in some way. Physicians may suffer vicariously from the traumas of their patients (Woolhouse, Brown, and Thind, 2012).

In his book *The Doctor and the Soul*, Victor Frankl (1973) has written of the importance of finding meaning in suffering. Frankl himself suffered greatly in a concentration camp during World War II but was able to find some meaning in his suffering. Almost any suffering can be tolerated if it can be imbued with meaning. Frankl tells the story of an elderly physician—a widower—who was very depressed by chronic illness and loneliness. Frankl asked him which he would have preferred: his present situation or for his wife to have been left alone and suffering. He began to see his suffering in a new light, as a burden he was carrying for his wife's sake after a long and happy marriage.

CASE 7.1

A woman with widespread metastases from carcinoma of the lung asked me if I (IRMcW) could assure her that she would not suffer. I told her that nobody could give her that assurance. Almost certainly, we would be able to relieve her pain, but suffering is intensely personal and not by any means synonymous with pain. There were many reasons for this woman to suffer. What we could say to her was that we would be sensitive to her sufferings, listen to her, be with her, and support her and her family during the last stages of her illness.

This woman was a widow who had lost her husband only 1 year earlier. She had two daughters, one in her twenties, the other in her teens, and suffered many anxieties about their future. She had paraplegia caused by spinal cord compression and had decided not to have surgery for this. The thoracotomy done for her primary tumor had been followed by respiratory failure, for which she had spent several months in the hospital. The steroids given for the spinal cord compression had given her a bloated appearance that caused her intense distress. She was so heavy that three nurses were needed to lift her. If she lay down, she became breathless and felt she was going to suffocate. Metastatic deposits in the cervical epidural space caused nerve root pain in the right arm, with progressive weakness and loss of function. A month before her death, she developed a pathological fracture of the femoral neck which caused severe pain on movement, uncontrollable by morphine. Because she was deemed unfit for surgical immobilization of the fracture, it was kept immobile by other means as far as possible, and she was moved with great care by a team of nurses.

The only way we could help this woman to bear her inevitable sufferings was to identify them and help her with them one by one. Her wheelchair mobility, and therefore her feeling of independence, was maintained until her fractured femur made it impossible. Discussions were held with the daughters and relatives about their future. In the course of these, the daughters became closer to each other than they had ever been before. One thing that always made the patient's eyes light up was to be complimented on her appearance. She would spend hours before her mirror and worked very hard to repair the ravages of her treatment. Her anxieties about suffocation were confronted. She had radiotherapy for the epidural metastases and morphine and a coanalgesic for her skeletal pain.

We cannot understand suffering until we realize that it is indivisible. Cicely Saunders (1984) uses the term "total pain" to express the fact that suffering is physical, mental, and spiritual. People suffer with their whole selves. The only way we can find out how they are suffering is to ask them. One of the most common errors we make as physicians is to treat pain but ignore other dimensions of suffering.

THE PHYSICIAN AS HEALER

All that a physician does for a sick person is dependent on the healing power of nature, expressed in the old principle of *vis medicatrix naturae*. Our therapies are designed to assist the patient's own healing powers and to remove the obstacles to healing. Lacerations heal when sutured, fractures heal when set and immobilized, and abscesses heal when drained. Before the advent of antibiotics, collapse therapy for pulmonary tuberculosis helped to remove an obstacle to healing by closing the cavities maintained by physical properties of the lungs. Antibiotics are of limited value when the immune system is impaired. General, nonspecific measures such as rest, nourishment, and relief of pain and anxiety are designed to strengthen the body's own healing powers. Our dependence on nature's healing powers becomes abundantly clear when we are dealing with a person whose immune system has failed or one who presents obstacles to healing that we cannot remove.

The healing powers of nature are not limited to physical wounds. A person is equally provided with powers to heal psychic wounds. Perhaps the most common example is the experience of bereavement. The natural response to bereavement and to other types of serious loss is a grieving process in the course of which the person experiences eventual healing, although, as with a physical wound, a scar remains. As with a physical wound or disease, healing may be inhibited. The healing of the psyche may be obstructed by various forms of self-deception, including the suppression from consciousness of painful or unwelcome feelings and experiences. In a bereaved person, the grieving process may be prolonged if the emotions of grief are suppressed. Shakespeare understood this well. In *Macbeth*, when MacDuff learns that his wife and children have been murdered, Malcolm says to him: "Give sorrow words. The grief that does not speak whispers the o'erwrought heart and bids it break." (Act 4, scene 3. Lines 13, 14).

What qualities do family physicians require as healers? First, we should be masters of those tools and techniques that fall within our own field. These are the therapeutic agents of healing at the physical level—the drugs, instruments, and manual skills. Among these are the skills of early diagnosis and rehabilitation. Much suffering can be avoided by good clinical practice. One of my (IRMcW) general practitioner father's aphorisms was "Rehabilitation begins at the time of the injury." Sometimes, the doctor has to help the patient to identify and work through problems that are inhibiting healing (see Case 9.6). Sometimes the doctor himself is adding to these problems (see Case 9.7). For patients who are struggling with progressive and permanent disabilities, there are many aids, ranging from mechanical devices to counseling services. The family doctor is unlikely to know them all, but at least he or she should know how a patient can gain access to them. Sometimes we deny patients access to services because in our egoism we cannot accept our own need of assistance.

Second, we should master the skills of healing at the mental level—the skills of communication: attentive listening, facilitation, and the provision of reassurance. Healing at the highest level, however, is not primarily a matter of technique. Techniques are certainly helpful, but they are not sufficient in themselves. For example, the best of listening skills will not be helpful if we do not believe that what patients are telling us is interesting and helpful. To be a healer for one's patients is to recognize and acknowledge their suffering, to understand the meaning the illness has for them, to be present for them in their times of need, and to give them hope.

Ian Gawler (1995), a long-term survivor of metastatic osteogenic sarcoma, describes five kinds of hope. One is the *absence of hope*—hopelessness—the belief that recovery is impossible. Even in cases of advanced cancer, Gawler urges doctors to leave patients with a little hope. Remarkable and unexpected remissions do occur. *Hope for survival* (the hope not to die) is a fragile stage and may lead to trials of alternative medicine. Patients need a lot of support at this time. In *hope for a better future*, patients are looking ahead to future plans and important events like a family anniversary or the birth of a new grandchild. This may be a time when short-term sacrifices are made in the hope of a better future: strict diets, for example. *Hope for spiritual realization* is the awakening to a deeper purpose in life that serious illness may provoke. The need here is for a doctor who will take this seriously. *Hope for the present moment* is the capacity for living in the moment by developing the practice of mindfulness: an awareness of experience from moment to moment that becomes so vivid that past and future lose much of their importance.

Recognition of a person's suffering sounds like such a simple thing, yet we hear so often that it is not forthcoming from doctors. In this regard, we cannot use lack of time as our excuse, for it is a question more of manner than of time. Patients are very quick to recognize indifference to their suffering in even the briefest of encounters. They are also very quick to recognize that a doctor senses their pain. In George Eliot's story "Janet's Repentance," Janet is in despair, abused by her husband and herself addicted to alcohol. In her despair she turns to the Reverend Tryan, a man who she senses has himself known suffering and despair:

He saw that the first thing Janet needed was to be assured of sympathy. She must be made to feel that her anguish was not strange to him; that he entered into the only half-expressed secrets, before any other message of consolation could find its way into her heart. The tale of Divine pity was never yet believed from lips that were not felt to be moved by human pity. (p. 81).

To understand the meaning of the illness for the patient one must listen to the story of the illness. " . . . illness in its immediacy is not simply an isolated physical event but rather it is an episode which is embedded in the unique life narrative of the patient. . . . present meaning is always constituted in terms of past meanings and future anticipations" (Toombs, 1992, p. 109). An understanding of the meaning of the illness for the patient is an integral part of the patient-centered clinical method (see Chapter 9). The doctor's interpretation should synthesize the pathological basis of the illness with the narrative context.

Listening to the story of the illness takes time, though less time in family practice than in other fields of medicine. The long-term relationships in general practice can give the doctor a prior knowledge of the patient's life story—a context into which each new event can be fitted. Often the doctor has been a witness to, or participant in, the story. However, our knowledge is never complete, and we are often surprised by the new understanding that emerges, even in patients we have known for many years.

To be present for patients in their times of need requires commitment and involvement. The healing relationship takes its place with those other human relationships where there is both commitment and involvement: husband–wife; parent–child; teacher–learner. A sufferer is not healed by a person who keeps his distance. As Toombs (1995, p. 98) puts it: "I don't want to be cared for by somebody who doesn't care about me." In the real world of conflicting obligations, one cannot always be present for those we care about. Even with our children, care must often be responsibly delegated. But there are times of great need when other obligations must be set aside. The need may only be for simple presence, as in a visit to a dying patient when everything else has been done. Some of the things I have regretted most have been those occasions when I have failed to realize the importance of presence. Sometimes one is forgiven for these failures, sometimes not.

Of course, the kind of involvement in the relationship between healer and patient is different from that in relationships where there is a kinship and emotional bond. There are both right ways and wrong ways for a healer to be involved. We will return to these presently.

As we listen to patients' stories, we are trying to form a picture of what life is like for them: of their own understanding of the illness, of their hopes and fears, of the disruptions in their social world, and of the strengths and resources they bring to bear in their struggle for wholeness. A well-timed question may help the patient to express these feelings, as well as assuring him or her of our interest. Toombs (1992, p. 106) says " . . . no physician has ever inquired of me what it is like to live with multiple sclerosis or to experience any of the disabilities that have accrued over the past seventeen years. Perhaps, most surprisingly, no neurologist has ever asked me if I am afraid, or, for that matter, even whether I am concerned about the future." She observes that "fears for the future are nearly always concrete. 'Will I be able to walk from my office to the classroom?' 'Will my illness be prolonged and prevent me from carrying out an important project?'"(p. 84). Concrete fears can always be addressed. Knowing this helps to remove our own sense of helplessness, which can make us afraid to ask the question.

Because each patient deals with an illness in his or her own way, listening to patients' stories is a matter of attending to particulars. This is in marked contrast to our diagnostic mode of thought in which we are trying to categorize the illness. Arthur Frank (1991, p. 48) writes,

> Caring has nothing to do with categories; it shows the person that her life is valued because it recognizes what makes her experience particular; . . .
>
> Care begins when difference is recognized. There is no "right thing to say to a cancer patient," because the "cancer patient" as a generic entity does not exist. There are only persons who are different to start with, having different experiences according to the contingencies of their diseases. The common diagnostic categories to which medicine places its patients are relevant to disease, not to illness. They are useful for treatment, but they only get in the way of care.

To be a healer is to help patients find their own way through the ordeal of their illness to a new wholeness. John Hull (1992, p. 133) writes in July 1985:

> I am developing the art of gazing with my hands. I like to hold and rehold and go on holding a beautiful object, absorbing every aspect of it. In a multicultural exhibition the other day, I was allowed to handle a string of beads, smooth and polished, and a South American water jar made from earthenware. There was a lovely, scraping sound when one rotated the lid of the jar, and thousands of tiny, tinkling hollow echoes were made when the full, round belly of the jar was touched with the fingernails.

Hull has long enjoyed the beauty of the English cathedrals. While he could see, his feeling for them was predominantly visual. After he became blind, he learned how their beauty could also be sensed through hearing and touch: the changing quality of sound as one moves through the building, the feel of the stone. He has now designed, with the help of others, acoustic and tactile guides for the blind in 17 English cathedrals, including Canterbury and York.

Suppose that we could, in a small way, help a patient in such a journey. Of course, only one in a million will take the path that Hull took. But each will have his or her own way, and perhaps it is the least articulate—those who do not write their stories—who need the most help.

INVOLVEMENT

Generations of medical students have been told, "Don't get involved: keep your distance." One of the assumptions of the conventional clinical method is that the correct attitude of the physician should be that of a detached observer. However, the teachers who gave this advice did not convey the complexity of the issue. They meant to say, we think, "Don't get emotionally involved." But they did not explain how to avoid this while maintaining the involvement necessary for healing. Neither did they admit that we can remain emotionally detached only by suppressing our feelings, a process that can seriously inhibit our capacity to heal. Our encounters with patients can provoke in us some very disturbing feelings, including those of fear and helplessness. One defense against these feelings is avoidance of the situations that provoke them—a common experience in the care of patients who are incurably or terminally ill. But in protecting ourselves, we deny our patients the care they have a right to expect from us. If we cannot be open to our own pain, how can we be open to the pain of others?

The question is better framed in two parts: "What is 'healing' involvement?" and "How do we avoid the pitfalls of emotional involvement?" Healing involvement can be expressed in two words: attention and presence. What it means to attend to a patient is conveyed by a story told in Jacob Needleman's book *The Way of the Physician* (1992). As a boy, he had to pay a visit to the family doctor, a longtime friend of the family who was like an uncle to him. As he was going into the waiting room, he passed the open door of an examination room where his "uncle," the doctor, was examining an obese old man. For a moment, their eyes met, but the doctor did not acknowledge him. Needleman went past the door again, hoping to get a smile from his uncle. Once again, there was no hint of recognition. At first he felt hurt, but then he understood that, for that brief time, the fat old man had the doctor's undivided attention: "you cared for that old man as much as you cared for me. Yet you were a friend of my family; you tousled my hair, you gave me candy, you called me by amusing names. But then and there you cared for that old man more than you cared for me." It was, says Needleman, a manifestation of "non-egoistic impersonal love" (Needleman, 1992, p. 16).

I (IRMcW) have never forgotten a brief experience I had as a medical student. When at home, I used to do rounds with the surgeon at the local hospital. After the round, he was asked to see an old vagrant from the workhouse, who was complaining of abdominal pain. The experience made a deep and lasting impression on me. The patient was exactly as one would have expected: his face red and blotchy; several days' growth of beard on his chin. For those few minutes, this old vagrant seemed to be the most important person in the world for the doctor. All his attention was focused on the old man, whom he treated with the utmost respect—a respect that showed in the way he talked and listened and the way he examined him. The word that perhaps describes it best is *presence*: for those few minutes, the doctor was a real presence in the patient's life.

The fact that this attention is non-egoistic and impersonal means that the doctor is at the same time involved and detached. When he has finished with one patient, he can transfer the same undivided attention to the next. It is not that feelings are absent, but that they are on a different level from egoistic emotions. It would be wrong, however, to suggest that the difference between the two ways of being involved is clear-cut. This is especially true for family doctors. The long-term relationships with patients often cannot be impersonal. Feelings of many kinds enter into these relationships, some of them helpful to healing, some of them harmful. It is when our egoistic emotions become involved that we encounter the pitfalls.

Egoistic emotions can enter into the relationship in many ways, some of them very subtle. Our helplessness in the face of suffering can make us afraid to recognize the sufferings of our patients; our openness to patients may be inhibited by our fears of what questions they will ask. We are capable of using our power to punish patients who anger us. Our therapeutic recommendations may be tinged with self-interest; our advocacy of our patients' interests may become a personal crusade in which their interests become secondary to our need to advance a cause. Work of healing with patients who have suffered childhood abuse has, in some overzealous hands, become a destructive process in which patients and their families have suffered. Sometimes, at a case conference, one becomes aware that the tone of the discussion has changed from one that is helpful to the patient in practical ways, to a dissection of the patient's soul from on high. Some of the great novelists teach us how subtle these pitfalls can be.

In *The Brothers Karamazov*, Dostoevsky describes how the young novice monk Alexey has tried to give money to a poor man who has been humiliated in public by Alexey's older brother. The man refuses the gift with indignation. Later Alexey is discussing with Lisa, an invalid girl, how he might get the man to take the money. "Listen Alexey," says Lisa, "don't you think our reasoning . . . shows that we regard him—that unfortunate man with contempt? I mean that we analyze his soul like this, as though from above? I mean that we're absolutely certain that he'll accept the money. Don't you think so?" Later in their discussion Alexey says to her, " . . . your question whether we do not despise that unhappy man by dissecting his soul was the question of a person who has suffered a lot . . . a person to whom such questions occur is himself capable of suffering."

In *Emma*, Jane Austen describes how, in a moment of truth, Emma Woodhouse realizes that "with insufferable vanity (she had) believed herself in the secret of everybody's feelings; with unpardonable arrogance proposed to arrange every-body's destiny." (p. 489). Instead of, as she thought, working for the good of her young friend Harriet Smith, she had in fact brought evil on her.

What makes the intrusion of egoistic emotions into the patient–doctor relationship difficult for us is the fact that they are so often at the unconscious level. In psychoanalysis, the process is referred to as transference and countertransference. "Transference in the clinical relationship denotes the patient's displacement and externalizing of internal issues onto the clinician; countertransference denotes the reverse" (Stein, 1985, p. 2). In analysis, the therapist deliberately does not respond intuitively to transference, because he or she wants the patient to face up to the immature response that the behavior represents. The therapist must try to identify responses arising from his or her own countertransference, so that he or she can avoid the harm that may be done if these feelings are acted out. It has taken a long time for us to realize that these notions apply to all therapeutic relationships, including those in family practice. Freud (Gay, 1989) described three types of transference. Negative transference is the direction of hostile feelings onto the analyst; in erotic transference, the analyst becomes the object of erotic love. Both of these obstruct healing and must be exposed and learned from. In the third type—sensible transference—the therapist is seen as a supportive ally in the process of healing. It is, said Freud, "essentially a cure through love."

In the long-term relationships of family practice, feelings may be expressed by both doctor and patient that are simply part of the relationship and have nothing to do with transference. When transference can be identified, it may not be harmful, as when a patient becomes temporarily dependent at a time of serious illness or crisis. On the other hand, all of us, at some time or other, act out our egoistic emotions in ways that are anti-therapeutic. How can we avoid these pitfalls? Only by striving for self-knowledge, that most difficult of all fields of knowledge—most difficult because it can be attained only by facing honestly those parts of our own nature that are most painful to acknowledge. Self-knowledge comes in a number of ways: sometimes at times of crisis, through illness, failure, or suffering; sometimes in moments of truth, such as one finds in the stories of the great novelists; sometimes in old age. In day-to-day experience, however, self-knowledge comes through attention to ourselves in the same way as we attend to our patients. By attending to our thoughts and feelings as they arise in us, we can become aware of them before they do harm " . . . it is a matter of emotions of man: how to control them, how to evoke the non-egoistic emotions, and how to free ourselves from the emotions that make wreckage of our lives individually and collectively. The question of human relationship is synonymous with the question of human emotions" (Needleman, 1992). Studying our own emotions should be the realm of psychology, but as Needleman (1992) and Bettelheim (1984) have observed, modern psychology is predominantly concerned with the study of other people's emotions. But psychology did not begin in modern times. All the great spiritual traditions have psychological theories as well as spiritual disciplines designed to do what Needleman describes. Though the disciplines differ in details, they are remarkably consistent in using contemplative methods of "mindfulness, awareness." These methods, or modifications of them, are now being used therapeutically.[2]

SPIRITUAL ASPECTS OF HEALING

It has become quite common to refer to the spiritual aspect of healing, sometimes in a superficial way that does not do justice to its importance. It may be seen, for example, as a category of problems—a fourth category to be added to the biomedical, psychological, and social. The spiritual then becomes another kind of problem-solving: an additional responsibility for the physician. We prefer to think of spirituality in healing in a much more specific sense. Spiritual experiences are those in which persons feel the presence of powers and influences outside themselves. The feeling is accompanied by a sense of awe and of deep meaning. The experience is at the root of all religions, though religious practice can, and often does, become completely separated from spirituality. Hawkins (1993, p. 60) observes that, paradoxically, the feeling that illness can be an occasion for spiritual growth is "strangely absent from religious pathographies, [but] ... present ... in a wide variety of pathographies that a, p. 60cknowledge no explicit religious referent."

The classical spiritual pathography is John Donne's *Devotions upon Emergent Occasions*, of which Hawkins (1993) writes:

> The organizing construct that explains the meaning both of the illness itself and of the various treatments to which Donne is subjected is religious belief. In accord with an underlying sacramentalism, all physical realities have a spiritual dimension and a spiritual analogue: illness is thus inherently meaningful and purposive. Not only is the physical dimension consistently interpreted as a metaphor for the spiritual, but physical realities are always subordinated to their spiritual counterparts. (p. 50)

Donne's illness teaches him that man is not separate from the cosmos: "No man is an island, entire of itself; every man is a piece of the continent, a part of the main." (Hawkins, p. 52)

In modern times, this sense is less likely to be expressed in strictly religious terms than in terms of cosmic consciousness: a feeling of connectedness with cosmic forces. It may be manifested in the scientist or naturalist as a feeling of awe in the contemplation of nature. In the physician it may be a sense of awe and reverence—perhaps largely unconscious—in the presence of the healing powers of nature. In older language it is the experience of being on holy ground. In *De Profundis*—a meditation on suffering—Oscar Wilde (1905, p. 5) wrote: "Where there is sorrow there is holy ground. Some day people will realise what that means. They will know nothing of life till they do." Vastyan (1981, p. 1) expresses a background to this feeling:

> "Healing" and "holy" have a common Old English root in our language. That common etymology well describes the older origin. From cover to cover, healing— holy healing—is the central concern of the Bible: the Jewish Bible, the Christian Bible. There we find a common insistence that healing springs from spiritual insight and spiritual action; that healing—all healing—is a holy task; that all healing has a holy source; that only the wounded can heal; that healing does not follow a path of upward mobility and autonomy and competition and minimum risk, but rather has a path of downward pilgrimage and sharing and community and maximum risk; that all who are touched in any way by the Holy are called to be healers; and that all who are healers, do the work of the Holy.

Does a physician who brings this quality to a relationship enhance it? One result is likely to be that patients feel able to be open about expressing their own spiritual experiences. Patients are very quick to sense when their experiences are being greeted by skepticism and disbelief. Perhaps also the sense of presence engendered by this quality plays some part in mobilizing the patient's own powers of healing.

Although this quality may be unusual today, there is reason to believe that it may have been present in previous generations, albeit at the subconscious and intuitive level. An account of Sir William Osler's visits to a child dying in the influenza pandemic of 1918 is an example:

> He visited our little Janet twice every day and these visits she looked forward to with a pathetic eagerness and joy. There would be a little tap, low down on the door which would be pushed open and a crouching figure playing goblin would come in, and in a high-pitched voice would ask if the fairy godmother was at home and could he have a bit of tea. Instantly the sick-room was turned into a fairyland, and in fairy language he would talk about the flowers, the birds, and the dolls who sat at the foot of the bed who were always greeted with, "Well, all ye loves." In the course of this he would manage to find out all he wanted to know about the little patient. . . . The most exquisite moment came one cold, raw, November morning when the end was near, and he mysteriously brought out from his inside pocket a beautiful red

rose carefully wrapped in paper, and told how he had watched this last rose of summer growing in his garden and how the rose had called out to him as he passed by, that she wished to go along with him to see his little lassie. That evening we all had a fairy tea party, a tiny table by the bed, Sir William talking to the rose, his "little lassie," and her mother in a most exquisite way; and presently he slipped out of the room just as mysteriously as he had entered it, all crouched down on his heels; and the little girl understood that neither fairies nor people could always have the colour of a red rose in their cheeks, or stay as long as they wanted to in one place, but that they nevertheless would be very happy in another home and must not let the people they left behind, particularly their parents, feel badly about it; and the little girl understood and was not unhappy. (Cushing, 1926, p. 1306)

At the time of this incident, Osler was near the end of his career. He was also deeply grieving the death of his only son in World War I. One feels Osler's total attention to the child and the sense of his presence she must have had. It seems that the healer and clinician were working together in perfect harmony, for he was at the same time absorbed in the patient and collecting the clinical information he needed. Nearly three centuries separate this account of an illness from that of John Donne, and the context has changed from a religious to a secular spirituality. Yet there are deeper resemblances. Just as for Donne every feature of his illness symbolizes some aspect of his spiritual life, for the mother there is a symbolic meaning in the last rose of summer. That Osler was not only a great clinician but also a great healer is evident from the accounts of his friends and colleagues. "[He] really brought Healing and Health, Life not Death," wrote one (Cushing, 1926, p. 1266). Although this quality in a clinician may be intuitive rather than consciously present, Osler was quite explicit in his teaching. In one address to students, he said:

> I would urge upon you . . . to care more for the individual patient than for the special features of the disease. . . . Dealing as we do with poor suffering humanity, we see the man unmasked, exposed to all the frailties and weaknesses, and you have to keep your heart soft and tender lest you have too great a contempt for your fellow creatures. The best way is to keep a looking glass in your own heart, and the more carefully you scan your own frailties the more tender you are for those of your fellow creatures. (Cushing, 1926, pp. 489–490)

THE MORAL DIMENSION

In all the great spiritual traditions, true spirituality shows itself in the conduct of life—likewise false spirituality. As Dante descends through the rings of the Inferno, encountering at each level greater depths of evil, the souls he meets are consumed by anger and hatred. In his journey through Paradise, he is met everywhere by the most exquisite courtesy. The moral life is a reflection of the spiritual life: the outer a reflection of the inner. The great spiritual masters have sometimes been accused of breaking the moral laws; the occasion, however, is always a call to a higher morality. The written code—the letter of the law—cannot always be applied literally; without the spirit, it becomes lifeless. The spiritual masters, however, are emphatic that true spirituality means, in the first place, living according to the law. The mistake made by some self-styled spiritual movements in the West has been to believe that spiritual growth comes from throwing off restraints and discipline. The opposite is true. The mastery of all true spiritual disciplines is a long and arduous process.

The reason for saying these things is the resemblance between religious experience and sickness. "Like the sick man, the religious man is projected on to a vital plane that shows him the fundamental data of human existence, that is, solitude, danger, hostility of the surrounding world" (Eliade, 1964, p. 27). Sacks wrote, after recovering from his illness, "I have since had a deeper sense of the horror and wonder which lurk behind life and which are concealed . . . behind the usual surface of health" (Sacks, 1984, p. ix).

This being so, it is not surprising that serious illness should often be the occasion for what may be a painful self-examination. Paul Tournier (1983), the Swiss general practitioner and psychotherapist, tells the story of a physician who consulted him at his wife's request after failing to recover completely after septicemia. The patient was full of remorse for the way he had spent his life and for betrayals he had not confessed to his wife. This remorse haunted him throughout his time in the hospital, and he would have liked to unburden himself to his doctors. In fact, he saw the illness as having deep meaning for him, as being a time for introspection and change. Although he was treated with great kindness, the talk during ward rounds was all of blood cultures and antibiotics. The doctors were surprised at how slowly he recovered from the illness. For all their kindness, they could not see the illness as having a deeper meaning for the patient. On leaving the hospital, the patient had refused convalescence and returned to his old defense mechanism of frenetic overwork. Healing did not take place until he found a physician who could reach his "moral loneliness."

The point here is not that physicians have any claim to be moral or spiritual teachers: it is simply that to be a healer, one must recognize and respond to all forms of suffering, at least by listening and comforting and, if not possessing the necessary experience ourselves, calling on others who have. "It is not a question of taking the clergyman's place, of teaching, preaching, indoctrinating, admonishing or proselytizing. . . . It is a question of perceiving the whole of our patient's suffering and of facing up to it without cowardice, without subterfuge. And if that suffering is a feeling of guilt, it is not enough to say that it is no longer in the doctor's sphere" (Tournier, 1983). To ignore spiritual suffering is to deny the wholeness of the person, to divide a person into compartments. As Tournier tells us, suffering knows no frontier. Physical illness is associated with spiritual suffering; spiritual suffering may be manifested as physical or mental illness. We do not have to be religious ourselves, in the world's sense of religious, and certainly not in the sectarian sense, to respond to a patient's sufferings, whatever their origin.

THE PEDAGOGY OF SUFFERING

The pedagogy of suffering means that one who suffers has something to teach—and thus something to give. "What is at issue is an ethic derived from a pedagogy of suffering that was stated in 1909 by Gyorgy Lukacs as he meditated the mysterious reciprocity between creative activity and the 'the primacy of ethics in life'" (Frank, 1997, p. 153). The impetus of ethics for Lukacs is loneliness; the pedagogy of suffering begins its teaching from a ground of loneliness seeking communion. Instead of one ethical person bearing all the weight of things, the weight is shared. Instead of bearing all the weight of medical decisions, the physician shares the weight with the patients he is responsible for, or the nurses he works with. The ethics that Lukacs recommends is exemplified by Dr. Hilfiker, who works, and lives with, the poorest of the poor in central Washington. Hilfiker does not work with the poor with condescension or with charity. He does it because of his brokenness. Having acknowledged his own brokenness, his service to the poor is that much easier, and he can receive support from his patients in return. Hilfiker titles his book *Not All of Us Are Saints* (1994). He works with the poor not because he is morally superior, but because he is needy. When will our medical profession have the grace to acknowledge this brokenness?

Jean Vanier (1988), the founder of *L'arche*, an organization to care for those with mental disabilities, makes the same point as Hilfiker. The mentally disabled give as much to their custodians as their custodians give to them. The Swiss cultural philosopher Jean Gebser sees our epoch as one in which our present ego-consciousness will give place to an openness that is founded on the transcendence of the ego. Ego-freedom is not so much a relapse into ego-lessness as a "deep affirmation of life, its forms and beyond all forms" (Fuerstein, 1995). Hilfiker and Vanier may be leading us along this path.

Because the pedagogy of suffering is taught in the testimony of illness stories, the kind of ethics it supports is a narrative ethic. Frank regards illness narratives as a postmodern development. In modern medicine, the physician took charge of the patients' illness and expressed it in medical terms; in the postmodern world, the patient insists on telling and re-telling his or her own story, even though there might still be a modern description supplied by the physician. "My concern," says Frank: "is with people's self-stories as moral acts, and with care as the moral action of responding to these self-stories" (Frank, 1997, p. 157). Narrative contributions can be made in this way to collaborative decision-making.

Steven Hsi (2004) was a family physician who personally experienced the modern healthcare system, its technical achievements, and its shortcomings. He has written a moving memoir of that experience and what he learned from it prior to his death. One insight he gained was the importance of physicians recognizing that, just like their patients, they too are vulnerable:

> Physicians erect great barriers to appear less vulnerable and it prevents us from reaching our own spiritual selves. The idea of humanity is very much tied in with vulnerability. To be truly human, to be part of the community, we have to recognize our helplessness in a lot of things and our dependence on other things and other people.

THE AUTHORITY OF THE HEALER

From the earliest times, healing has been associated with power and authority. In traditional cultures, shamans are persons who have acquired power and knowledge by going through an intense initiatory experience. Whether selected by inheritance or personal vocation, the shaman is not recognized as such until he has received two kinds of teaching: an ecstatic experience (altered state of consciousness), through which he has learned the mysteries of human destiny; and didactic instruction in the theory and practice of healing. The ecstatic experience often followed an ordeal, such as a period of isolation or a serious illness. The ecstatic "journey" of the soul to the underworld changes the person forever, and confers on him the power of healing. "The shaman is the great specialist of the human soul" (Eliade, 1964). The shaman has experienced serious illness or existential crisis himself, has looked death in the face, and has recovered. Eliade suggests that the ecstasy of the shaman is an archetype of "gaining existential consciousness" (p. 394). In Greek mythology, the archetype is expressed in the stories of Chiron the wounded healer, Orpheus's journey to the underworld, and the death and resurrection of Aesculapius. In modern times, any manifestation of the archetype is likely to be overlaid by layers of culture and history that separate us from the ancient world.

Modern medicine has valued and emphasized technical knowledge, almost to the exclusion of the esoteric knowledge gained by reflection on the deep experience of life and death that medicine can provide. Its muted manifestations can be seen, perhaps, at the margins: in the hospice movement, in the literature on illness and healing, or in music therapy, described by one of its practitioners as "a contemplative practice with clinical implications" (Schroeder-Sheker, 1993).

The shaman is a person set apart in his society as a manifestation of the sacred, a person who, by unusual means, has "experienced the sacred with greater intensity than the rest of the community" (Eliade, 1964). For

Needleman (1992), the generation of physicians preceding our own "was one of the last surviving traces of the sacred in our world." Perhaps this is what Robert Louis Stevenson meant when he said that the physician "stands above the common herd . . . almost as a rule." (As quoted by Osler,1906) Among the classes of humankind thus distinguished by Stevenson were also the soldier, the sailor, and the shepherd—all of whom experience life and nature in the raw (or did, until our own time). It is doubtful whether Stevenson would have said this of the modern physician. Our technologies often distance us from the realities of human experience. Needleman was astonished to find that the physicians he encountered had seldom been present at a patient's death.

Of all fields of medicine, perhaps family medicine and psychiatry can best preserve and cultivate this power of healing. Bettelheim (1984) has reminded us that the term we translate into English as *psyche* was the German *seele* in the writings of Freud—more accurately translated as "soul." The logotherapy of Victor Frankl (1973) is a direct outcome of his experience as a prisoner in Auschwitz. However, the successes of pharmacotherapy seem to be leading psychiatry in another direction. Although affected by modern trends, family medicine retains a closeness to the realities of human life, an experience captured vividly in Berger and Mohr's book *A Fortunate Man* (1967).

To value the power of the healer may seem to be at variance with the modern reaction against the authoritarian attitudes of physicians. On closer examination, however, it is clear that we are dealing with two different kinds of authority. The modern reaction is against physicians who disempower patients by making decisions for them. The power and authority of the healer is of an entirely different order, mobilizing the patient's will to live and releasing the powers that he or she alone possesses.

NOTES

1. The extract is from *Touching the Rock* by John Hull, copyright ©1992 by John M. Hull. Reprinted by permission of Pantheon Books, a division of Random House.
2. One example is the work of Jon Kabat-Zinn at the University of Massachusetts Medical Center, described in his book *Full Catastrophe Living: Using the Wisdom of Your Body and Mind to Face Stress, Pain and Illness* (New York: Bantam Doubleday Dell, 1990). The role of mindfulness in medicine has been the object of increasing interest since that volume was published. See, for example, Ludwig DS, Kabat-Zinn J, Mindfulness in medicine, *JAMA* (2008), 300(11):1350–1352.

REFERENCES

Austen J. Emma. Open Road Integrated Media. New York.
Baron RJ. 1985. An introduction to medical phenomenology: I can't hear you while I'm listening. *Annals of Internal Medicine* 103:606.

Berger J, Mohr J. 1967. *A Fortunate Man: The Story of a Country Doctor*. London: Allen Lane.

Bettelheim B. 1984. *Freud and Man's Soul*. New York: Vintage Books

Cassell EJ. 1990. *The Healer's Art*. Philadelphia, PA: Lippincott.

Cassell EJ. 2013. *The Nature of Healing: The Modern Practice of Medicine*. New York; Oxford: Oxford University Press.

Cushing H. 1926. *The Life of Sir William Osler*. New York: Oxford University Press.

Eliade M. 1964. *Shamanism: Archaic Techniques of Ecstasy*. Princeton, NJ: Princeton University Press.

Eliot G. 1883. *Janet's Repentance: Scenes of a Clerical Life*. Norman L. Munro. New York.

Frank A. 1991. *At the Will of the Body*. Boston, MA: Houghton Miffin.

Frank A. 1997. *The Wounded Storyteller: Body, Illness and Ethics*. Chicago: University of Chicago Press.

Frankl VE. 1973. *The Doctor and the Soul: From Psychotherapy to Logotherapy*. New York: Vintage Books.

Fuerstein G. 1995. *The Structures of Consciousness, the Genius of Jean Gebser*. Lower Lake, CA: Integral.

Gawler I. 1995. The five stages of hope: How to develop and sustain hope—an essential pre-requisite for profound healing. In: Gawler I, ed., *Proceedings of the Mind, Immunity and Health Conference: Psychoneuroimmunology and the Mind–body Connection*. Yarra Junction, Victoria, Australia.

Gay P. 1989. *Freud: A Life for Our Time*. New York: Anchor Books.

Hawkins AH. 1993. *Reconstructing Illness: Studies in Pathography*. West Lafayette, IN: Purdue University Press.

Hilfiker D. 1994. *Not All of Us Are Saints: A Doctor's Journey with the Poor*. New York: Hill and Wang.

Hsi, S. 2004. *Closing the Chart: A Dying Physician Examines Family, Faith, and Medicine*. Albuquerque: University of New Mexico Press.

Hull JM. 1992. *Touching the Rock: An Experience of Blindness*. New York: Vintage Books.

Kleinman A, Kleinman J. 1997. The appeal of experience; the dismay of images: cultural appropriation of suffering in our times. Chapter 1 in Social Suffering. Kleinman A, Das V, Lock M, eds., Berkeley: University of California Press.

Lifton RJ. 1967. *Death in Life: Survivors of Hiroshima*. New York: Random House.

Needleman J. 1992. *The Way of the Physician*. London: Penguin Books.

Osler W. 1906. *Aequanimatas*. McGraw-Hill Book Company. New York.

Price R. 1994. *A Whole New Life*. New York: Atheneum Macmillan.

Sacks O. 1984. *One Leg to Stand On*. London: Gerald Duckworth.

Sacks O. 1989. *Seeing Voices*. Berkeley; Los Angeles: University of California Press.

Saunders C. 1984. The philosophy of terminal care. In: Saunders C, ed., *The Management of Terminal Malignant Disease*, 2nd ed. London: Edward Arnold.

Schroeder-Sheker T. 1993. Music for the dying: A personal account of the new field of music thanatology—history, theories, and clinical narratives. *Advances* 9(1):36.

Shea G. 2013. *Song Without Words: Discovering My Deafness Halfway Through Life*. Boston: De Capo Press.

Stein HF. 1985. *The Psychodynamics of Medical Practice*. Berkeley: University of California Press.

Stetten D, Jr. 1981. Coping with blindness. *New England Journal of Medicine* 305:458.

Toombs SK. 1992. *The Meaning of Illness: A Phenomenological Account of the Different Perspectives of Physicians and Patients*. Dordrecht: Kluwer.

Toombs SK. 1995. Healing and incurable illness. *Humane Medicine* 11(3):98.

Tournier P. 1983. *Guilt and Grace*. San Francisco, CA: Harper and Row.

Vanier J. 1988. *The Broken Body: The Journey to Wholeness*. New York: Paulist Press.

Vastyan EA. 1981. *Healing and the Wounded Healer*. Philadelphia, PA: Society for Health and Human Values.

Wilde O. 1905. *De Profundis*. London: Methuen.

Woolhouse S, Brown JB, Thind A. 2012. "Building through the grief": Vicarious trauma in a group of inner-city family physicians. *Journal of the American Board Family Medicine* 25(6):840–846.

CHAPTER 8

୶

Patient–Doctor Communication

M any of the errors in medical practice have their origins in a failure of communication. The doctor either fails to understand the patient's meaning or fails to convey his or her own meaning. These misunderstandings cause frustration for doctors and patients, with all that follows in lowered morale, patients' dissatisfaction, ineffective medicine, conflict, and litigation. Effective communication is fundamental. If we have not understood the patient's problem as the very first step, everything that follows in investigation and treatment may be wrong. Even when diagnosis and therapy are technically correct, the way in which they are communicated to patients has important implications for their response. Moreover, communication is the essence of a therapeutic relationship.

In family practice, communication between doctor and patient has some important special features. Most of these can be summed up in one word: context. Communication usually takes place between a doctor and patient who know each other, who have shared previous experiences, and have other relationships in common, for example with other family members. It takes place, very often, over extended periods of time, and in the different environments of office, home, and hospital. It is important, therefore, for us to understand how context influences and enhances communication.

Most consultations between doctor and patient begin with the patient's account of his or her symptoms. In many cases, these will eventually be supplemented by other data. However, as we have seen, a very high proportion of patients have symptoms without physical signs or abnormal investigations. Even when signs and abnormal tests are found, the correct diagnosis is more likely to depend on the history than on the examination and investigation. This is particularly so in general practice. An understanding of the patient's symptoms is, therefore, fundamental.

Symptoms are the patient's description of what he or she perceives to be abnormal sensations. By definition, they are subjective and not open to verification by empirical methods. There is no objective test by which we can verify that a patient is actually feeling a pain. This is not to say, however, that we cannot apply rigorous methods to understanding the meaning of a patient's symptoms. The methods are those of attentive listening, clarification of meaning through dialogue, and avoidance of selection bias.

Symptoms are a form of communication—the way in which a patient conveys feelings of illness, distress, or discomfort. Symptoms are the information on which we base our understanding of the patient's problem. The starting point is the information received by the patient in the form of messages transmitted from his or her nervous system. Information about bodily functions is constantly being transmitted via the nervous system and by chemical transmitters to the brain—information that provides the basis for the body's self-regulation. Normally, we are unaware of these messages. The signals that lead to an adjustment in heart rate, blood pressure, or posture are, under usual circumstances, received and acted on below the level of consciousness. Nor are we normally aware of bodily functions like digestion and respiration. In unusual circumstances, signals reach consciousness and must be interpreted or decoded. How the signals are decoded depends on a number of factors, including the person's past experience and culture. These all form the context within which the messages are transmitted and interpreted.

Because the memory of a significant experience has an affective component, the interpretation is both cognitive and affective.

Let us suppose that the constancy of the background feeling is broken by a sensation of chest pain on waking one morning. At first there is a moment of anxiety; then a fall the day before, when a blow was received on that part of the chest, is remembered. This explanation is accompanied by a feeling of relief. On the other hand, no such explanation may be available. Perhaps the memory instead is of a colleague who had a severe heart attack accompanied by chest pain. The anxiety results in a visit to the doctor. The presenting complaint is probably the pain, not the anxiety. But things can be even more complicated. Even though the anxiety is not expressed in words, it may be expressed in bodily ways—facial expression, gestures, heart rate, and so on. An observant physician may recognize the emotion from these signs.

To complicate things even more, the original change in body state may itself be the bodily expression of an emotion. In a remarkable book, Siri Hustvedt clearly illustrates this point. She initially dealt with her father's death in a business-like way: "When the time came, I didn't weep. I wrote. At the funeral, I delivered my speech in a strong voice, without tears" (Hustvedt, 2009, p. 2). Two and one half years later, however, while delivering a speech to him at the dedication of the planting of a tree in his honor, she began to shake uncontrollably, from the neck down. Attempting to understand the peculiar symptoms that she experienced, she investigated the history of hysteria, conversion disorders, and the emerging neurosciences (Hustvedt, 2009).

> From the chin up, I was my familiar self. From the neck down, I was a shuddering stranger. Whatever had happened to me, whatever name would be assigned to my affliction, my strange seizure must have had an emotional component that was somehow connected to my father. The problem was that I hadn't *felt* emotional. I had felt entirely calm and reasonable. (Hustvedt, 2009, p. 7)

Expressions of grief may be expressed cognitively, emotionally, and somatically. The puzzlement often felt about bodily experiences of emotion lies in the Western cultural divide between the mind and the body (see Chapter 5, "Philosophical and Scientific Foundations of Family Medicine").

Information is provided by signals that convey differences from the usual state of affairs. The information level of a signal is directly related to its capacity to surprise the receiver. A person who usually coughs up some mucoid sputum in the morning gets no information by looking at his sputum. If one morning it is bloodstained, he does get information. The information conveyed by the bloodstained sputum will depend on the context within which the message is received. A person who believes that blood in the sputum always means cancer will decode the message differently from the person who does not connect the blood with cancer. A person who coughs up blood for the first time will decode it differently from a person who has coughed up blood before. A person who wakes with a headache after an excess of alcohol gets little information. A person who wakes with a headache "out of the blue" gets a lot more information, especially if he has never suffered from headaches before.

We know from population surveys, and from our own experience, that information arising from differences in our inner state is a daily occurrence. We all experience minor aches, pains, and discomforts of various kinds: headaches, muscle pains, dyspepsia, fatigue, itching, insomnia, irregularity of bowels or menses, and so on. The fact that a person consults a physician means that he has interpreted the information as a departure from his usual pattern, or as a signal that is outside his frame of reference. This interpretation varies enormously from one person to another. There is no clear relationship between the severity of the symptoms and the decision to consult (see Chapter 3). A common defense against unwelcome information is denial. It is not uncommon for people to explain away symptoms like anterior chest pain that they know may indicate myocardial infarction. People have a great capacity for self-deception. On the other hand, there are those whose tolerance is low and who consult for very minor ailments. There may, of course, be a very good reason for consulting, as with the person who comes with vague chest pain after a friend has died of a myocardial infarction.

This initial decoding of information we will call the first gate: the gate where information from bodily feelings is interpreted and acted on in illness behavior (see Chapter 3). Symptoms admitted through this gate may be acted on in different ways. For some, self-care will be tried, at least for a time; others will rely on advice from family, friends, or members of the person's lay referral system. The decision to consult a physician may be an individual one or may be made with the assistance of family and friends. Sometimes it is on the insistence of family and friends.

This decision brings us to the second gate. Having decided to see a doctor, the person must then decide how to code his or her symptoms for transmission to the physician, including what language to use and which symptom or problem to mention first. The decision is influenced by many factors. Very seldom is there a single symptom or problem; usually there are many. Often there are also emotions related to the symptoms: anxieties, fantasies, fears. How can the patient convey how he or she feels? At this gate we encounter the complexities and difficulties of doctor–patient communication. First the patient has to code the information in verbal form. How well he or she can do this depends on the availability of a language and his or her own familiarity with it. For some symptoms a well-understood language is quite readily available. The message is coded in words that have a direct causal relationship with the sensation the patient is trying to communicate. There may also be a clear and direct relationship between the symptom and a diseased state, such as the one between anginal pain and ischemic heart disease. Other sensations and feelings are much more difficult to put into words: vague illness and distress, changes of mood, unhappiness, anxiety, grief, self-doubt, guilt, and remorse. These difficulties are so great that some very sick people do not consult physicians. It is not uncommon for severely depressed people to never consult a physician (see Chapter 13, "Depression"; Hannay, 1979). It seems that disorders that threaten the integrity of the personality are particularly difficult to find expression for.

The relationship between the presenting complaint (what the patient states is the reason for visiting the doctor) and the principal problem (as defined by the physician) has been examined in different settings. Burack and Carpenter (1983) found that agreement between complaint and problem was 76% when the problem was perceived by the physician as somatic in nature, but only 6% when categorized as psychosocial in nature. In a geriatric clinic, the concordance between the chief complaint and principal problem was greatly enhanced by the additional information provided by caregivers, and sometimes was essential to arriving at a correct understanding of the problem (Duke, Barton, and Wolf-Klein, 1994). Beckman and Frankel (1984) found no relationship between the order in which a patient's complaints are presented and the medical significance that the physician attaches to them. Through the medium of the Internet and direct-to-consumer advertising, patients now often approach their physician expressing medical terminology rather than communicating their actual symptoms (Achkar, 2006), and this can be very misleading, causing inappropriate investigations, treatments, and delays in diagnosis. It is important that the physician ask about the actual symptoms that the patient is experiencing and then listen carefully to his or her response (Brandt, 2007).

To overcome these difficulties of expression, patients find other ways of coding their message. This means using an indirect, rather than a direct, form of communication. When patients express personal distress through bodily symptoms, they are not inventing the symptoms, or imagining the sensations. They are simply selecting the aspect of the illness experience that they can most easily put into words. A patient who cannot find words for his or her feeling of despair may express the problem in terms of a familiar symptom like headaches, which may be an effect of the problem but are not the core of it. It is much easier to talk about headaches than about despair. In indirect communication, the patient may express meaning by using metaphors or nonverbal forms. Metaphors, according to Jeremy Campbell (1982), "place the familiar in the context of the strange"—or, one might add, the strange in the context of the familiar. The message is in the context. A patient with a chronic disease, who is also in personal distress, may communicate this distress in the form of a visit for the disease (Case 8.1).

It is a universal experience that words are inadequate to express feeling: " . . . words, like nature half reveal and half conceal the soul within," (p. 965) wrote Tennyson in *In Memoriam*. In all cultures, the deepest feelings are expressed in dance, drama, poetry, and other forms of symbolism. Many patients who come to see us are in the grip of powerful emotions, so it is not surprising that indirect communication is common in family practice.

Problems that arouse shame or guilt—like family and sexual problems— may be communicated indirectly. The problem may be introduced in the context of a visit for a "checkup" or for an unrelated problem. A woman suffering from dyspareunia may say that she has come for a routine

---

CASE 8.1

A patient with multiple sclerosis came with the usual symptoms of her disease. The distress she was trying to communicate was caused by her husband's refusal to countenance birth control. This problem was related to the disease, in that she felt unfit to manage another child, but only indirectly.

examination. If asked directly about difficulty with intercourse, she may deny problems. Then, in the course of the pelvic examination, she may ask, "Should it hurt there when I have intercourse?" Note that the problem is framed in the form of a question (a common form of indirect communication) and that the most sensitive issue is raised during the physical examination.

If the context is a visit for another problem, mention of the most sensitive problem is likely to be left to the last. This has been called the "exit problem" or "doorknob comment"—the one that is not mentioned until the patient is getting up to leave, sometimes introduced by the words "By the way, Doctor." The exit problem is usually the main reason for the patient's visit.

Indirect communication protects us against rejection or embarrassment. If a patient requests a sickness absence note for an illness he is recovering from and the request is refused, he loses face. If he first complains of symptoms and allows the doctor to assess his illness, then asks for the note as an afterthought, refusal causes much less embarrassment.

A patient may introduce an embarrassing subject by hinting. A hint is somewhat ambiguous and does not reveal the problem all at once. If the physician responds to the hint, the patient still has the choice of how much to reveal (Case 8.2).

How a patient codes personal distress for transmission to the physician depends also on his or her perception of how the physician will receive the information. A doctor who is perceived by the patient as working in the context of physical pathology is likely to receive messages about personal distress coded in the language of physical symptoms. A doctor who is perceived to be patient centered, encouraging the expression of feeling, is more likely to have personal distress conveyed to him or her directly. Given the difficulty of finding words for distress, it is not surprising that patients often complain first of bodily symptoms (see Cases 4.1, 8.3, 9.1). This is often referred to as *somatization*. If it is persistent, it is known as *somatic fixation*. There is a category of *somatic symptom disorders* in the *Diagnostic and Statistical Manual*.

CASE 8.2

The wife of a soldier who had been away from home was disturbed to find that he had pubic lice on his return. He attributed them to dirty blankets provided in his billet. Instead of saying what was on her mind, she asked, "Can you get crab lice from bedclothes?"

SOMATIZATION TO MEDICALLY UNEXPLAINED SYMPTOMS (MUS)

Somatization is defined as the process by which emotions are transduced to bodily symptoms, for which medical aid is sought. In its original formulation, somatization was related to the psychoanalytic concept of *conversion*: the transduction of a psychological conflict into bodily symptoms. In psychoanalytical theory, conversion was viewed as a defense mechanism by which the patient unconsciously avoided having to deal with the internal conflict and gained some protection from threatening circumstances through bodily symptoms (secondary gain). The symptoms of conversion were therefore forms of communication, rather than the experience of physiological disturbances. The concept has now been expanded to embrace any bodily manifestation of distress. The classical manifestation of conversion hysteria is now uncommon, and most bodily manifestations of distress are compatible with physiological correlates of emotion. However, the implication of personal gain remains. The term *somatization* is unfortunate in that it suggests that the process is abnormal and that the patient is the agent of the transduction. It is therefore difficult to avoid the implication that the patient is morally responsible for his or her own illness, especially when there is the added suggestion that the illness enables him or her to avoid responsibilities. The idea of somatization, therefore, always has the potential for putting the doctor and patient in conflict.[1]

Using the term *medically unexplained symptoms* (MUS) has the advantage of avoiding the notion that patients are in some way, either consciously or unconsciously, provoking the experience of emotions in the body. It also more accurately places the issue on the inadequacy of the diagnostic categories used in medicine. It is estimated that between 25% and 50% of all symptoms presented to physicians in primary care have no medical explanation (Peveler, Kilkenny, and Kinmonth, 1997).

It is normal to feel emotion in the body.[2] The problem is not the bodily expression of emotion but the patient's inability to make the connection between the emotion and the bodily sensations. In many patients, the understanding lies just below the level of consciousness, and the connection is soon made, given the right approach by the physician. Some patients, however, are resistant to any suggestion that their symptoms are the bodily expression of emotion. McDaniel, Campbell, and Seaburn (1990) describe this somatic fixation as "a process whereby a physician and/or a patient or family focuses exclusively and inappropriately on the somatic aspects of a complex problem." This formulation of McDaniel, Campbell, and Seaburn thus recognizes that the family may reinforce the patient's fixation and that the doctor's biomedical bias may result in unnecessary investigations and therapies.[3] The physician, too, is thought to have a role to play in avoiding somatic fixation through the appropriate use of consultation skills and a healthy patient–doctor relationship (Grol, 1981).

Yet it has been found that 2.5% of patients presenting with MUS meet the definition of chronicity (Verhaak, Meijer, Visser, and Wolters, 2006). Epstein and colleagues found that when physicians were faced with a new patient with MUS, they scored lower on measures of patient-centeredness (Epstein, Shields, and Meldrum, 2006). This means that those patients who stand to benefit a great deal from a patient-centered approach may not be helped, leading to their symptoms becoming chronic. We must change our concepts around the false dichotomy of mind and body to improve on this.

CONTEXT

"All communication necessitates context ... without context there is no meaning," wrote Gregory Bateson (1979, p. 16). One of the most difficult things for a physician is knowing what context to use in decoding the patient's message. The context we all internalize in the course of our training is the classification of diseases according to their organic pathology. If a patient is using symptoms as a form of indirect communication for a problem of living, correct decoding requires the physician to identify the context as a personal one. If the physician decodes the message using the context of physical pathology, the result may be a spurious diagnosis, with all its consequences. If the patient is also misreading the context, as is sometimes the case, the possibilities of misdiagnosis are even greater.

For family physicians, it is not sufficient to have one internal context for decoding patients' messages. They need to be very receptive to those information cues that indicate what context the patient's message is encoded in. These cues are referred to by Gregory Bateson as *metamessages*, messages that make other messages intelligible by putting them in context. Many of the illnesses encountered in family practice can only be understood by understanding their context. As in all human communication, decoding is not a once-and-for-all process. The decoder makes hypotheses, which he or she then proceeds to check by questions and observations.

In *Much Ado About Nothing*, Shakespeare provides an amusing example of the effect of a change of context on meaning.

Beatrice and Benedict have a teasing relationship, vying as to who can be more insulting to the other. Benedict's friends deceive him into thinking that Beatrice is really in love with him. No sooner has he come to believe this than Beatrice enters and says:

Against my will I am sent to bid you come in to dinner.

Instead of the usual insulting reply, Benedict answers:

Fair Beatrice, I thank you for your pains.

Beatrice: I took no more pains for those thanks than you take pains to thank me: if it had been painful I would not have come.

Benedict (after Beatrice has left): Ha. "Against my will I am sent to bid you come in to dinner," there's a double meaning in that. (Act 2, scene 3, lines 206–210).

[She really loves me.]

As with diagnoses, so with therapy; to be successful the physician has to work in the right context. To treat at the level of symptoms, when the problem is in the doctor–patient relationship, or the way a person's life is organized, will lead only to frustration. Shifting the attention from one context to the other may of course be a very difficult process, especially when the patient himself has decoded his illness incorrectly. Conversely, trying to shift the attention to the personal context when the problem *is* the symptom also leads to frustration. In patients with chronic headache, for example, the problem may be the symptom itself, and the attitudes and coping mechanisms developed by the patient. Even if the headaches originated in a problem of living, an attempt to shift the focus to this context after the symptom has become autonomous is usually not helpful.

CUES TO CONTEXT

The following cues should alert the physician to the possibility that he or she should be working in the personal and interpersonal rather than the clinical—pathological context:

- Frequent attendances with minor illnesses
- Frequent attendance with the same symptoms or with multiple complaints (Case 8.3)

CASE 8.3

A well-dressed young man of 19 came for the third time in 1 year with intercostal pain and tenderness. His age suggested that his problems might be those common to adolescence. When encouraged to talk, he revealed such despair that he had twice called the suicide prevention service. His father had died, he was unable to communicate with his mother, and he had no siblings or close friends. He was almost totally without supporting relationships at a critical stage in his development (see also Case 8.1).

- First attendance with a symptom that has been present for a long time
- Patient-initiated attendance with a chronic disease that does not appear to have changed
- Incongruity between the patient's distress and the comparatively minor nature of the symptoms
- Failure to recover in the expected time from an illness, injury, or operation
- Failure of reassurance to satisfy the patient for more than a short period
- Frequent visits by a parent with a child with minor problems (the child as a presenting symptom of illness in the parent)
- An adult patient with an accompanying relative
- Inability to make sense of the presenting problem.

CULTURE AND CONTEXT

One of the most important determinants of a person's interpretation of his or her illness and the expectations of the physician is the culture or subculture to which he or she belongs. Kleinman, Eisenberg, and Good (1978) have referred to this as "the cultural construction of clinical reality." It is difficult for physicians to accept that their construction of clinical reality, based on pathology, is only one of many possible constructions. If the patient's construction is different, and no attempt is made to reconcile the difference, the probable outcome will often be a breakdown of communication and a failure of treatment.

These difficulties are at their greatest when there is a very wide cultural gap between doctor and patient, as, for example, when the doctor is from the dominant culture and the patient an immigrant from a different ethnic and language group. It is a general principle of human communication that difficulties in communication increase with the cultural distance between the participants (Bochner, 1983). The difficulties arise both in verbal and non-verbal communication. It can be difficult to "read" the behavior of a person from a very different culture. It is difficult, for example, to detect depression in a patient from a widely different culture (see Chapter 13, "Depression"). Cultural differences are not only ethnic. Subcultural groups defined by age, social class, sex, education, occupation, or region may also experience cultural distance from each other, and therefore difficulties in communication. Medicine itself is a subculture with its own set of unstated assumptions and expectations. A patient entering this subculture is therefore in the same position as a traveler visiting a strange country. This puts the patient at a social disadvantage, as well as being made vulnerable by his or her illness and lack of medical knowledge. It is therefore the doctor's responsibility to be aware of potential communication difficulties and to do everything possible to mitigate them.

Although the process is difficult, a strange culture can be learned. The main problem confronting the learner is that the rules governing behavior in a culture are not explicit. Indigenous members of a cultural group learn the rules implicitly, beneath the level of awareness. Unless they have the rare ability to view their own culture from outside, indigenous members of a culture are not even aware that their behavior is governed by rules. The same applies to the assumptions of a culture: rarely are these made explicit. In the subculture of medicine, our own assumptions about what a disease is are not made explicit, and many physicians remain unaware that they are assumptions.

An illustration of the implicit rules governing behavior is the question of when a person may be addressed by his first name or by his last name without the title "Mr." The rules for first naming are quite different between Europe and North America. Yet, for a visitor, it is not easy to discover what the rules are. They are even different between occupation and age groups within the same culture. An elderly lady in my practice (IRMcW) was outraged at receiving a letter from the practice nurse, addressing her by her first name. To a young person in our culture, using first names is a sign of friendliness; to many older people it is an invasion of privacy. Using a person's last name alone is not an uncommon practice among European men. In North America, it would be considered impolite in some circles.

How can family physicians prevent failures of communication? They can make a practice of ascertaining patients' expectations in any clinical encounter. They can try to elicit patients' explanatory model of illness and the meaning their own illness has for them. These are important principles in the clinical method described in Chapter 9. Kleinman, Eisenberg, and Good (1978) suggest a set of questions designed to elicit the patient's explanatory model: What do you think has caused your problem? Why do you think it started when it did? What do you think your sickness does to you? How severe is it? What kind of treatment do you think you should receive? Other questions are designed to elicit the patient's therapeutic goals and the cultural meaning of the illness: What are the most important results you hope to receive from this treatment? What are the chief problems your sickness has caused you? What do you fear most about it?

These questions are designed to be tailored to the individual patient. The problem with direct questions, however, is that so often they do not elicit the information we need. We certainly need to have them available in our clinical method; even if we do not ask them of the patient, we should ask them of ourselves; but much of the information we seek will only come by attentive listening and responsiveness to the subtle cues by which patients convey their meaning. Unfortunately, physicians often don't respond to cues (Levinson,

Gorawara-Bhat, and Lamb, 2000), though recognizing and responding to cues is necessary for successful patient–doctor encounters (Gask and Underwood, 2002). They represent an invaluable tool for the family physician (olde Hartman and van Ravesteijn, 2008).

Physicians can also try to make their own expectations and assumptions explicit. If there are conflicts between their own expectations and those of the patient, they can deal with them wherever possible by negotiation rather than by confrontation. They can also try to coach their patients in how to be more effective in the subculture of medicine. Taking this approach, Greenfield, Kaplan, and Ware (1985) coached patients to ask questions and to negotiate medical decisions with their physicians. When compared with a control group receiving a standard educational session, these patients were more involved in the interaction with the physician and were twice as effective in obtaining information from him.

Family physicians as teachers of their patients will only be effective if they model the behavior they are trying to teach. For example, telling the patient to ask questions will not help unless the physician is open to receiving the questions, listens carefully to them, and takes them seriously.

HIGH- AND LOW-CONTEXT CULTURES

In his book *Beyond Culture*, anthropologist Edward Hall (1977) draws a distinction between high- and low-context communication. A high-context communication is one in which most of the information is in the context. The receiver of the information must, of course, be "programmed" to receive this information from the context. Because the context is usually implicit, rather than explicit, this implies a sharing of assumptions. A low-context communication is one in which most of the information is in the explicit code. The language of science and technology is low context. A paper on mathematics, physics, engineering, or immunology can be understood by a specialist in the field from any part of the world, regardless of context. The language of diplomacy is high context: the diplomat on the spot is usually much more reliable in decoding diplomatic messages than the bureaucrat in a distant office who has no knowledge of the country from which the message comes.

Similarly, cultures can be viewed as high, medium, or low context. In a high-context culture, much communication takes place implicitly. For this to occur, there must be a high level of mutual understanding and sharing of assumptions. High-context cultures, therefore, tend to be marked by long-term human relationships, homogeneity, and a low level of social mobility. Low-context cultures, on the other hand, tend to be complex, technologically advanced, and subject to rapid change.

Another perspective on these communication differences is provided by the Canadian scholar Harold Innis (1951), known for his theory of the bias of communication. This can be stated as follows. The things we pay attention to are strongly influenced by our technology of communication. Oral forms of communication favor continuity over time in communities bound together by custom, tradition, and kinship. Visual forms of communication favor the development of codified rules and laws, specialization, fragmentation, and bureaucracy. The act of translation from oral to written form involves abstraction. Much of the contextual richness of the original data is lost in the process.

Innis maintained that once we know the dominant communication technology of a culture, we will know the shaping force of its entire structure. The dominant technology produces a bias in the culture, of which the culture is usually not aware. The danger is that the bias may become so overwhelming as to be destructive. Communication technologies such as the Internet have profound effects on what and how we think and contain hidden assumptions about how the human mind works, and they have the ability to subtly shape our thinking processes (Carr, 2010).

If we view medicine from these perspectives, we believe that we see many of its subdivisions moving toward the low-context end of the spectrum. Attention is paid less to the patient's story than to the data abstracted from him or her: the computer printout, the biochemistry panel, the scan, the echocardiogram. There are only a limited number of things we can attend to at one time. If we have our attention fixed on a monitor, it is unlikely that we are listening with attention to the patient. Increasing specialization, in large and bureaucratic institutions, reduces the opportunities for long-term relationships to develop. A family practice that remains faithful to its origins should, on the other hand, be high-context. In a practice where the population is relatively stable, and the physician and patients are members of the same community, long-term relationships can develop, with all that this implies in shared assumptions.

Conveying and receiving information through context, Hall observes, is a way of dealing with information overload. If more information is carried in the context, less has to be carried in the coded message. It is a common experience that the better a physician knows the patient, the less need he or she feels for large quantities of data. There is no significant relationship between quantity of data and quality of care. But there are pitfalls in relying too much on the knowledge that comes from a long-term relationship. Sometimes it leads to unjustified assumptions that preempt communication. The fact that family practice is usually high-context may account for economies of time made by the family physician. In other words, time spent in building relationships may be time saved in communicating about episodic problems.

DIFFICULT RELATIONSHIPS

We are indebted to Dr. W. W. Weston for many of the observations in this section. Weston defines a difficult patient as one with whom the physician has trouble forming an effective working relationship. The long-term relationships with patients in general practice make this a particular problem for family physicians. Because therapeutic success depends so much on the relationship between doctor and patient, the inability to form a therapeutic relationship is usually a source of much frustration for the doctor. Paradoxically, failure of the relationship does not necessarily lead to its termination, so that dealing with the problem is a continuing struggle.

Difficult patients fall into a number of categories:

Patients who have developed a "somatic fixation," that is, who express personal distress in the form of somatic symptoms and refuse to believe that no organic disease is present. These are patients we perceive as working in the wrong context. They seek answers from the medical system and the answers they get are negative: negative tests and failed therapies. The medical system often fails them by reinforcing their context error. Negative answers usually do not deter them from seeking yet more tests and consultations with specialists. Little wonder that these patients often end up having unnecessary surgery.

Patients who abuse themselves with drugs or alcohol, or who use their diseases in a self-destructive way—for example, diabetics who induce attacks of ketoacidosis

Patients who have become dependent on prescription drugs

Patients who make excessive demands on us by frequent visits, out-of-hours calls, pressure for tests, medications, or referrals

Patients who move from doctor to doctor or who go to several doctors for the same problem, perhaps playing one off against the other

  Seductive patients

  Angry patients

  Some patients fall into more than one of the above categories.

Certain cues may alert the physician to a problem—or a potential problem—in his or her relationship with a patient. Some of these have already been described as cues to a context error.

A new patient who comes after leaving another physician (perhaps a whole series of them) and is extravagant in his praise for you, while expressing great hostility toward the former doctor. There may be immediate demands for action in the form of referrals or prescriptions.

Frequent visits for problems that never respond to treatment; persistent complaints of symptoms with repeatedly negative tests and unhelpful consultations with specialists. This was called by Balint (1964) "the fat envelope syndrome" after the bulging charts accumulated by these patients. These patients have also been called "heartsink patients"—identified by the feeling they evoke in the doctor (O'Dowd, 1988).

Disagreements over prescription drugs. These patients may be quite content as long as they receive their monthly prescription. Often this is requested by mail or phone, so that personal contact with the physician can be avoided. The relationship is placid on the surface but only remains so as long as the doctor confines questions to safe topics and does not try to change or discontinue the medications (Balint et al., 1970). The medication may be taken for a spurious diagnosis that goes back many years and for which no evidence can be found in the record.

Cues from our own feelings. Weston enjoins us to be curious about it when a patient becomes special to us in some way—evoking feelings of anxiety, pressure, boredom, or frustration—or when we particularly want to please and impress a patient.

Grant (1996) has observed that these relationships often become self-fulfilling prophecies. What patients fear most about the relationship is what they invite by their behavior. The doctor falls into the trap of responding automatically to the behavior, rather than to the patient's needs. What the patient fears most may be rejection. But his or her behavior, paradoxically, invites rejection, and the doctor, if unreflective, responds accordingly. After describing three examples, Grant (1996) writes:

> . . . it was almost a relief to acknowledge them as heartsink patients. It was much more of a challenge to acknowledge that I was part of the problem, part of a heartsink relationship. It was relatively easy to identify their contradictory behavior—it was much more difficult to acknowledge my destructive responses. And yet, they could not be denied. I rejected a man who feared rejection; I ignored a woman who feared not being heard; I fought for control with a man who feared losing it. Their behaviors as supplicant, martyr, and adversary, contradicted their needs. My impulsive responses, as tyrant, bored bystander and antagonist, reinforced their fears. It was only when I was able to look more critically at my own and my patients' behavior, as clinical data, without shame or blame, that I was able to formulate responses that stood a chance of breaking the heartsink cycles and of rewriting scripts that had been written many years before.

There is no easy solution to these difficulties. Physicians who can correctly identify the problem, however, and avoid the many pitfalls, may not only save themselves much frustration, but also in some cases help their patients, if in no other way than protecting them from harm.

Here are some general guidelines:

Try to avoid somatic fixation by dealing with it when it first occurs. If it is already established, try to shift the context by focusing on the patient as a person: life history, expectations, feelings, and relationships. Try to respond to the inner pain, of which the symptoms may be an expression.

Be cautious in prescribing narcotics for chronic or recurrent pain. Try to protect patients from harm in a medical system that is oriented toward physical pathology (from unnecessary tests, medication, or surgery).

Be alert for countertransference reactions in yourself, for example by responding to a needy patient with excessive attempts to please and pacify.

Do not overreact if a patient tests the relationship. Patients who have difficulty forming a relationship with a doctor usually have problems with other relationships, too. Sometimes they have experienced a whole series of rejections and betrayals. Their provocative behavior may be a way of testing the doctor to see if he or she will respond with a rejection, like everybody else. If the doctor can avoid this temptation, the ensuing relationship may be the patient's first experience of trust.

Be prepared to set limits—to the amount of time for visits, to the number of visits, and so on.

Involve colleagues in your management plan: the practice nurse and receptionist, and colleagues who take calls for you, will need to know what you expect of them. They may also have a useful contribution to make.

If conflictual relationships become persistent and pervasive in your practice, seek consultation or supervision.

Do not make things worse by being a "difficult" doctor. Sometimes the patient seems to be difficult, but the difficulty is really with the doctor, as in Case 8.4.

CASE 8.4

A resident expressed frustration with an elderly diabetic who had persistent glycosuria but would not cooperate in attempts to monitor his blood sugar or adjust his insulin. Eventually the resident was able to see that the problem was her own inability to accept the limited goals that were quite acceptable to the patient, and quite reasonable from his point of view.

INTERVIEWING

Interviewing[4] is a process by which one person, usually a professional, reaches an understanding of another, usually a patient or client. The same principles apply to any kind of interviewing, medical or nonmedical. Medical interviewing provides the context for history taking—the collection of information about the patient's problem. Interviewing is a process of communication, both verbal and nonverbal. It is much more than asking questions and receiving answers. "The question-and-answer technique may be of some value in determining favored detergents, toothpaste and deodorants," wrote Studs Terkel (1975, p. xxv), "but not in the discovery of men and women." It is this "discovery of men and women" that is the aim of interviewing. Questions must of course be asked, but what questions are asked, how they are asked, and how the answers are received will determine whether the interview achieves its aim.

Although the principles of interviewing are universal, their application in the conditions of family practice requires some comment. Even if family physicians are good managers, they cannot avoid working under pressure. In a normal working day, time for a lengthy interview is difficult to find. But there is a paradox here. If time in the short term is at a premium, in the long term it is abundant. Because of the continuing relationship, family physicians have ample opportunity to "discover" the men and women who are their patients. This has several implications. First, it means that physicians do not need to devote time to establishing rapport at every visit. Rapport has already been established and needs only to be maintained. Second, they start out with some personal knowledge of the patient. Third, the process of "discovery" does not need to be hurried.

The lack of short-term time exposes the family physician to certain pitfalls. Rather than giving the patient time to express himself or herself, the physician may resort to the question-and-answer method from the beginning of the interview. Although this may shorten the interview, it is often false economy, for the patient may then keep returning at intervals. One longer interview that accurately identifies the problem may take up less time than the aggregate of several shorter interviews that fail to do so. In their study of doctor–patient interviews in general practice, Byrne and Long (1976) found that dysfunctional interviews were significantly shorter than satisfactory interviews, and that less time in these interviews was devoted to finding out why the patient had come. Physicians who engage their patients in a patient-centered manner are more flexible, altering their manner in keeping with the patient's cues (Stewart, Brown, McWhinney, et al., 2014). Some visits are for routine items; others are much more laden with meaning (Miller, 1992). The skilled clinician is always alert to the nuances of the patient's presentation and adjusts her approach accordingly.

LISTENING

The greatest single fault in interviewing is probably the failure to let the patient tell his or her story. So often the talk is dried up by questions that divert the flow of conversation, by changes of subject, or by behavior in the physician that expresses lack of interest (thumbing through the records or glancing at a wristwatch). At the beginning of an interview, the physician should try, by every means possible, to encourage the patient to tell her own story in her own way.

Listening to the patient with undivided attention is a very difficult discipline. It requires intense concentration on everything the patient is trying to say, both verbally and nonverbally, overtly and through those very subtle cues by which patients convey meaning. It is so very easy to focus only on the content of a patient's utterance, and not on how it is said. If a patient with advanced cancer says, "I seem to have needed a lot more morphine recently," the physician can reply, "Yes, your needs have increased," or he or she can say, "Does that concern you?" The second response will probably lead to an unfolding of why the patient raised the issue. Possibly the patient views increased needs as the beginning of the end.

Attentive listening requires us to empty ourselves of personal concerns and distractions, and to set aside, for the moment, our preconceptions and frames of reference. Carl Rogers (1980) puts it very well:

I am now much more sensitive to the times when my emotions or fatigue make me a poor listener, for I find that my own inner hurts and anxiety, even suppressed, interfered with my really listening to another. (p. 45).

This kind of sensitive, active listening is exceedingly rare I our lives. We think we listen, but ver rarely do we listen with real understanding, true empathy. Yet listening of this very special kind, is onef the most potent forces for change that I know (p. 135).

Doctors, often, are not good listeners. We frequently interrupt. In one study, the average interval between the patient beginning to tell his story and the doctor interrupting was 18 seconds (Beckman and Frankel, 1984). A more recent study (Marvel, Epstein, Flowers, and Beckman, 1999) suggests that the situation may have slightly improved, with first interruption occurring after 23.1 seconds. Pursuing our own train of thought, we may not even hear the crucial remark:

Patient: And I often feel I could cry.

Doctor: Does the pain go anywhere else?

Questions from patients are often ignored or sidetracked. Interviews tend to be dominated by questions from the physician. There is a place for serial questions in the search for information, but simply asking questions is not a way of getting to know and understand a patient. It is a common experience to find that a patient who replies "no" when asked if he or she has any worries turns out to have major personal problems. So common is it that questions like "Have you any worries?" are of little value. Michael Balint wrote: "If you ask questions, you will get answers, and nothing else." One of the most common errors in interviewing is asking a question, then providing the answer before the patient has time to respond:

Doctor: How are you sleeping? All right?
Patient: Yes.

With very sick or elderly patients, the response may be a long time in coming. The doctor may have to listen in complete silence for up to a minute. Restraining oneself from interrupting in these circumstances is extremely difficult. An elderly man was dying of prostate cancer. His pain was under good control but he seemed to be very depressed:

Doctor: How do you feel today, Mr.?
Patient (pause of about a minute, then): Everything seems hopeless.
Doctor: Is any situation completely hopeless? Is there nothing you can hope for?
Patient: I would like to see my children settled.

Open expression by the patient can be encouraged by facilitation. This is a communication, not necessarily verbal, that encourages the patient to continue. A common example of this is repetition of the patient's last words:

Patient: I felt so awful. (Pause)
Doctor: You felt awful?

Gestures can have the same effect—leaning forward, closer to the patient, or slowly nodding the head. As in the example given earlier, silence can be facilitating.

If questions are needed, open-ended questions encourage expression by the patient more than closed questions. Consider the difference between "Where is your headache?" and "Could you tell me about your headache?" There is a place for both types: closed questions are for getting very specific information about the problem, and open-ended ones for reaching an understanding of the patient.

In some cases, expression by the patient may be helped by feedback of an observation in their behavior. In this way, the physician helps the patient face up to some aspect of his behavior, for example, "You look upset," or "You seem to be angry."

The effect of this is to bring feelings into the open, where they can be more effectively dealt with. The effect may be a flood of tears, or an outburst of anger. Whatever form it takes, emotion in the consulting room should be accepted and acknowledged without surprise or embarrassment, for it deepens insight and changes the level of the relationship. Crying can be responded to with empathetic listening and by reassurance that crying is nothing to be ashamed of. Relatives of the dying, for example, sometimes need permission to cry, especially if they are men who have been brought up to believe that men do not cry.

Anger is more difficult to deal with, especially if it is directed against the physician or one of his colleagues. Anger is natural in anybody whose life is disrupted by serious illness in herself or her family. If the physician can acknowledge the anger, without becoming angry himself or herself, the patient may come to an understanding of his or her feelings. If the physician has provoked in some way the patient's feelings, he or she can acknowledge the anger and explore the reasons for it. In family practice, actual or perceived delays in diagnosis may be a cause of anger. Given the insidious nature of many diseases, none of us can escape this at some time or other. Sometimes, the patient's anger is accompanied by the physician's feeling of discomfort and guilt. Often these feelings are acted out by doctor and patient avoiding each other. They are much better brought into the open and discussed.

The expression of feeling is often helped by touch. Little is said about touch in medical education. The hidden message is that touching patients is not permissible, except in the physical examination. Yet it has often been our experience that touching has helped patients to express their feelings.

> A 40-year-old woman dying of cancer seemed to be full of pent-up emotions. She complained of being "beside herself," but could not say why. She did not cry or express feeling of any kind. I (IRMcW) was sitting by her bedside encouraging her to talk without success. Then I (IRMcW) reached across and held her hand. Almost immediately she started to cry and express her feelings.

Touching, however, is not always appropriate. When and how to touch are questions requiring sensitive judgment of the patient's needs. In the following case, touch was misinterpreted by the patient and had negative results.

> I was discussing the question of resuscitation and artificial life support with a woman with advanced amyotrophic lateral sclerosis. During the discussion I (IRMcW) put my hand on her hand as it lay paralyzed across her chest. After I left her room, the nurse told me that she had become upset. The nurse assumed that the cause of her distress was the subject of our discussion but found that it was my touching her hand that had upset her. She had interpreted this as an expression of sympathy and did not want people to feel sorry for her.

CONNECTIONAL MOMENTS

Sometimes the obstacle to genuine communication between doctor and patient is the doctor himself or herself. A patient is not likely to open his heart to a doctor who is detached and objective. True reciprocity may come only when the doctor has shown that he or she, too, is human. Paul Tournier tells the story of a surgeon whose son died of a sarcoma. One day he was visiting a patient in the very room where his son had died. The patient was an old lady, inconsolable over the death of her daughter and bereft of the will to go on living. He tried to console her, to no avail. Then he said to her "Do you know, my son died in this room." The next day, the old lady dressed, put on her makeup, and walked out of the hospital.

In their book *Six Minutes for the Patient*, Michael and Enid Balint (1973) have described this sudden change in the relationship between doctor and patient as the "flash." Suchman and Matthews (1988) describe these as connectional experiences: moments of closeness and intimacy. They seem to occur when we cross the professional/patient boundary and begin to relate to a patient as a fellow human being. It may not be possible to make them happen, but we can probably prepare ourselves for them by avoiding the things that inhibit them. These seem to be our preoccupation with theory or the need to be "doing" something—though not knowing what to do or say—rather than simply being with the patient.

EMPATHY

Empathy is the capacity to enter into another person's experience. For the physician, it is the capacity to sense what it is like to be the patient: to experience illness, disability, depression, and so on. On other occasions, it may be the capacity to sense what it is like to be the person caring for the patient. This may seem like an impossible task. Some experiences are so different from the common run that nothing can prepare one for them. Many people have described bereavement in these terms. William Styron (1992) said the same about severe depression.

While accepting this, Toombs (1987) maintains that the alienation from the body experienced by the sick is accessible to others through everyday experience of the body as object. We all experience bodily symptoms, discomforts, and limitations, which, if reflected on, can open us to the experience of being alienated from one's own body. We can all gain some intimation of the difference between unconsciously "living" our bodies, and becoming aware of them as objects apart from ourselves. This understanding can be enriched by reading patients' narratives of illness and listening to their stories with openness to their experience.

Rudebeck (1992, p. 59) regards the capacity for bodily empathy as central to the general clinical competence of the family practitioner. Although empathy is usually understood as the professional route for the understanding of emotions, he observes that bodily processes play a part in the transfer of emotions from person to person. "Perception and intuitive imitation of facial expression and bodily posture are supposed to lead to an 'affective resonance,' including also a neuro-hormonal state. . . ." Thus bodily empathy is a route to the understanding of both the emotions and bodily experiences. The neurologist, Damasio, provides the neurobiological evidence for rooting emotions in the physiological processes of the body (Damasio, 2003). They are indeed two sides of the same coin. As Rudebeck also observes, the physical examination is an important vehicle for the exercise of bodily empathy.

The development of a capacity for bodily empathy requires a change in our perception of the clinical task. In the conventional clinical method, symptoms are conceived as avenues to the diagnosis of a patient's disease. We need also to see the patient's bodily discomforts as experiences to be understood in their own right (Rudebeck, 1992).

KEY QUESTIONS

Even after listening attentively and responding to all the cues given by the patient, we may still feel that some things have been left unsaid. We need questions that will help a patient to express himself or herself, perhaps by clearing away some inhibition.[5] It is sometimes said that asking questions about sensitive issues is an invasion of privacy. This can only be so if the question is poorly worded and if questioning is pursued against the patient's wishes. Even if a key question produces no response, it does at least convey to the patient that the doctor is open to such issues. Sometimes, as in the following case, failure to ask a sensitive question may have unfortunate consequences. The patient was a young woman who had just been released from prison to a halfway house. She complained of sore throat and fatigue and I (IRMcW) suspected early mononucleosis. I (IRMcW) asked no questions about her experience of prison or her feelings about her situation. The same evening she attempted suicide. She had been sentenced to prison for infanticide.

BREAKING BAD NEWS

Giving patients bad news is so difficult that we are often tempted to shy away from the task. We are afraid of being too frank; we fear the questions we might be asked; and we are afraid of the emotions that may be unleashed. There are many defense mechanisms we can invoke to avoid dealing with our fears. We can disguise the truth ("I think we got it all out"). We can put off the evil hour ("Let's do some more tests"). We can fail to respond to the subtle ways in which the patient opens the subject ("I seem to be getting weaker." "How are you sleeping?"). We can avoid the patient altogether, either by not visiting or by taking care not to see him alone. Nowhere have these defense mechanisms been better described than in Tolstoy's story "The Death of Ivan Illich."

We do not believe there is a single physician who has not used one of these maneuvers at some time or other, or who has not made mistakes in breaking bad news. It is something one has to struggle with. We have found some general principles to be helpful:

Never tell the patient something that is not true. At the same time, do not tell him more than he wants to know. The truth will emerge sooner or later, and, when it does, patients who have been lied to and misled will feel betrayed. Not surprisingly, the result is usually irreparable damage to the relationship between doctor and patient, and often damage to family relationships as well.

Applying these principles is not easy. How do we discover what the patient wants to know? First, we can find out what the patient knows, or at least suspects, already. Patients usually know much more than we think they do. In her study of patients dying of cancer, Elizabeth Kubler-Ross (1969) found that most patients knew that they were dying and did not need to be told. What they needed was the opportunity to discuss their feelings openly and without evasion. We find that the question "What is your understanding of your illness?" usually gives us a good insight into what the patient knows.

We find it helpful to let the patient ask the questions, so that we can follow where he or she leads:

"Do you have any questions about the gland that was removed from your neck?"
"Yes, what did it show?"
"You know why it was removed?"
"Yes, it was to see if the cancer had spread from my lung."
"Yes. It did show that there is cancer there. Is there anything you wanted to ask me about that?"
"Does that mean that the cancer is all through me?"
"No. It does mean that it has spread from the lung to the lymph glands, but your bone scan was normal—no sign of spread there—and there isn't any sign of spread elsewhere. With the chemotherapy you are starting, we are hoping that you will get a remission of the disease. Do you know what I mean by a remission?"
"Yes—the disease being arrested for a time."

"That's right. Any other questions at this point?"

"Not just now; I did have some, but I've forgotten."

"All right. I'll be back to see you on Thursday, so make a note of any other questions and we can discuss them then."

In this case, the patient already knew that he had cancer. When a serious diagnosis is being conveyed for the first time, one can get a feeling for how much information the patient wants by asking, "Are you the kind of person who likes to know all the facts?" When giving bad news for the first time, sometimes when it is not expected, pain is not avoidable. What can be avoided is any unnecessary addition to the patient's burden by insensitivity. Patients sometimes complain that information is given to them in a brutal fashion, as in the following instance, recounted to me by a patient:

"We've got the results of your tests and they show that you've got cancer of the kidney."

"What's going to happen to me?"

"We are going to have to remove your kidney."

"When will that be?"

"Tomorrow morning."

The pain of devastating news is mitigated somewhat if the doctor shows consideration for the patient's feelings, takes time to answer questions, and assures the patient of continuing support. Do not give bad news, then walk away. If possible, sit down with the patient. Take time. When you leave, try to ensure that there is somebody else with the patient. Assure the patient that you will see him or her again soon and will continue your support. Bad news should be given only in the context of a continuing, supportive relationship.

An openness to indirect communication is especially important when talking to patients with devastating illness. Rather than asking, "Am I going to die?" patients, for understandable reasons, may ask, "Is it serious?" or "Why do I feel so tired?" The temptation to evade the issue is great, for example:

"Why do I feel so tired? I've no energy."

"Let's do a blood test. Maybe your electrolytes are out of balance." Instead of

"Do you understand about your illness?"

"Yes, I know I have cancer."

"The disease itself will make you feel tired and lacking in energy."

"Does that mean it is progressing?"

"It is a progressive disease, so we must expect that. How rapidly or slowly it will progress I can't tell you. However, there are ways we can help the tiredness."

"How?"

"By relieving pain, by making sure you get a good night's sleep, by attending to your diet."

One of the ways people deal with devastating news is denial. Such is our capacity for denial that a person may not even remember being told that he or she has a fatal disease. Denial may precede the gradual acceptance of the facts, or it may be maintained to the end. When faced with denial, it is not our place to try to break it down. An individual's way of dealing with the crisis must be respected. There is no reason, however, that we should enter into the process of denial ourselves by reinforcing unrealistic expectations. If patients who are denying their illness ask questions, we should reply honestly.

When a patient's family learns that the prognosis is serious, they may insist that the patient not be told. This may be based on their loving understanding of the patient's wishes. On the other hand, it may be more an expression of their own fears. It places the doctor in a dilemma. How can we reconcile our secondary responsibility to the family with our primary obligation to be truthful to the patient? Our response to this is to tell the family that we will not impose the truth on the patient, but that we will not lie if the patient asks us questions. We also try to get family members to see what a strain this deception will put on their own relationship with the patient. The patient, who will almost certainly know that he or she is dying, will feel increasingly lonely and isolated, unable to share his or her feelings with those who are close to him or her.

The words we use in talking to patients will depend on the culture we are working in. Some words, in some cultures, may be so emotive that we cannot use them. Some words have associations for a patient that are quite different from the associations they have for us. I (IRMcW) once told a patient at a postpartum visit that she had superficial phlebitis in a varicose vein. Her husband came to see me later in great distress. His wife had seen her mother die of a pulmonary embolism arising from thrombophlebitis of the leg.

In some cultures, *cancer* is such a word. Other words have to be used as substitutes, but we should not see this as an excuse for using words that are evasive. If the patient uses an emotive word first, then we know that we can use it ourselves, remembering to ask what the word means to them:

"Is it cancer, doctor?"

"Yes, it is cancer. What is your understanding of that?"

"Does that mean I am not going to get better?"

"No. With this type of cancer you have a good chance of getting better."

If patients ask us how long they have to live, we never give them a specific time period. We do not think we should ever do so. Prognosis is a much less precise art than diagnosis. We are almost certain to be wrong, often by weeks, sometimes by months and years. The effects on patients and their families are usually negative. Hope diminishes, and they become increasingly anxious as the stated time approaches. The last guiding principle in giving bad news is to try to find some reason for hope in every patient. Even if it is not hope for survival, it may be hope for living until a task is completed or a grandchild born, or hope for a period of remission, or for a peaceful death without pain (Chapter 6).

REASSURANCE

As Kessel (1979) has written, "The utterance of reassurance should be as planned and deliberate as the use of any other medical skill." Although it is not possible to provide specific rules for the application of this skill, there are some principles that, if followed, will help the physician to be more effective in his reassurance and to avoid some errors and pitfalls.

1. The essential basis for effective reassurance is a trusting relationship between patient and doctor. The family physician starts out with the great advantage of having in many cases already established this relationship.
2. If reassurance is to be specific, the physician must know what the patient's anxieties are. Only then can he or she take the necessary steps to achieve reassurance. If a man with chest pain is worried about lung cancer, he will not be reassured if the physician tells him—on the basis of an ECG—that he does not have coronary heart disease. Specific reassurance requires that his anxiety be identified and the investigation directed toward it.
3. Premature reassurance is ineffective and may be interpreted by the patient as a rejection. The patient must be convinced that the physician has obtained the information necessary for reassurance. If a patient says, "Do you think this pain is anything to worry about?" it may be tempting to say, "No, it's nothing to worry about." It may be better, however, to say "It doesn't sound like anything serious, but before telling you there's nothing to worry about I'd like to ask you some more questions and examine you."
4. When reassurance can be given with confidence, it should not be delayed. A patient coming to hear the results of tests has little thought for anything but the news he or she is about to hear. Questions about how the patient is feeling will attract only partial attention. Better to start straight away with "Well, Mr. Smith, your X-rays are fine."
5. The patient's complaints—and his or her perception of them—should be taken seriously. It is very disturbing for a patient to be told, "There is nothing wrong with you." It suggests that he or she is malingering. Better to say,

"I can assure you that your symptoms are not due to cancer or any other serious disease." If this can be followed by a description of what is producing the symptoms, so much the better.

6. Some hope should always be given. This does not have to be false hope. Patients do not always want to be reassured that they will recover from their illness. They may have accepted permanent disability and need to be assured only that they will still be able to go for a walk, do their gardening, or engage in some other activity they enjoy. Even in terminal illness, the assurance that they will not suffer pain may be a source of comfort.

7. Emphasis should be given to the hopeful aspects of the condition. To say "Eighty percent of patients get back to normal activity with this disease," sounds very different from "Twenty percent of patients have some residual disability after this disease." The information is the same, but its effect on the patient can be quite different. We are sometimes so hesitant and negative in our reassurance, even with diseases carrying a good prognosis, that the patient is left in doubt and anxiety.

8. When the nature of the disease is explained, everyday language should be used, with checks to see that the patient has understood. We often forget that words we use every day have no meaning at all for many patients. I (IRMcW) once observed a resident explaining to a patient about the need for surgery for an aortic aneurysm. When the doctor had finished, the patient asked, "What is an aorta?"

The above principles apply to the assurance of patients with what we may call "normal" anxiety: the anxiety that a person naturally feels when faced with the threat of death or disability. With abnormal anxiety, reassurance is ineffective, for it will not relieve the anxiety. In these patients, anxiety is part of a more deep-seated disorder and must be dealt with differently.

DEPENDENCE

The long-term nature of the doctor–patient relationship in family practice means that some patients may become frequent attenders because of their dependency needs. Not all dependency is pathological. We are all dependent on others for support. At some times in our lives we have special needs, especially at times of crisis, grief, and illness. It is natural that many people turn to their family physician then. K. B. Thomas (1974) has used the term "temporarily dependent patient" for patients who come mainly to be supported during a period of stress, often only for one visit. Nigel Stott (1983) speaks of the "refuge role" of the family physician. Physicians also have their dependency needs. We have a need to be seen as a good doctor, to be sought after and liked by our patients.

It is not easy to avoid pathological dependency. When in doubt, most of us would probably risk dependency rather than fail to support a patient who really needed our help. No family physician can avoid having some patients who are chronically dependent. The most we can do is to be aware of the risk of pathological dependency in our patients and ourselves and to avoid fostering it.

NOTES

1. This issue is discussed in LJ Kirmayer's essay, Mind and body as metaphors: Hidden values in biomedicine. In: Lock M, Candon D, eds., *Biomedicine Examined* (Ondrecht: Kluwer, 1988).
2. The idea of somatization is only conceivable in a culture that views diseases as entities and assigns a different status to illnesses with no verifiable physical pathology. In medical traditions with a unitary view of illness—such as Ayurvedic and Chinese medicine—the idea of somatization would make no sense. See Horatio Fabrega's essay, Somatization in cultural and historical perspective. In: Kirmayer LJ, Robbins JM, eds., *Current Concepts of Somatization* (Washington: American Psychiatric Press, 1991). For a fuller discussion of these implications, see my (IRMcW) article, The importance of being different, *British Journal of General Practice* (1996), 46:433–436; and McWhinney IR, Epstein RM, Freeman T, Rethinking somatization, *Annals of Internal Medicine* (1997), 126(9):747–750.
3. For a good practical approach to somatic fixation, see <AU: please add author's name.>Integrating the mind-body split: A biopsychosocial approach to somatic fixation. In: McDaniel S, Campbell T, Seaburn D, eds., *Family Oriented Primary Care*, 2nd ed., chap. 19 (New York: Springer Verlag, 2005).
4. A number of comprehensive texts on interviewing are available. See, for example, Lipkin M, Carroll RM. Frankel R, Putnam S, eds., *The Medical Interview: Clinical Care, Education and Research* (New York: Springer Verlag, 2011); Enelow A, Forde DL, Brummel-Smith K, *Interviewing and Patient Care*, 4th ed. (New York: Oxford University Press, 1999); Coulehan JL, Block MR, *The Medical Interview: Mastering Skills for Clinical Practice* (Phildelphia: F. A. Davis, 2005).
5. For a strategy designed to systematically develop key questions see Malterud K, Key questions: A strategy for modifying clinical communication. *Scandinavian Journal of Primary Health Care* (1994), 12:121–127.

REFERENCES

Achkar E. 2006. The death of the chief complaint or how GERD replaced heartburn. *American Journal of Gastroenterology* 101:1719–1720.

Balint M. 1964. *The Doctor, His Patient and the Illness*. London: Pitman.

Balint M, Hunt J, Joyce R, Marinker M, Woodcock J. 1970. *Treatment or Diagnosis: A Study of Repeat Prescriptions in General Practice*. London: Tavistock Publications.

Balint M, Balint E. 1973. *Six Minutes for the Patient*. London: Tavistock Publications.

Bateson G. 1979. *Mind and Nature: A Necessary Unity*. New York: E. P. Dutton.

Beckman HB, Frankel RN. 1984. The effect of physician behaviour on the collection of data. *Annals of Internal Medicine* 101:692.

Bochner S. 1983. Doctors, patients and their cultures. In: Pendleton D, Hasler J, eds., *Doctor–Patient Communication*. London: Academic Press.

Brandt LJ. 2007. The lament of the chief complaint: Not one, not always, but a good conversational start. *American Journal of Gastroenterology* 102:485–486.

Burack RC, Carpenter RR. 1983. The predictive value of the presenting complaints. *Journal of Family Practice* 16:749.

Byrne PS, Long BEL. 1976. *Doctors Talking to Patients*. London: Her Majesty's Stationery Office.

Campbell J. 1982. *Grammatical Man: Information, Entropy, Language and Life*. New York: Simon and Schuster.

Carr N. 2010. *The Shallows: What the Internet Is Doing to our Brains*. New York: W. W. Norton.

Damasio A. 2003. *Looking for Spinoza: Joy, Sorrow and the Feeling Brain*. New York; London: Harcourt.

Duke WM, Barton L, Wolf-Klein GP. 1994. The chief complaint: Patient, caregiver and physician's perspectives. *Clinical Gerontologist* 14(4):3–11.

Epstein R, Shields CG, Meldrum SC, Fiscella K, Carroll J, Carney PA, Duberstein PR. 2006. Physicians' responses to patients' medically unexplained symptoms. *Psychosomatic Medicine* 68(2):269–276.

Gask L, Usherwood T. 2002. ABC of psychological medicine: The consultation. *BMJ* 324(7353):1567–1569.

Grant N. 1996. Heartsink relationships: Self-fulfilling prophecies and how to avoid them. Unpublished manuscript.

Greenfield S, Kaplan SH, Ware JE, Jr. 1985. Expanding patient involvement in care. *Annals of Internal Medicine* 102:520.

Grol R. 1981. *To Heal or to Harm: The Prevention of Somatic Fixation in General Practice*. London: Royal College of General Practitioners.

Hall ET. 1977. *Beyond Culture*. New York: Anchor Press/Doubleday.

Hannay DR. 1979. *The Symptom Iceberg: A Study in Community Health*. London: Routledge and Kegan Paul.

Hustvedt S. 2009. *The Shaking Woman or A History of My Nerves*. New York: Picador.

Innis HA. 1951. *The Bias of Communication*. Toronto: University of Toronto Press.

Kessel M. 1979. Reassurance. *Lancet* 1:1128.

Kleinman A, Eisenberg J, Good B. 1978. Culture, illness and care: Clinical lessons from anthropologic cross-cultural research. *Annals of Internal Medicine* 88:251.

Levinson W, Gorawara-Bhat R, Lamb J. 2000. A study of patient cues and physician responses in primary care and surgical settings. *Journal of the American Medical Association* 284(8):1021–1027.

Kubler-Ross E. 1969. *On Death and Dying*. New York: Macmillan.

McDaniel S, Campbell TL, Seaburn DB. 1990. *Family-Oriented Primary Care: A Manual for Medical Providers*. New York: Springer Verlag.

Marvel MK, Epstein RM, Flowers K, Beckman HB. 1999. Soliciting the patient's agenda: Have we improved? *Journal of the American Medical Association* 281(3): 283–287.

Miller WL. 1992. Routine, ceremony, or drama: An exploratory field study of the primary care clinical encounter. *Journal of Family Practice* 34(3):289–96.

O'Dowd TC. 1988. Five years of heartsink patients in general practice. *British Medical Journal* 297:528.

Olde Hartman T, van Ravesteijn H 2008. "Well doctor, it is all about how life is lived": Cues as a tool in the medical consultation. *Mental Health in Family Medicine* 5:183–187.

Peveler R, Kilkenny L, Kinmonth AL. 1997. Medically unexplained physical symptoms in primary care: A comparison of self-report screening questionnaires and clinical opinion. *Journal of Psychosomatic Research* 42(3):245–252.

Rogers C. 1980. *A Way of Being*. Boston, MA: Houghton-Mifflin.

Rudebeck CE. 1992. General practice and the dialogue of clinical practice. *Scandinavian Journal of Primary Health Care*. Supplement 1.

Stewart M, Brown JB, Weston WW, McWhinney IR, McWilliam CL, Freeman TR.2014. *Patient-Centered Medicine: Transforming the Clinical Method*, 3rd ed. London; New York: Radcliffe.

Stott NCH. 1983. *Primary Health Care*. Berlin: Springer Verlag.

Styron W. 1992. *Darkness Visible: A Memoir of Madness*. New York: Vintage Books.

Suchman A, Matthews D. 1988. What makes a doctor–patient relationship therapeutic? Exploring the connectional decisions of medical care. *Annals of Internal Medicine* 108:125.

Tennyson A. *In Memoriam* in The College Survey of English Literature Eds. Witherspoon, Whiting, Millett, Shepard, Hudson AP, Wagenknecht E, Untermeyer L. Harcourt, Brace and Company, New York. 1951.

Terkel S. 1975. *Working*. New York: Avon Books.

Thomas KB. 1974. The temporarily dependent patient. *British Medical Journal* 1:1327.

Toombs SK. 1987. The meaning of illness: A phenomenological approach to the patient–physician relationship. *Journal of Medicine and Philosophy* 12:219.

Verhaak PF, Meijer SA, Visser AP, Wolters G. 2006. Persistent presentation of medically unexplained symptoms in general practice. *Family Practice* 23(4):414–420.

CHAPTER 9

⌒∿⌒

Clinical Method

This chapter describes a clinical method that we believe to be both appropriate and necessary for family practice: the patient-centered clinical method. Its essence is the physician's attempt to fulfill a twofold task: understanding the patient and understanding his or her disease. From this understanding flows the process of therapy for both patient and disease. The process of diagnosing disease has been central in medical education for many years. So prominent has it been that students could be excused for thinking that this process was synonymous with clinical method. Understanding the patient and what the illness means to the patient has tended to be an afterthought, something added on after the diagnostic task has been completed. The patient-centered clinical method provides an integrated and systematic method for bringing together the patient and the disease.

For several reasons, family medicine has been at the forefront of attempts to develop a reformed clinical method. No disease-specific diagnosis is possible in 25%–50% of patient visits to family physicians. Only by understanding the patient and the patient–doctor relationship can we gain insight into these problems. Even when a physical diagnosis can be made, successful therapy often requires an understanding of the context of the disease. In Chapters 6 and 7 we have seen how important an understanding between doctor and patient is for healing. Other fields of medicine face these issues, too, but few to the same extent as family medicine.

The conceptual distinction between illness and disease helps us to understand the nature of the task (Fabrega, 1974). Illness is the patient's personal experience of a physical or psychological disturbance. It includes patients' sensations and feelings—especially their fears—disabilities and discomforts, attitudes toward their condition and toward the physician, the effect of the condition on their activities and relationships, the reasons for coming, their expectations, and their ideas. Disease is the pathological process physicians use as an explanatory model for illness. In family practice, we often encounter illness without a discernible pathological process—illness without disease. Illness without disease may be simply the inability of our existing methods to identify pathology. Disease and illness belong to two different universes of discourse: one to the world of theory, the other to the world of experience. In the vernacular, "illness is what you have when you go to the doctor; disease is what you have when you've seen the doctor." Illness and disease also belong to different levels of abstraction[1] and have different levels of meaning. Illness is the meaning for the patient's life; disease is the meaning in terms of pathology. All significant illness is multilevel,[2] and the patient-centered method aims to understand the illness at all its levels, from pathology to thoughts and feelings.

THE CONSULTATION

The consultation or clinical encounter—whether it takes place in the consulting room, the home, or the hospital—is the context for the patient-centered clinical method. In family practice, each consultation is one episode in a continuing relationship. There is much to be learned from consultation analysis, but we must always remember that in most cases, a single consultation is not the beginning or the end of the story for patient or doctor. Each new consultation carries over memories of previous ones; many consultations have some unfinished business to be taken up in due course. Some of this common memory of previous encounters is entered in the record and is available if the patient sees another doctor. Much of it, however, is tacit information that cannot easily be expressed in words.

A consultation may take many forms, in addition to the common one of presentation and assessment of a new complaint. It may be for follow-up of chronic illness, preventive procedures, counseling, the communication of test results or consultants' reports, examinations for administrative purposes, and so on. The patient may be alone or accompanied by a spouse, parent, adult child, or friend. In some cases, the consultation may take the form of a family conference. Some have more to do with the pastoral than the clinical aspect of general practice.

Some observers have classified consultations in terms of the process (Marinker, 1983; Miller, 1992). Miller describes four types: routine, drama, ceremony (transitional), and ceremony (maintenance). Routines are everyday family practice problems—acute infections, minor trauma, need for reassurance—that by mutual agreement are dealt with simply and rapidly. Dramas are encounters involving uncertainty, conflict, emotion, lack of common ground, family discord, or diagnosis of an illness with grave implications. Doctors try to recognize dramas early. Often, however, they unfold in the course of a routine visit. The doctor's aim in these cases is to allow the drama to start and to "buy time." This is accomplished by following four steps: the patient must know that the doctor believes him or her; the doctor must address the patient's greatest fears; he or she should perform some physical examination; and he or she should give the patient hope and something to do before the next visit. These consultations Miller describes as transitional ceremonies, whose purpose is to provide a transitional explanation and protect the patient from harm until a longer visit can be arranged.

Maintenance ceremonies are consultations that have settled into a regular, recurring pattern. These may be dramas that have resolved into a period of adjustment, visits for control of a chronic disease, or a periodic need for support and reassurance. Others are visits that physicians find disturbing: patients with chronic symptoms that do not respond to treatment, people with self-destructive tendencies, and those whose wants cannot be satisfied. Ceremonies are so called because of their ritualized, symbolic character. The same ritualized conversation, examination, or therapy may take place at each visit. Miller suggests that the physician in these consultations is acting like a shaman (see Chapter 7).

The type of consultation is usually identified by the doctor in its early stages. Typing depends on answering a number of questions: Why did the patient come? What does he or she want? What are the doctor's intuitive feelings based on past encounters? What mode of communication is the patient using?

THE HISTORY OF CLINICAL METHOD

Crookshank (1926) has described the development of diagnosis in terms of a tension between two schools of thought: the natural or descriptive and the conventional or academic. The natural, concerned with the organism and disease, attempts to describe the illness in all its dimensions, including its individual and personal features. The conventional, concerned with organs and diseases, attempts to classify and name the disease as an entity independent of the patient. The tension between these two schools of thought in each era of medicine has its counterpart in the controversy between the Coans and Cnidians in ancient Greece, the Coans being the natural, the Cnidians the conventional diagnosticians. The rival schools of Cos and Cnidus were said by "Boinet to stand for "the two great doctrines which recur ceaselessly across the centuries." (Crookshank, 1926, p. 995).

Each of the schools of thought is associated with a different theory of disease. The Coans saw the essential unity of all disease, with various presentations depending on personal and environmental factors; the Cnidians were concerned with the diversity of diseases and the distinctions between them. For the Coans, the purpose of diagnosis was descriptive—an assay of the patient's state. The classical account is given in the First Epidemics of Hippocrates, in which he says that he framed his judgments by paying attention to

> what was common to every and particular to each case; to the patient, the prescriber, and the prescription; to the epidemic constitution generally and in its local mood: to the habits of life and occupation of each patient; to his speech, conduct, silences, thoughts, sleep, wakefulness, and dreams—their content and incidence; to his pickings and scratchings, tears, stools, urine, spit and vomit; to earlier and later forms of illness in the same prevalence; to critical or fatal determinations; to sweat, chill, rigour, hiccup, sneezing, breathing, belching; to passage of wind, silently or with noise; to bleedings; and to piles. (Crookshank, 1926, p. 995).

For the Cnidians, the purpose of diagnosis was to classify the patient's illness in accordance with a taxonomy of diseases. To them, diseases had a reality independent of the patient. The Coans, on the other hand, did not separate the disease from the person, or the person from environment. The Coans employed individual description, the Cnidians abstraction and generalization. These differences were also reflected in attitudes toward therapy. The Cnidians employed the specific remedy deemed efficacious for the named disease. The Coans treated each patient individually and symptomatically, attempting to assist nature in restoring the functional unity of the organism. The Cnidians prescribed remedies, the Coans a regimen.

The differences between these two schools of thought are summarized in Table 9.1. Each has strengths and weaknesses. The strength of the conventional approach is its explanatory and predictive power in certain types of illness. Its weakness is that the schema used by physicians may so influence them that they miss individual features of the illness. There is an instructive parallel with art. In his book *Art and Illusion*, Gombrich (1960) discusses the

Table 9.1. DIFFERENCES BETWEEN THE COAN AND
CNIDIAN SCHOOLS OF THOUGHT

Cos	Cnidus
Organisms and illnesses	Organs and diseases
Individual description	Classification
Concrete	Abstract
High-context	Low-context
Holistic	Reductive
Regimen	Specific remedy

use of formulas in the training of artists, such as the schema for drawing the human head. The problem is that the schema may so influence artists' perception that they fail to notice the particular features of the head they are drawing. Using such a schema can block the path to effective portrayal unless it is accompanied by a constant willingness to correct and revise. Artists should use a schema only as a starting point that they will then clothe with flesh and blood. Similarly in medicine, a diagnostic schema should not be an end in itself, but a starting point that the physician will then clothe with flesh and blood.

The strength of the natural approach is its concreteness—the richness of its descriptions. Its weakness is that a distrust of classification and a focus on symptoms may lead to a failure to explore the origins of illness in more depth. The natural method suffers also because it is difficult to articulate. Natural diagnosticians tend to teach by example rather than by the spoken word.

The tension between the two schools of thought can be discerned in other ages. During the Renaissance, it was reflected in the controversy between the Hippocratists and the Galenists, summed up by Crookshank (1926) as one between a system founded on experience and a system founded on reason. In the seventeenth century, conventional diagnosis was greatly advanced by the work of Sydenham, who in turn was influenced by the Swedish biologist and systematizer Linnaeus, and by the philosopher John Locke. Like the best physicians in all ages, Sydenham had in him something of the natural and something of the conventional diagnostician. He was critical of the theoreticians who interpreted illness by reference to a priori theories that had little relation to clinical observation. Sydenham's method was to observe and record the phenomena of illness at the bedside, and this earned him the name "the English Hippocrates." On the other hand, he believed strongly in the existence of distinct disease entities, comparing them to the botanical species described by Linnaeus.

Using this method, Sydenham was able to separate a number of infectious diseases into distinct categories: measles, scarlet fever, smallpox, cholera, and dysentery. He distinguished gout from rheumatism and was the first to describe chorea. Sydenham followed the course of diseases over time and was therefore able to test his categories for their predictive power. This correlation of clinical categories with their course and outcome—the study of the natural history of disease—was an important innovation that was not followed by his immediate successors. Eighteenth-century physicians did continue to produce classifications of disease, but these were "uncorrelated catalogues of clinical manifestations . . . lacking the prognostic or anatomic significance that would make the results practical or useful" (Feinstein, 1967, p. 77). English physicians, on the whole, displayed little enthusiasm for these classifications and continued to regard diagnosis as a process applicable to persons rather than to diseases.

Early in the nineteenth century, clinical method took a sharp turn toward conventional diagnosis. The impetus for this turn came from the innovations of the French school of clinician-pathologists, who began to turn their attention to the physical examination of the patient. New instruments such as the Laennec stethoscope revealed a new range of clinical information. At the same time, clinicians examined the organs after death and correlated symptoms and physical signs with postmortem appearances. The result was a radically new classification of disease based on morbid anatomy—far more powerful than the nosologies of the eighteenth century. English physicians were so impressed with the result that they were soon converted to the new system. "To interpret in terms of specific diseases [became] almost the only duty of the diagnostician" (Crookshank, 1926, p. 940). Prior to this, the differentiation between mind and body, between anatomical changes and functional symptoms, was much less clearly delineated. For example, the term *angina* was originally a ". . . free-standing symptom-based functional disorder—a characteristic pattern of chest pain symptoms not connected to one organic lesion . . ." and eventually became known ". . . as symptom of a specific, anatomically defined disease: coronary artery obstruction leading to myocardial infarction." (Aronowitz, 2001, p. 84).

In the course of the nineteenth century, the new system led to the clinical method that has dominated medicine in our own day. The emergence of the method has been described by Tait (1979) in a study of clinical records at St. Bartholomew's Hospital, London, dating back to the early nineteenth century. The modern structure first appeared about 1850 in reports of necropsies. Then the physical examination and, in the 1880s, the medical history began to be recorded in their modern form. By the end of the century the evolution of the method as we know it was complete. The record was divided into presenting complaint, history of present condition, systems inquiry, and so on. The method aimed to provide students with a conceptual structure within which they could work rationally and methodically toward their goal—the formulation of a diagnosis in terms of organic pathology. For this purpose the student doctor's clinical attention was directed and made selective in character. In particular, its concentration on the special points needed to achieve a diagnosis in pathological terms did result in a relative neglect of the psychological and social aspects of illness (Tait, 1979).

In the early twentieth century, textbooks on clinical diagnosis began to appear. In 1926, Crookshank commented that these "gave excellent schemes for the physical examination of the patient, whilst strangely ignoring, almost completely, the psychical." (p. 941). The turn toward conventional diagnosis had gone so far that the other part of the clinician's task had been all but forgotten. Conventional diagnosis in its modern form is strictly objective. It does not aim, in any systematic way, to understand the meaning of the illness for the patient or to place it in the context of his or her life story or culture. The emotions are excluded from consideration; the physician is encouraged to be objective and detached. The objectivity of the method fits well with its nineteenth-century origins: it is, indeed, a product of the European Enlightenment.

The conventional method has been brilliantly successful in paving the way for the great therapeutic advances of the twentieth century. The application of these therapies required a diagnostic method with high predictive power. With its predictive power based on organic pathology, enhanced by new diagnostic technologies such as imaging, endoscopy, and chemistry, the new method provided that. Paradoxically, it is probably the successes of medical technology that have exposed so vividly the limitations of the modern method. Concentration on the technical aspects of care tends to divert us from the patient's inner world. The complexities and discomforts of modern therapeutics have, at the same time, made it even more important for us to understand the patient's experience.

Besides providing predictive power, the conventional method did two things that no clinical method had done before. It provided the clinician with a clear injunction: conduct the clinical inquiry in this way and you will either arrive at a physical diagnosis or exclude organic pathology. And it provided clear criteria for validation: the pathologist told the clinician whether he or she was right or wrong. The clinicopathological conference became the epitome of the process.

ATTEMPTS TO REFORM THE MODERN METHOD

As the limitations of the modern conventional method have become apparent, attempts have been made to develop new models.

In the 1950s, Michael Balint, a psychoanalyst, began to work with groups of general practitioners to explore the patient–doctor relationship. He was struck by the inadequacies of the conventional method for reaching any deep understanding of the patient's illness. The need was to listen, not to ask questions. Balint (1964) developed the concepts of attentive listening and responding to a patient's "offers" as means of reaching an understanding of his or her illness. He distinguished between traditional diagnosis, the search for pathology, and overall diagnosis, the attempt to understand the patient and the patient–doctor relationship. Balint also spoke of physicians themselves as powerful diagnostic and therapeutic tools and of the need to understand how to use them—hence the importance of self-knowledge in physicians.

In the 1970s and 1980s, George Engel (1980), from his experience as both internist and psychiatrist, developed the influential biopsychosocial model described in Chapter 6. This model requires the physician to consider and integrate information from several levels of the hierarchy of systems: from the *milieu intérieur*, from the person, and from the interpersonal level.

Kleinman and his colleagues (1978) have drawn attention to the frequency with which patients have explanatory models of illness that are discordant with the biomedical model. If the physician fails to explore the patient's understanding of illness, and to negotiate some rapprochement between the two models, the outcome is likely to be unsatisfactory. Although illustrated most vividly when the physician and patient come from different cultures, discordance can occur even within the same culture. Kleinman and his colleagues recommend a series of questions designed to attain this level of understanding, followed by an explanation of the doctor's interpretation of the illness, and, if necessary, a negotiation between the two views of clinical reality.

All these models have been attempts to develop a framework for a more patient-centered clinical method. So far, they seem to have had limited impact on clinical method as taught in the medical schools. One reason, we believe, is that they do not fulfill the requirements so successfully met by the conventional method. They do not provide a clear and relatively simple injunction to the physician, and they do not provide criteria for validation.

The method described here uses insights provided by Balint, Engel, and Kleinman, but goes further. It specifies the clinical task in simple terms and establishes criteria for validation. It was formulated as a clinical method and evaluated by Joseph Levenstein and a group of colleagues at the University of Western Ontario (Brown et al., 1986; Levenstein et al., 1986). The team has almost three decades of experience in developing, researching, and teaching the method (Stewart et al., 2014). The method has four integrated components:

1. Exploring health, disease, and the illness experience;
2. Understanding the whole person;
3. Finding common ground with the patient about the problem and its management;
4. Enhancing the patient–doctor relationship.

It is important not to think of the patient-centered method as a strictly defined process, with sequential stages and standardized procedures and interviewing styles. If the flow of the consultation is to follow the cues given by the patient, its course will depend on how and when these cues are given, and will vary from patient to patient. As with the conventional method, the main criterion of success is the outcome. Did the doctor reach an understanding of the patient's expectations and feelings and the social context of the illness? Was the clinical diagnosis correct? Was there an attempt to reach common ground? Did the therapeutic plan follow logically from the process? If the answer to any of these questions is "no," then one can look at the process to identify errors. If the answer to all of them is "yes," one may still examine the process for what may be learned from it, but whether certain items are right or wrong is unlikely to be a profitable discussion. Attempts to evaluate the consultation process in terms of right and wrong, without regard for the outcome, are liable to end in controversy; experts can often be found to differ. As with any practical art, there may be wrong ways of making a diagnosis or understanding a patient's illness, but there is no single right way.

THE PATIENT-CENTERED CLINICAL METHOD

Every patient who seeks help has expectations, based on his or her understanding of the illness. All patients have some feelings about their problem. Some fear is nearly always present in the medical encounter, even when the illness may seem to be minor: fear of the unknown, fear of death, fear of insanity, fear of disability, fear of rejection.

Understanding the patient's feelings, fears, ideas, expectations, and the impact of the illness on his or her daily functioning is specific for each patient. The meaning of the illness for the patient reflects his or her own unique world. Frames of reference from biological or behavioral science come from the doctor's world, not the patient's. They may help the physician to explain the problem, but they are not a substitute for understanding each patient as a unique individual.

The patient-centered clinical method, like the conventional method, gives the clinician a number of injunctions. "Ascertain the patient's expectations" recognizes the importance of knowing why the patient has come. "Understand and respond to the patient's feelings" acknowledges the crucial importance of the emotions. "Make or exclude a clinical diagnosis" recognizes the continuing power of correct classification. "Listen to the patient's story" recognizes the importance of narrative and context. "Seek common ground" enjoins us to mobilize the patient's own powers of healing. To these, we would add two others: "Monitor your own feelings." They may give you some vital cues; on the other hand, they may be anti-therapeutic (see Figure 9.1), and "pay attention to the patient–doctor relationship."

The key to the patient-centered method is to allow as much as possible to flow from the patient, including the expression of feeling. The crucial skills, described in Chapter 8, are those of attentive listening and responsiveness to those verbal and nonverbal cues by which patients express themselves. Failure to take up the patient's cues is a missed opportunity to gain insight into the illness. If cues do not provide the necessary lead, a question may help the patient to express feelings: "What is your understanding of your illness?" "What is it like for you to . . .?" or "Are you frightened . . .?" "What was going on when the symptoms started . . .?"

The following reconstructed example contrasts a visit that was not patient-centered with one that was patient-centered, for the same problem.[3]

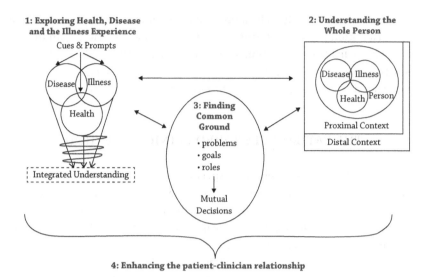

Figure 9.1:
The patient-centered clinical method applied. (Stewart M, Brown JB, Weston WW, McWhinney IR, McWilliam CL, Freeman TR. 2014. *Patient-Centered Medicine: Transforming the Clinical Method.* 3e Oxford UK, Radcliffe Medical Press Ltd.

A 55-year-old female patient has been told, 1 week ago by a replacement doctor, that her breast cancer has recurred. She returns to her family doctor for the initiation of her next phase of care.

Approach That Is Not Patient-Centered

Doctor: Um, Mrs. Collins, I believe we were to talk about, about ahem, your biopsy, is that right?

Patient: Yes, I came in to see earlier Dr. Armstrong in an appointment and he gave me my results a week ago.

Doctor: Um. Yeah, I remember that now . . .

Patient: Um, before we begin. It's just um, I've been on the Internet a lot this week, and talking to a few people and they made some suggestions about alternative procedures or treatments that might exist and . . .

Doctor: Excuse me.

Patient: Suggesting about fat and

Doctor: Let's find out exactly what's going on before you start thinking about all sorts of alternatives. . . . Um, I think the important thing now is to go over these plans. Are you clear on exactly what this means?

Patient: Um. I think I am, but I'd appreciate it if you could reiterate it to me.

Doctor: Basically, it means the cancer has recurred on the area of your chest wall and the biopsy was taken. Um, and what we have to determine now is whether that's the only recurrence or whether it has spread elsewhere in your body.

Patient: Um, you think it may have spread elsewhere?

Doctor: I don't know if it's spread elsewhere. So then we have to find that out and um, to do that, the first thing I'd like to do is just go over how you've been feeling in general the last little while. For example, how's your appetite been?

Patient: Well, this past week has been terrible. Uh, my husband's away and my only child, I have a daughter who's pregnant. I haven't told any of them about this. So, I'm not sleeping. I'm not eating and I feel terrified. . . .

(The doctor asks about cough, shortness of breath, nausea, vomiting, bowel movements, and pain in the abdomen.)

Patient: Um, my stomach hurts all the time.

Doctor: Any particular place? . . .

Patient: I, I really don't know. What does this got to do with any of this?

Doctor: Well, it's important to know the state of your health. So that's what I'm trying to establish so that we can go ahead and determine the best way to treat you. Um, Alright. You know when we're finished discussing these issues, I'm going to examine you. But um, in the mean time I think it's important we get some further tests and try and . . . once we do that we can discuss the treatment.

Patient: Treatment . . . What do you mean treatment?

Doctor: Well, treatment for your cancer. A lot will depend on whether it's localized or whether it's spread out.

Patient: Okay. Um, are you sure there's nothing else I can be doing right now? This is all so hard. I, I wasn't prepared for this. Is there something I could have done differently to have prevented this?

Doctor: There's nothing you can do to prevent this. Nothing you can do to prevent anyway. The important thing is to find out exact state of the cancer so that we can determine optimal treatment. And that's . . .

Patient: Are you talking about chemotherapy again?

Doctor: Ah, well chemotherapy is possible. It depends on where the tumor is. And we really prematurely discussed that and I just want to establish we don't know. There's so many treatment options depending on the nature of the cancer. And we don't know that.

Patient: I don't want to die right now. I have a granddaughter coming and I want to do things with my husband. I, I just don't want to die right now.

Doctor: Mrs. Collins, of course you don't. I think what you really need is to get some help. And I have here a couple of organizations that can be very helpful for you. The Canadian Breast Cancer Foundation, got their phone number. The Canadian Cancer Society has a self-help group. Why don't you take these brochures and give them a call and um forget the tests. I'll get my secretary to book them. And I'll see you as soon as we get them.

Patient: Okay.

Doctor: So, all clear now?

Patient: I suppose so.

The Patient-Centered Approach

Doctor: Good morning, Mrs. Collins.

Patient: Good morning, Doctor.

Doctor: This must have been a terrible week for you.

Patient: It's been dreadful, absolutely.

Doctor: Can you tell me a bit about it?

Patient: Well, of course, Dr. Armstrong gave me the news last week.

Doctor: Yes, I know.

Patient: And, ah, I wasn't expecting this, but, ah three years ago I went through it and I guess this is my worst nightmare. I, I'm a wreck. I haven't slept, I haven't eaten. Sam's in Europe on business. I haven't talked to Helen, I don't want to upset her, she's four months pregnant. And I just feel like my world is falling apart.

Doctor: Have you talked to Sam?

Patient: No I haven't, ah, other than on the phone. I haven't told him. I haven't told him . . . I don't want to worry him I guess. There's no point. He's got things to do.

Doctor: But if he had cancer, wouldn't you want to know? . . .

Patient: Perhaps, perhaps you're right. Listen um, during this week though, because I'm at home alone, I've been doing some reading and doing some Internet searches and there's a lot of talk in alternative medical circles about shark's cartilage, perhaps too much fat in the diet. Is there something I could have done, is there something I can do now, um, is there anything at all I can do to feel like I am in some control here?

Doctor: Okay. So you've been doing a lot of reading and been preparing stuff over the Internet.

Patient: Yeah.

Doctor: Look, ah with respect . . . I don't think you've done anything to bring this on. The issue of alternative medicine and what to do about it is not something that I'm very familiar with but I think that at times it's very helpful to people. But I would suggest we might just put this on hold for a short period of time until we really clarify what's going on.

Patient: Okay.

Doctor: I think we could, because I think the issue now is, as you know, the biopsy showed that the cancer had reoccurred on the chest wall.

Patient: Yeah.

Doctor: And one of the issues that we have to address is, has it spread anywhere else? Now it may well not have . . . but I think it's important that we make sure because how we treat you is going to depend on the results of that sort of . . .

Patient: Treatment, what do you mean?

Doctor: Well, there are a variety of ways of treating breast cancer which has recurred . . . (Pause and seeing her shoulders slump). That is certainly not the kind of thing I hope you have to have.

Patient: (Crying) I just don't know why?

Doctor: I know.

Patient: This is just so wrong. It's just the wrong time. I don't want to die. I, I want to live to see my grand daughter. I want to retire with my husband. I want to do everything that I've worked all my life to do.

Doctor: Mrs. Collins, I wish I could tell you 100% that you are not going to die of this cancer. And even if we find out that the tumor has spread, there are excellent treatments that can give you many years of usable life. But I can't tell you that for sure or not because I don't know the extent to which the tumor has spread. If not . . .

Patient: How do I find out the extent to which it's spread? What do we do?

Doctor: Well, we do three things . . . (Doctor enumerates the three things). But what I'd like you to do is tell me how you've been in general, not in the last week, because obviously the last week everything's been chaos. But before that, were you feeling reasonably well before you . . .

Patient: Yeah, reasonably well.

Doctor: Okay. Had you lost any weight?

Patient: No, not that I, no I don't think so.

Doctor: Was your appetite okay?

Patient: Good, normal.

Doctor: No nausea or vomiting?

(Doctor covers the history and several tests.)

Doctor: Now, when is Sam coming back?

Patient: He should be by the end of the week.

Doctor: Why don't you call him? (pause) Or would you like me to call him?

Patient: Um, That might work better, I don't want to right now. (sigh) Oh, God, I'll do it. I'll do it.

Doctor: My guess is he will want you to share this with him and I'm sure he'll want to be here to help you out.

Patient: I guess I just kept hoping it would go away. Denial again, I guess.

Doctor: Okay. Um, is there anything else right now that I can do to help you out?

Patient: Well, I guess just . . . no . . . I mentioned the alternative things and you said that we can proceed on some of that according to the results, is that . . .

Doctor: Well, yeah, I thought that when we . . . By all means, you know, look up what you want and if there's anything in particular that you wish to pursue, I'd appreciate if you'd bring it to me . . .

Patient: Okay . . .

Doctor: And, I'd really like to see you later this week. I won't have the test results but this is a pretty stressful time.

Patient: Yeah.

Doctor: I think it will help to talk a little bit more about how you're feeling and what we can do about it.

Patient: Okay, thank you.

In the example of not being patient-centered, the physician initially cuts off the patient's ideas about alternative treatments. He states his agenda and preempts the patient's description of her terrible week, her isolation from her family, and her feelings of terror. When the patient questions the relevance to her concerns of the physician's history-taking, the physician ignores the cue and defends his approach, continuing to the end in an unfeeling manner.

In the patient-centered example, the physician immediately acknowledges the patient's suffering. The physician allows the consultation to be guided by the patient's issues, her husband's absence, and her search for control through considering alternative treatments. He responds to her emotions, after which she expresses a readiness to discuss the history, tests, and treatment. He ends with an offer of a return visit to talk about her feelings.

The patient-centered approach is also illustrated in Case 9.1.

The process in this case is shown as a flow diagram in Figure 9.2. In addressing the patient's agenda, the physician is formulating and testing hypotheses based on the cues he or she receives and on the previous knowledge of the patient or of the symptoms. To an experienced physician, some symptoms are associated with particular fears, such as the fear of

---

CASE 9.1

An elderly woman complained of a suffocating feeling in the chest, occurring in the early hours of the morning, which was relieved to some extent by sitting by an open window. She first came in the middle of a busy office session when time was short. Given the above cues, the doctor formed a first hypothesis of nocturnal cardiac asthma, and after a physical examination revealed no signs to support the diagnosis, sent the patient for a chest X-ray. When this too was normal, he asked the patient to come in for a longer interview.

On this occasion he obtained the following history. Her main complaint was of very active peristalsis and abdominal discomfort occurring at night and keeping her awake. After lying awake for hours she would get more and more tense, get a suffocating feeling, and have to get up and go to the window. The abdominal symptoms had been present for 20 years, but the insomnia was of more recent origin. Many years previously she had had a cholecystectomy, which failed to relieve her symptoms, and a mastectomy for carcinoma. She had a fear of surgery and on direct questioning admitted to an anxiety that her abdominal symptoms might be due to cancer. She had been widowed several years and lived in an apartment by herself. Recently her landlord had raised her rent without giving her any notice. Her two children were both married and living away. Recently, her daughter had moved near her after living away for some years. During the interview, she expressed hostility toward her landlord, who, she felt, had been very unfair to her.

---

cancer. This knowledge may enable the physician to identify the patient's fears very rapidly. But we must always guard against the fallacy of treating a hypothesis as an assumption. In the previous example, the doctor-centered physician assumed without attempting validation that the main item on the patient's agenda was to follow-up on her surgery. This is a common pitfall with doctor-initiated visits of all kinds (Stewart, McWhinney, and Buck, 1979).

Five questions are commonly asked about the patient-centered clinical method. First, is it always necessary to use the method? Suppose the problem is very straightforward: an injury, for example, or an uncomplicated infectious disease. The answer is that we do not know unless we ask. Patients have fears and fantasies even about common and minor problems. In emergencies, of course, the medical priority must take precedence, as in the above-mentioned clinical example. But when these needs have been met, no patient is in greater need of being listened to than the one with sudden and severe acute illness or trauma.

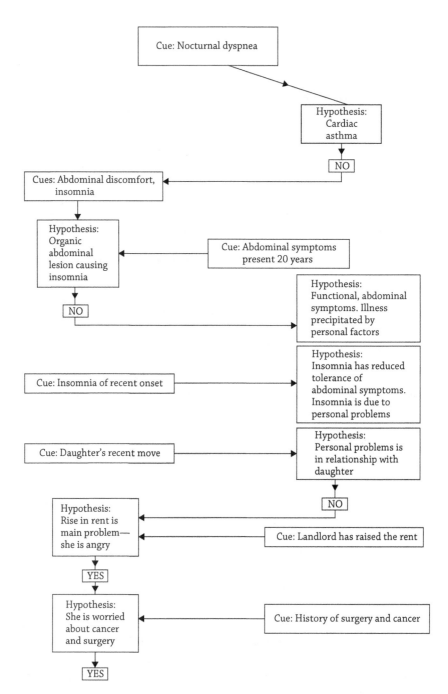

Figure 9.2:
Flow diagram to illustrate hypothesis testing in Case 9.1.

Second, what if there is a conflict between the patient's expectations and the medical assessment? Suppose, for example, that a patient wishes to manage his diabetic ketoacidosis without admission to the hospital. The physician must then try to reconcile the two conflicting views. The more the physician can understand about the reasons for the patient's position, the more chance there will be of a satisfactory conclusion. The reluctance to go into the hospital, for example, may be caused by a feeling of responsibility for a child or elderly parent. In some cases, there will be an irreconcilable conflict, as in a demand for a narcotic drug, and the physician will have to refuse to meet the patient's expectations. In the more usual situation, doctor and patient have different interpretations of the illness or conflicting notions about its management. The patient, believing that the pain indicates an organic disease, cannot accept the doctor's view that this is not the case. The doctor is reluctant to prescribe oxycodone tablets for a patient who finds they relieve his periodic headaches. Our contribution to reconciling conflicting views is threefold. First, we can acknowledge the validity of the patient's experience and take his or her interpretation seriously, even if we cannot accept it. Second, we can be aware of the danger that our own prejudice, rigidity, dogmatism, or faulty logic may be the cause of the difference. A mild narcotic used occasionally by a sensible person may be an appropriate remedy for headaches. The patient's interpretation of his or her symptoms may be more correct than the physician's. Third, we can make sure that the patient has all the information we can provide. Conversely, some humility may be called for, as when a very well-informed patient knows more than we do about his or her condition.

The third common question is whether there is a risk of invading the patient's privacy. Suppose the patient does not want to, or is not ready to, reveal her secrets? If privacy is invaded, then the method has been misunderstood. The essence of it is that the doctor responds to cues given by the patient, allows and encourages expression, but does not force it. If cues are not given, feelings are explored with general questions that invite openness. If the patient does not wish to respond, the matter is not pursued. At least the doctor has indicated that such matters are admissible.

Fourth, what about the time problem? How can we afford the time to listen to the patient? It is difficult to answer this, because little research has been done on the relation between consultation time, clinical method, and effectiveness. From work done so far, we can say tentatively that patient-centered consultations take a little longer, but not much longer, than doctor-centered ones. Beckman and Frankel (1984) found that when patients are uninterrupted, their opening statements lasted only 2.5 minutes on the average. Stewart et al. (2014) reported that 9 minutes or more was the critical duration for patient-centered consultations. What we do not know is how much time is saved in the long run by an early and accurate identification of the patient's problems. Our hunch is that the patient-centered clinical method will prove to be a time-saver in the long run.

Fifth, what if the doctor opens up a host of psychological, emotional, and social problems that he or she is not able to deal with? This is closely related to the time issue, but it is also the case that sometimes physicians eschew emotionally laden encounters in the midst of a busy day. Physicians, by their nature feel compelled to offer an intervention, but for some human suffering, such as great and tragic loss, no effective intervention is available. In these situations, simply bearing witness to the suffering is what is needed.

Sixth, a patient-centered clinician does not ignore medical knowledge of disease processes and treatments. This basic knowledge is necessary, but not sufficient, in making a diagnosis. What is required is an integrated understanding of the whole person at all levels (biological, psychological, social, and spiritual). The challenge for the physician is to know at which level(s) to intervene at any given time, keeping in perspective that, over time, all levels need to be considered for a full understanding.

It is important to distinguish between active and passive listening. Attentive listening, as described on, is not a commitment to listen indefinitely to a rambling monologue. That would be passive listening. A flow of words usually expresses something, even if its significance is the feeling rather than the content. A response to the feeling may enable the patient to express herself in a different way. Making a home visit to a 90-year-old man with lung cancer, I (IRMcW) was detained by his wife, who went on at great length about what she tried to get her husband to eat. Eventually I broke off the conversation and left. As I was driving away, the penny dropped. Surely she was trying to express her feeling of impotence at being unable to care for her husband in the way she believed to be best.

VALIDATION

The ultimate validation of a diagnosis in the conventional clinical method is the pathologist's report. In the clinico-pathological conferences modeled by *The New England Journal of Medicine*, a clinician is presented with a case report and develops a differential diagnosis, which is then confirmed (or otherwise) by a pathologist. The clinico-pathological conference can be regarded as the quintessence of the conventional method. Other forms of validation are available, notably the response to therapy and the outcome of illness.

The ultimate validation of the patient-centered method is also the patient's report that his or her feelings and concerns have been acknowledged and responded to. This may be ascertained by qualitative studies and by periodic surveys of patients, using validated questionnaires such as the one produced by Stewart et al. (2014). In the normal course of practice, validation comes from the natural history of the illness and the patient–doctor relationship. If common ground has been attained, therapy is likely to go more smoothly, reassurance to be more effective, and the relationship to be free from tension.

Physicians wishing to have some external validation of their clinical method may choose to have their consultations evaluated by an observer using one of the rating scales developed for this purpose (Brown et al., 2001). If these are used as a basis for coaching by an experienced teacher, they can be a source of valuable insights. It is difficult for any of us to be fully aware of recurring faults in our clinical practice. Until the coming of audio and video recording technologies, the consultation—the central event of family practice—remained hidden from view. After-the-fact reporting of the process could not possibly convey its nuances. An observer in the same room was liable to change the process, and discussion afterward was limited by the inability to verify the observer's recollection of the process by recourse to a recording. Thanks to the evolving technology, all of us can now develop as clinical artists in the way that artists have always learned—by submitting our work to the judgment of a respected teacher.

LEARNING THE PATIENT-CENTERED METHOD

It is important to distinguish between the process by which physicians learn a clinical method and the process by which they practice it. To assist learning, the process is broken down into a number of rules, tasks, and stages. A systematic review of 43 randomized studies designed to train providers in how to share control and decision-making with patients (elements of the patient-centered method), found that short-term training (less than 10 hours) was as effective as longer training (Dwamena, Holmes-Rovner, Gaulden, et al., 2013). However, learning these components is not the same as acquiring the process itself. No list of components can include all the tacit knowledge that can only be acquired by experiencing and "dwelling in" the process. One problem faced by the student is that it is impossible to be aware of the components and the whole process at the same time. Polanyi (1962) has clarified this issue by distinguishing between focal and subsidiary awareness. Focal awareness is awareness of the process as a whole. Subsidiary awareness is awareness of the components.

Riding a bicycle can be described in terms of rules for correcting imbalance and of the adjustments made by the body in response to changes in equilibrium. Learning the rules, however, is not the same as riding a bicycle, because the rules cannot embody all the tacit knowledge involved in performing the task. To perform the task, one must be focally aware of the whole process while remaining only subsidiarily aware of the components. Focusing on the components may actually cause one to fall off the bicycle. Similarly, when practicing a clinical method, one cannot do so while trying to keep in mind the subsidiary rules and components. These can be learned beforehand and referred to afterward, but in the performance of the task they must remain at the level of subsidiary awareness. The tension between these two levels of awareness, and the need to alternate between them, can be difficult for students at first. When the skill is acquired, the tension resolves. The doctor "dwells in" the process, and focal awareness is maintained throughout. Subsidiary awareness is brought into being only when teaching the skill to somebody else or when reviewing one's own process after the fact.

Case presentations are an important learning and teaching tool and were recognized as such in the late nineteenth century by Walter Cannon (1890). The traditional format of the case presentation has evolved over the century since that time, taking into account new and emerging ideas such as the problem-oriented medical record (Weed, 1969) and the biopsychosocial model of Engel (1977). Presentation of case histories are an important part of the medical training of students and residents, and it has been pointed out that the decisions of what material to present and its organization are powerful reinforcements of a particular worldview (Anspach, 1988). Typically, the conventional case history leaves out the more personal aspects of the patient, including the lived experience of the individual. There is an overwhelming focus on the disease to the exclusion of everything else. Attempts to correct this imbalance include the use of patient stories to increase physician empathy (Charon, 1986; Donnelly, 1989). Narrative-based medicine has developed an extensive literature (Greenhalgh and Hurwitz, 1998; Charon, 2001).

The Clinical Crossroads section of the *Journal of the American Medical Association* has been a welcome change to the usual case history and includes the patient's firsthand account (Winker, 2006). The patient-centered case presentation has been used to reinforce the patient-centered approach in the education of residents in family medicine (Freeman, 2014). It explicitly requires the presenter to address a couple of areas not found in the conventional case history. These include the patient's illness experience with an appropriate quotation, if possible, and comment on the patient–doctor relationship and whether common ground was achieved. By placing the patient at the core of the report, the patient-centered case presentation reinforces the primacy of the person rather than the disease. Without sacrificing the information found in the conventional case history, it supports the values inherent in the patient-centered method.

Case books are another way of describing and reinforcing the principles of the patient-centered method (Borkan, Reis, Steinmetz, and Medalie, 1999; Brown, Stewart, and Weston, 2002).

EVALUATION OF THE PATIENT-CENTERED METHOD

Some studies have been critical of the patient-centered clinical method, but have misunderstood the method. For example, in one study (Lussier, Richard, 2008), patients were asked to choose their preference from several consulting styles, one of which was the patient-centered method. Patients were then numbered according to their preferred style. The authors inferred that some patients do not want the patient-centred clinical method. This is not correct. The physician conducts the consultation in accordance with the cues he or she receives from the patient. There are no "styles" of clinical method, any more than there are styles of biomedical approach. Patients are not given a choice between what tests they have.

In contrast, Little et al.'s (2001a, 2001b) series of studies in the United Kingdom revealed that over 75% of patients wanted a patient-centered approach. In addition, patients valued highly all three of the components studied. In the Patient-Centered Care and Outcomes Study, patients frequently expressed elements of the illness experience such as ideas (89%), expectations (72%), problems with functioning (57%), context issues (55%), and feelings (42%) (Stewart et al., 2014).

Recent reviews of outcome studies of patient-centered care, measured in a variety of ways, have revealed benefits to the doctor, the patient, and the system. Benefits to doctors include higher doctor satisfaction, better use of time, and fewer complaints from patients. Benefits to patients include higher patient satisfaction and better patient adherence (Stewart et al., 2003, chapter 17). Benefits to the system include fewer diagnostic tests, fewer referrals (Stewart et al., 2000), and fewer return visits (Campbell et al., 2005). The method has been found to be associated with significantly lower costs to the healthcare system (Stewart, Ryan, and Bodea, 2011).

However, the most stringent validation is the patient self-report and patient health status. Studies have found patient-centered care to correlate with patient self-report and patient health status in a cohort study (Stewart et al., 2000) and to influence patients feeling better in a randomized controlled trial (Stewart et al., 2007).

The systematic review by Griffin et al. (2004) found that most of the 35 interventions—to improve patient-centered care—increased scores on patient–doctor communication, and slightly more than half improved patient's health, such as resolution of symptoms, headache, sore throat, anxiety distress, and physiologic status.

Furthermore, studies confirm the positive influence of patient-centered care internationally, in Spain (Moral, Almo, Jurado, and de Torres, 2001), South Africa (Henbest and Fehrsen, 1992), and China (Ge and Stewart, 2006).

THE PATIENT-CENTERED METHOD IN FAMILY PRACTICE

Like the conventional method, the patient-centered method is applied some-what differently in each field of medicine. Because family doctors are available for all types of problems, they can make no prior assumptions about why the patient has come (the reason for the encounter). Nor can they assume that the first problem presented is the main problem. In the early part of the consultation, therefore, they will be forming hypotheses about the patient's reason for coming and the patient's expectations, while formulating the problem to be addressed. The hypotheses will be based on cues from the patient's expressions and body language, as well as any intuitions from previous knowledge of the patient. As the patient talks, the doctor will be assessing the significance of the presenting symptoms. On this assessment will depend hypotheses about whether the symptoms signify a minor clinical problem, a major clinical problem (perhaps urgent), a problem of living presenting as symptoms, or a need for reassurance.

Putting all these together into a global assessment, the physician should have an idea of what course the consultation is likely to take. The original hypotheses, of course, may be wrong, and it may take an unexpected turn. In Cases 9.1 and 4.1, the initial hypothesis of an urgent clinical problem proved to be incorrect, and the focus shifted to the patient's emotions and relationships. In Cases 8.1 and 8.3, the mode of presentation, together with the doctor's previous knowledge of the patient, pointed to emotional distress. In Case 4.3, the symptoms and the doctor's knowledge of the family correctly indicated stressful family relationships. In Case 4.2, early hypotheses of a major psychiatric disorder proved incorrect on testing.

There is no predetermined order in the consultation. It does not flow in a uniform fashion from history of present condition through to systems inquiry and examination. The order is mutually guided by the patient's presentation and the doctor's response. It is an important principle of the patient-centered method that the doctor should in most cases allow the patient to determine the flow. "I think I can feel a lump in my breast" will lead very quickly to a history, and examination, followed by an exploration of the patient's feelings and fears. For a skin rash, history, examination, and exploration of feelings will probably occur together. The physical examination reveals more than physical signs. From the beginning of the consultation, the doctor is noting the patient's body language: posture, gait, movements, and facial expressions. Bodily habitus is often reflective of the multiple contexts in which people live, their social position, and the material conditions of their lives (Gatrell and Elliott, 2009, p. 19). Sometimes, the deepest feelings are not expressed until a painful area is palpated. Rudebeck (1992) writes,

When moving from dialogue to examination it is assumed that the symptom has been quite well defined by the doctor. However, the patient continues to present her symptoms by vegetative and muscular reactions, by the look of her face, by gestures and bodily posture.

It is not uncommon that spirit and meaning enter into communication precisely at the moment of examination. The doctor must not abandon the patient at this point and turn his attention to the possible disease.

Nor is therapy left only to the end. The whole consultation is part of the therapeutic process.

SYMPTOMS

Symptoms are the patient's way of expressing his or her experience of the illness. A bodily sensation, with its affective coloring, is translated into language. Because patients describing their own symptoms are saying something about themselves, their language always has an expressive as well as a literal meaning. The important meaning may be the literal one, or the expressive one, or both. Symptoms that fit closely with a well-defined disease category have a literal meaning in terms of physical pathology. Experience that is difficult to articulate may only be understood by attending to the expressive language. A terminally ill patient's pain may be expressed only by a furrowed brow or a groan when the patient is turned. In a patient with headache, key information may be expressed by the quivering lip, which soon gives place to tears if the response is appropriate.

Rudebeck (1992, p. 48) distinguishes between the symptom and the symptom presentation: "Doctors never meet symptoms that are adjusted to suit their knowledge, but human beings, who in their *symptom presentations* try to communicate discomforting or worrying signals from within their own bodies" . Symptoms are abstractions. As such they are detached from the acts through which the patient presents them." Rudebeck postulates that the ability to grasp the meaning of the symptom presentation is a fundamental skill of general practice. A key element in general clinical competence, it is "a basic ability to grasp the character of patient's problems and needs, useful in a vast number of patient–doctor interactions." Symptoms described in medical textbooks are abstractions. The doctor does not face abstractions, he or she

faces a human being who in her *symptom presentation* tries to communicate an experience which is often quite personal, since body and self are inseparable. A symptom gives rise to reflections and fantasies, which in important ways decide how the symptom will be presented. . . . The first and very basic question of general practice is therefore: Who is this person presenting this symptom? . . .

A symptom is no longer an evident expression of disease, but a bodily experience which might be an expression of disease (p. 31).

CLINICAL DIAGNOSIS IN FAMILY PRACTICE: THE GRAMMAR OF CLINICAL PROBLEM-SOLVING

This section deals with the physician's conventional task of clinical problem-solving and decision-making, with particular reference to family practice. Although discussed in this separate section, the process is integral to the patient-centered method described earlier.

Although the general principles of problem-solving and decision-making are the same in all branches of medicine, each discipline has its own way of applying them. The differences between disciplines are the result of differences in the problems they encounter and in their roles within the healthcare system. The problem-solving strategies of family physicians have evolved in response to a number of special features of family practice. Some of these features are shared with other primary care disciplines, especially those providing continuity of patient care.

For many years, medical thinking about the diagnostic process was dominated by a fallacy. The fallacy was that physicians make diagnoses by collecting data in routine fashion, by history-taking and examination, then by making deductions from the data. Studies of clinicians' thinking have now shown that this is not how physicians solve clinical problems. They do it in the way everybody else solves problems, in science and in everyday life. Early on in the process, they form hypotheses based on the available evidence. They then proceed to test their hypotheses by the selective collection of data from the patient's history, clinical examination, and laboratory investigation. This is known as the hypothetico-deductive approach to problem-solving. It may not be the only approach. In some situations, clinicians may use reasoning that is purely deductive, such as "since this male patient is 16 years of age, we need not consider prostatic hypertrophy as a reason for his urinary symptoms." We suspect, however, that this type of thinking plays a relatively small part in most fields of medicine.

Although clinical problem-solving is better taught nowadays, some important aspects are still not made explicit. The setting in which instruction takes place is often the medical department of a tertiary-care hospital. It is natural for the student to assume that the methods appropriate to this setting can be transferred unmodified to any other medical context. As we will see, this is not the case. The sensitivity, specificity, and predictive value of clinical data and tests vary greatly with the prevalence and distribution of illness in the population, and therefore with the setting in which the physician is working. Moreover, how we perceive and interpret the world is shaped by our mental constructs. We see what we know. A student who learns clinical problem-solving in a tertiary-care hospital will tend to have a frame of reference appropriate for patients with serious and well-defined diseases in their later stages. If the student uses this frame of reference for solving problems in family practice, he or she will get into difficulties, the kind of difficulties described so well by James Mackenzie many years ago:

> I had not long been in the practice when I discovered how defective was my knowledge. I left college under the impression that every patient's condition could be diagnosed. For a long time I strove to make a diagnosis and assiduously studied my lectures and textbooks, without avail. . . . For some years I thought that this inability to diagnose my patients' complaints was due to personal defects, but gradually, through consultations and other ways, I came to recognise that the kind of information I wanted did not exist. (Moorehead, 1999, p. 40).

A frame of reference will have to be learned, one that will take into account problems rarely encountered in the tertiary-care hospital. Learning a new frame of reference is one of the objectives of vocational or postgraduate residency training. Family physicians of previous generations did this by trial and error—a slow and painful process. Thanks to progress in describing the principles and methods of family practice, it is now possible to acquire this knowledge in a much shorter time and with less risk to ourselves and our patients. Even so, the transition from one context to another can be difficult, as many residents find when they experience family practice for the first time. The trauma is lessened if a student's early experience of clinical problem-solving has taken place in a variety of contexts ranging from primary to tertiary care.

This section takes an analytical approach to clinical method, including quantification in some places. One might question whether this is necessary or even wise. Medicine has had many brilliant diagnosticians who worked intuitively, without being able to make their thinking explicit. Is it necessary to understand the theory of diagnosis and decision-making in order to be a good clinician? For most physicians, we believe it is. We learn and grow as clinicians mainly by examining our errors. Error, like uncertainty, is inherent in medicine. If we are going to learn from our errors, we need to be able to analyze our decision-making so that we can pinpoint where the error occurred and why. It is rather like learning to write. We do not usually think in terms of grammar when we write something: as long as it reads well and expresses what we want to say, we do not need to. But if what we have written looks wrong or conveys the wrong meaning, then we have to get down to the business of analyzing our sentences and thinking about our tenses and subordinate clauses. The theory of clinical decision-making is a grammar we can use to gain insight into our own thought processes, and to understand our errors so that we can avoid them in the future. It may be true to say that one can be a good intuitive clinician without having any insight into the clinical process. It is also true that the greatest clinicians in medical history—the Sydenhams, the Laennecs, the Oslers of medicine—have taken a deep interest in the theory of medicine.

There are other reasons for family physicians to take an analytical approach to clinical method. We sometimes receive well-meaning but ill-conceived advice from physicians in other branches of medicine about adopting certain procedures into our practices. The advice is ill-conceived if it falls into the error of extrapolating from one clinical context to the other without supporting data from family practice. When given this kind of advice, we usually feel intuitively that it is wrong. It is not easy, however, to put this feeling into words, particularly when the person offering the advice has all the authority of being an expert in the field. How much better, both for ourselves and for the expert, if we can say exactly why the advice is erroneous.

New tests, procedures, and therapies are constantly being introduced. We rely on specialists to recommend them to us, but we need also to be critical of them. We need to know what kind of questions to ask our colleagues. How will the test change the relative likelihood of the diagnosis in this patient? What is its predictive value? What is its risk?

The reader will notice that we tend to use terms such as *problem-solving* and *decision-making* rather than *diagnosis*. *Diagnosis* is a time-honored word, but it is—somewhat ambiguous. To some physicians, it has meant diagnosis of a disease; to others, diagnosis of a patient. In its modern sense, *diagnosis* is the assignment of the patient's illness to a category that links the symptoms with a pathological process and, in some cases, with a specific cause. It is in this sense that we will use the term here. Problem-solving and decision-making both have wider scope than diagnosis. The solution to a patient's problem may have very little to do with the diagnosis, as in Case 9.2.

Decisions must be made at all stages of the clinical process. The process of making a diagnosis is itself a series of decisions. In addition, decisions must be made before diagnosis, and often without a diagnosis. For family physicians, one of the most common and most difficult decisions is the one demanded by a night call: Should I see the patient now, or give advice on the phone and see the patient in the morning? In family practice, as we will see, it may be necessary to go straight from assessment to decision-making without diagnosis.

THE FAMILY PRACTICE CONTEXT

The pattern of illness in family practice is similar to the pattern of illness in the community—not identical, but similar. This means that there is a high

---

CASE 9.2

Sarah is an 88-year-old woman who has been a widow for the past 20 years. She came to her family physician with complaints of frequent urination. A quick urinalysis noted that there was glucosuria, and subsequent culture found no evidence of infection. A fasting blood sugar was undertaken and found to be 10 mmol/L. The results were explained to her and a treatment plan outlined to which she readily agreed. There were no other illnesses identified. Her family physician started her on metformin and made arrangements for her to attend a diabetic education clinic. A month later her blood sugars were normal, but on the follow-up visit, she discussed the need to dispose of her personal belongings and her desire not to have extreme measures taken in the event of a heart attack or stroke. Her physician noted the dramatic change in her normally optimistic demeanor and inquired about it. She related to him that she considered the diagnosis of diabetes to be fatal and that she recognized the need to "get things in order." Her physician emphasized that diabetes was a controllable chronic disorder that would require some changes in her life, but need not be considered fatal. Further discussion revealed that she had attended her older sister in the last year of her life as she died due to complications of diabetes. She and her physician discussed the differences between her sister's experience and the expectations of the course of events for her. In this case, the physician's perspective was that the disease was a manageable phenomenon. From the patient's perspective, it had grave symbolic significance. This was only understandable after learning of her previous experience with it.

---

incidence of acute, short-term illness, much of it transient and self-limiting; a high prevalence of chronic illness; and a high prevalence of illness unrelated to identifiable organic pathology. Contrary to the conventional view, patients do not usually present with either physical or psychological problems; they come with problems that are often a complex mixture of physical, psychological, and social elements.

Diseases that are common in a referral practice or tertiary-care hospital may be rare in a general practice, and vice versa. It is often astonishing for new students in family practice to realize that they could go years without seeing a patient with leukemia or systemic lupus erythematosus. Put in technical terms, the population at risk for a family practitioner differs greatly from the population at risk for a referral specialist. The probability that the family physician will encounter certain diseases differs greatly from the probability that the specialist will encounter them. In technical terms, again, the prior probabilities of diseases are very different in family practice. This does not mean that family physicians never think of uncommon diseases. Under certain conditions—given certain presenting symptoms—a rare disease may be the first hypothesis. It does mean, however, that other things being equal, they will usually consider the most likely disease first. This may sound obvious, but it is important. Failure to think in this way can result in unnecessary and inappropriate investigation.

Because of their role as primary physicians, family practitioners tend to encounter illness in its earliest stages. Early diagnosis is a special responsibility, especially in those diseases where early treatment makes a difference to prognosis. The family physician, therefore, has to be especially alert to the clinical data that distinguish serious and life-threatening illness in its early stages from less serious illness. This presents a problem. The symptoms, signs, and tests that identify diseases in their early stages are often different from those that identify them in their later stages. The sensitivity and specificity of signs and tests vary with the stage of the disease. As we will see later, this creates pitfalls for those beginning in family practice after experience that has been limited to in-hospital medicine. Textbooks of medicine are of little help, for they do not usually tell one how to diagnose disease in its earliest stages.

The differences in prevalence of disease between family practice and specialized practice have another consequence. The predictive value of a test varies with the prevalence of the disease in question. Why this is so will be explained later in this chapter. It means that the same test may be useful for diagnosis in tertiary care, but useless—and perhaps harmful—in family practice, and vice versa.

Another feature of the family practice context is that the illness encountered is usually undifferentiated and unorganized. By an undifferentiated illness, we mean one that has not previously been assessed, categorized, and named by a physician. In the process of diagnosis, the physician interprets the raw data presented by the patient, adds the data acquired by his or her own search, and tries to fit the illness into a disease category within his or her own frame of reference. In this way, many patients presenting to family physicians have their raw illnesses differentiated into well-known disease categories.

On the other hand, many patients have illnesses that defy this kind of differentiation. There are at least five reasons why this should be so. First, an illness may be transient and self-limiting, creating a functional disturbance that clears completely, leaving no evidence on which a diagnosis can be based. These illnesses are usually brief, but not invariably so. Sometimes a patient may suffer for months from an illness that eventually clears without ever having been diagnosed. Second, an illness may be treated so early that it is aborted before it reaches the stage of a definitive diagnosis. Many cases of pneumonia are probably aborted in this way by giving antibiotics to patients with fever, cough, and minimal chest signs.

Third, there are, at the edge of every disease category, borderline and inter-mediate conditions that are difficult or impossible to classify. Because family physicians see all variants of disease, they are especially liable to encounter milder variants and borderline conditions that may never reach the specialist.

Fourth, an illness may remain undifferentiated for many years before its true nature unfolds in time. It may be years before a transient blurring of vision is followed by other evidence of multiple sclerosis.

Fifth, an illness may be so closely interwoven with the personality and per-sonal life of the patient that it defies classification. Patients with chronic pain often present examples of this type of illness.

Estimates of how much illness in family practice remains undifferentiated—even after assessment—vary from 25% to 50%. The exact figure will obvi-ously vary with the duration of observation and the criteria adopted for differentiation.

The fact of persistently undifferentiated illness has many implications for the clinical method in family practice. The key to its understanding may be the diagnosis of the patient as a person or the patient–doctor relationship, rather than the disease—hence the importance of the patient-centered clini-cal method. The importance of time in revealing a diagnosis makes clinical observation an important tool in the family physician's armamentarium, and one that he or she has excellent opportunities to use. Given the elusiveness of diagnosis, moreover, the family physician frequently must ask the question "When do I stop the investigation?"

The concept of the organization of illness is an important one for family medicine. As we have seen in Chapter 7, when patients first present their problems to a physician, they often do so in a fragmented and oblique man-ner. Several problems are often presented at one visit; the most important one for the patient may not be presented first; for many reasons, problems may be expressed in indirect rather than in direct literal language. Although the patient may have his or her own explanation for the illness, it is probably not organized in terms of a medical frame of reference. Once the patient has been through the physician's assessment process, all this changes. Unless the patient's own frame of reference is very resistant to change, he or she will tend to see the illness in a different light. Instead of having troublesome pain, the patient will now have a gallbladder problem or a duodenal ulcer. By the very direction of the inquiry, the doctor will have taught the patient which symp-toms are medically significant and which are not. This is an illustration of the fact that one cannot observe nature without changing it. It is an awesome responsibility for the family physician. As the first doctor to see the patient, he or she has great power to change the way the patient perceives and orga-nizes the illness.

Giving the illness a name has great symbolic significance. It may be a great relief for a patient to know that the illness is a familiar thing, not some vague menace. It may have an important legitimizing function. Patients with chronic fatigue syndrome describe receiving a diagnosis as a turning point in their illness. At last, their suffering is taken seriously by family and friends. On the other hand, the name given to the illness may be so terrifying that the word should not be spoken unless support is at hand.

Organizing and naming the illness (diagnosing the disease), when based on good clinical evidence, confers great benefits. It has great explanatory and predictive power, adding meaning to the patient's experience. On the other hand, diagnosis based on spurious clinical evidence has potential for harm in fostering somatic fixation.

We must also consider the importance of time in the family practice context. The patient–doctor relationship is usually a long-term one. This makes for pitfalls that are less of a problem in other fields of medicine (see Chapter 8). It also has many advantages. Observation of the patient over time can be a powerful test of clinical hypotheses, provided, of course, that there is no risk attached to waiting or that the risk of waiting is less than the risk of active investigation. Because the relationship is continuing, the family physician need not be in a hurry to solve all the patient's problems, unless, again, there is a risk attached to delay. The difference in the time scale between tertiary-care medicine and family medicine is one of the most difficult things for beginners in family medicine to grasp. The use of time to validate hypotheses can save many unnecessary investigations in self-limiting illnesses.

CLASSIFICATION

One of the objectives of the clinician is to place the patient's illness into its correct disease category. In modern times, in fact, this has been viewed as the chief objective. Classification has five very important results:

1. By using their knowledge of the natural history of the disease category, clinicians can predict the outcome of the illness, if untreated.
2. They can make inferences about the cause or causes of the illness.
3. Armed with this knowledge, they can prescribe the specific therapy for the disease.
4. They can make inferences that go beyond the evidence of their senses—for example, about the state of the internal organs.
5. By using the common nomenclature of medicine, they can communicate their findings to other clinicians and provide the patient with a name for his or her disease.

If, for example, a patient with fatigue, pallor, and loss of weight is classified as having pernicious anemia, the clinician can predict that he or she will die if untreated and will respond rapidly to injections of vitamin B_{12} and can infer that he or she is deficient in intrinsic factor.

Classification is a very powerful tool. The successful application of technology to medicine depends on it, for unless we can predict the outcome of untreated illness, we cannot know whether our interventions are effective. Unless we can classify illness correctly, we cannot be specific in our application of therapeutic technologies.

Disease categories vary greatly in their predictive power. In giving pernicious anemia as an example, we chose a particularly powerful one. Others have very little power. "Low back syndrome," for example, tells us very little about the prognosis of the condition or its pathological basis. Such categories are sometimes no more than a restatement of the patient's symptoms. As we have seen, our system for classifying diseases is based on the linkage of symptoms and signs with pathological data. Our categories are mental constructs that we create for their explanatory and predictive power. As our investigative and therapeutic technologies become more precise and effective, some of our old categories change and some new ones are called into being. An example of such changes is the evolution in understanding of what was originally known as Stein-Leventhal syndrome, which was thought to consist of subfertility and ovarian cysts. It is now understood to be a much wider metabolic and hormonal disturbance with epigenetic and environmental components. It is only since the advent of coronary angiography and bypass surgery that we have had a precise anatomical classification of ischemic heart disease. The category "polymyalgia rheumatica" was unknown until the 1950s, when steroids had recently become available. One sometimes reads editorials in medical journals that ask whether or not such-and-such a category is an "entity." This question betrays confusion about what a disease category is; the questioner is guilty of the fallacy of treating a mental construct as if it had a concrete existence. The question should be "Does such-and-such a category have good predictive and explanatory power?"

Besides using the common disease categories, family physicians use other types of category to help them in dealing with early and undifferentiated illness. In a patient with acute abdominal pain, for example, the doctor's first task may be to place the patient into one of two categories: "probably acute abdomen" or "not acute abdomen." If the latter, then the physician can discontinue the search and observe the patient, expecting the illness to be minor and self-limiting. In these cases, the physician can achieve the objective by defining what the patient does *not* have—the so-called eliminative diagnosis (Crombie, 1963).

Other clinical dichotomies are exemplified in Figure 9.3. Although patients may be usefully categorized in this way, one must always bear in mind that the patient's problems may fall in both categories, for example, upper and lower respiratory tract infection. It need hardly be said that such categorization is

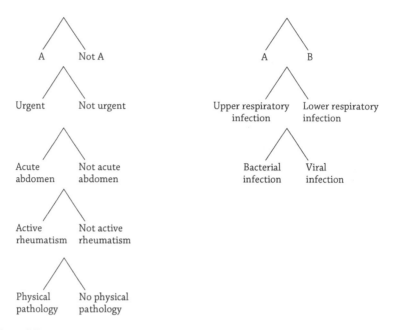

Figure 9.3:
Examples of broad categories used in family practice.

only a starting point, leading to further steps toward a more precise clinical diagnosis or a better understanding of the patient. One thing to remember about these binary categories is that the tests that are useful for distinguishing between them are different from the tests that are useful for making more precise diagnoses. This is often forgotten in the teaching of clinical method. The erythrocyte sedimentation rate, for example, is a very useful test in family practice for assessing patients with aches and pains and older patients with headache. It is of little or no value in distinguishing between different categories of inflammatory disease of connective tissue.

Another use of categorization by family physicians is the movement from assessment to decisions, without an intervening stage of diagnosis in the conventional sense. Howie (1973) has described how family physicians base their management decisions in acute respiratory illness on the presence or absence of certain clinical features rather than on the diagnostic label applied. His study encompassed 62 practices and 1000 patients with respiratory illness. Cough and chest signs were present in 163; of these, 152 (93%) received an antibiotic. The presence of cough and chest signs had, therefore, a predictive value for antibiotic treatment of 93%. Twelve different diagnostic labels were applied to the 163 patients. Five of the labels had a predictive value of only 45%. It appears that the physicians were placing the patients into one of two treatment categories (antibiotic/no antibiotic) based on clinical data. The actual name given to the condition was comparatively unimportant and probably was given as an afterthought.

In dealing with this type of illness, the strategy used by the physicians makes a lot of sense. The distinction between different types of respiratory illness in their early stages (tracheitis, laryngitis, bronchitis, coryza) is arbitrary and of little value. Waiting for definitive pneumonia or bronchitis to develop may lead to a more precise diagnosis but is not good medical practice.

While maintaining a proper respect for the power of diagnostic categories, we should also not become their prisoners. Some categories in common use have very little predictive value. An example is the distinction between common migraine and tension headache. Rather than spending time trying to make this distinction, we might be better employed in listening to the patient. We must also keep in mind the limitations of classification. Categorization is a generalizing process that works by ignoring individual differences. Precise categorization is not a substitute for understanding the individual features of the patient and his or her illness.

THE PROBLEM-SOLVING PROCESS

Figure 9.4 shows a model of the process of clinical problem-solving based on the work of Elstein, Shulman, and Sprafha (1978), with modifications. When presented with a problem, the clinician responds to cues by forming one or more hypotheses about what is wrong with the patient (Figure 9.5). The clinician then embarks on a search (the history, examination, and investigation) to test the hypotheses. In the course of the search, he or she looks for positive (confirming) and negative (refuting) evidence. If the evidence refutes the hypothesis, it is revised and the search begins again. The process is a cyclical one, with the clinician constantly revising, testing, and further revising the hypothesis, until it is refined to the point at which treatment decisions seem justified. Even after this point, the clinician must still be prepared to revise the hypothesis if the progress of the patient is not as predicted.

CUES

When a patient presents his or her problem, the physician is faced with a plethora of data: from what the patient says, from the physician's own observations, from his or her previous knowledge of the patient, from the relatives, from other physicians who have seen the patient, or from other members of the healthcare team. There is so much information that the physician cannot deal with all of it. Moreover, the different items of information are not of equal value. The physician therefore responds to certain items of information that have a special meaning for him or her. We call these cues. The information in the cue may be useful for a number of reasons. It may help the physician to

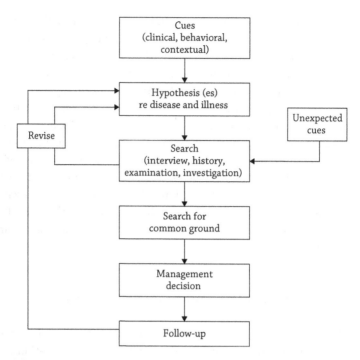

Figure 9.4:
A model of the diagnostic process.

identify and solve the patient's problem; it may help him or her to understand the context of the problem; or it may help him or her to understand the patient.

A cue may be a symptom, sign, statement, or an aspect of the patient's behavior. It may be something that is known about the patient, such as age, previous history, or ethnic origin. It may be a contextual cue, such as when a teenaged girl is accompanied by her mother or a patient tolerates a symptom

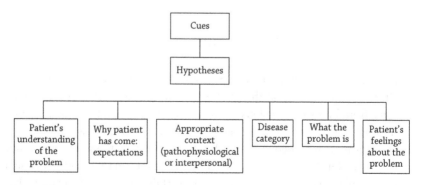

Figure 9.5:
Variety of hypotheses formed by the family physician.

for 20 years before presenting it. It may be a subjective cue, arising from the doctor's personal feelings, such as "This patient makes me feel depressed."

As well as identifying cues, the physician also assesses their significance; he or she attempts to grasp the meaning of the symptom presentation. The physician responds not only to individual cues, but to patterns. The patient's symptoms form patterns or clusters that the physician can relate to similar patterns presented by patients in his or her past experience. For the experienced clinician, pattern recognition is an important factor in the formation of hypotheses (Case 9.3).

Cues may be certain or probabilistic. A certain cue enables the physician to say with certainty what is wrong with the patient. This is what we usually mean by a spot diagnosis. The rash of herpes zoster is an example. Certain cues are rare in family practice, as they are in most fields of medicine. Most cues are probabilistic; that is, they may indicate a number of different conditions with varying probabilities. The physician can therefore only formulate hypotheses about what is wrong with the patient. The hypotheses then have to be tested by a search for further information.

Of all the cues presented to family physicians, symptoms are the most frequent. In the early stages of illness, and in the varieties of illness seen by the family physician, signs are less frequently available. The family physician is especially concerned with two aspects of a symptom: first, its capacity to bring the patient to see the doctor (i.e., its significance for the patient). This has been called by Feinstein (1967) the "iatrotrophic stimulus." For example, hemoptysis has greater power as an iatrotrophic stimulus than does cough. Also important are the sensitivity, specificity, and predictive value of the symptom in the early stages of illness. These terms will be defined later in this chapter when we discuss the search. All of them are measures of how effective a symptom or test is in identifying a disease and in discriminating between it and other diseases or a state of health.

CASE 9.3

A second resident in family medicine approached one of us (TRF) to describe a 6-year-old boy he had just seen, and he was puzzled about the case. He described a child with fever, red eyes, swollen, cracked lips, and with the tips of the fingers red and exhibiting desquamation. Recalling a single case seen in his own training, the preceptor asked, "Do you think it could be Kawasaki's?" This was met by a querulous look. "Let's go see him together." The child did indeed have Kawasaki's disease and was referred to a local pediatric hospital for further investigation of cardiac function. Though rare in general practice, suspicion of diagnosis by pattern recognition is possible.

HYPOTHESES

Investigators of the clinical process have found that clinicians form their first hypothesis very soon after the patient has presented the first problem (Elstein, Shulman, and Sprafha, 1978). Hypothesis formation is a mark of the clinician's creativity. We do not know how clinical hypotheses are generated, any more than we know how they are generated in scientific discovery. They are certainly not the result of linear logic; they seem to spring into consciousness as we respond to the cues. Experience is certainly a factor; the incoming information is matched with other information stored in our mind's filing system. Generally speaking, the greater the clinician's experience in his or her field, the more powerful will be the hypotheses. It does depend, however, on what use the physician has made of his or her experience. There is a well-known comparison between a physician who has 20 years of experience and one who has 1 year of experience 20 times.

The clinician usually has between two and five hypotheses at any one time; to handle more than six is difficult for the human mind. As old hypotheses are discarded and new ones called up, the clinician can consider many more in the course of the investigation.

The hypotheses are placed in ranking order, based on two main criteria: probability and payoff. Payoff is an indication of the consequences of diagnosing or not diagnosing a disease. The more serious a disease and the more amenable to treatment, the greater the positive payoff of making the diagnosis and the greater the negative payoff of missing it. If a disease has a high payoff, it may be ranked high on the clinician's list, even though it has a low probability. In a child with abdominal pain, for example, acute appendicitis may be ranked high—even though of low probability—because of the high positive value of an early diagnosis.

If considerations of payoff do not arise, the hypotheses are ranked in order of probability. Note that this is not the prior probability (the prevalence of the disease in the practice population) but the conditional probability (the probability of the disease, given the patient's symptoms). A synonym for conditional probability is predictive value: the predictive value of symptom x for disease A. As we have seen, predictive value varies with prevalence. Because of differences in disease prevalence, there may be a big difference between the predictive values of the same symptom in family and specialty practice. For example, in a patient with fatigue but with no other presenting data, the first-ranking hypothesis would usually be depression. For a hematologist, the first-ranking hypothesis might be a blood disorder. Each would be correct in its own context, given the differences in predictive value of the symptom of fatigue. Similarly, our first-ranking hypothesis in a patient with headache might be different from that of a neurologist.

How much does the ranking order matter? It matters because the order of hypotheses determines the search strategy. If depression is the first-ranking hypothesis, we would begin by seeking evidence of depression. If our hypothesis is supported, one would test it further by ruling out other causes of fatigue—usually by a few simple and economical tests and by continuing observation over time. If the first hypothesis is a blood disorder, one would begin by seeking evidence for this and would consider depression as part of the routine inquiry. Again, each search strategy would be appropriate in its context. However, a search strategy based on erroneous ranking (assuming payoff factors are not operative) can lead to a waste of resources and—here tests carry a risk—harm to the patient.

Before we leave hypotheses, two fallacies must be mentioned. The first is that the family physician always thinks of common diseases first. This is not necessarily so; it depends entirely on the cues. If the cues are highly probabilistic, such as fatigue, this will hold true. If, on the other hand, the cue indicates a rare disease with relative certainty, this will be the physician's first hypothesis. If a hypertensive patient complains of attacks of sweating and flushing, for example, the first hypothesis may be pheochromocytoma, even though the physician may see only one case in his or her entire lifetime.

The second fallacy is that diagnosis in family practice is different from diagnosis in other fields of medicine because it is probabilistic. All clinical diagnosis is probabilistic. Where family practice differs is in the relatively low levels of probability at which many decisions must be made. This is because of the early stage at which disease is seen, not—as is sometimes suggested—because of lack of time to pursue a more specific diagnosis.

THE SEARCH

The purpose of the search is twofold: to test and validate the physician's hypotheses, and to bring to light new and unexpected cues. These purposes are fulfilled, respectively, by the directed and the routine search.

The Directed Search

Because the purpose of the directed search is to test the physician's initial hypothesis, it follows that the search strategy will vary with the hypothesis. In selecting a search strategy, the family physician has to make two kinds of choices: which tests to use and what the extent of the search should be.

The word *tests* embraces history questions, items of physical examination, and laboratory and imaging investigations. Tests are selected according to two kinds of criteria. First, the capacity of the test to change the prior or pretest probability that the patient has or has not the disease in question; second, the risks and benefits of doing the test. The measures used to determine the usefulness of a test are its sensitivity, specificity, and predictive value.

Box 9.1

SENSITIVITY, SPECIFICITY, AND PREDICTIVE VALUE OF THE MONOSPOT TEST FOR INFECTIOUS MONONUCLEOSIS (IM) IN PATIENTS WITH SORE THROAT (PREVALENCE OF IM IN PATIENTS WITH SORE THROAT = 20/1000)

Infectious Mononucleosis
Monospot Test

	Present				Absent
Positive	17	a	b		69
Negative	3	c	d		911
	20				980

$$\text{Sensitivity} = \frac{a}{a+c} \times 100 = \frac{17}{20} \times 100 = 85\%$$

$$\text{Specificity} = \frac{d}{b+d} \times 100 = \frac{911}{69+911} \times 100 = 93\%$$

$$\text{Predictive Value Positive} = \frac{a}{a+b} \times 100 = \frac{17}{17+69} \times 100 = 19\%$$

Sensitivity expressed as a percentage is therefore

$$\frac{a}{a+c} \times 100$$

Another way of putting this would be

$$\text{Sensitivity} = \frac{\text{True positives(TP)}}{\text{True positives (TP)} + \text{False negatives (FN)}} \times 100$$

One way of understanding these indices is by means of a 2 × 2 table, illustrated in Box 9.1. In Box 9.1, the boxes have been completed for the monospot test in infectious mononucleosis. The sensitivity of the test is

$$\frac{17}{17+3} \times 100 = 85\%$$

Patients with the disease (infectious mononucleosis) are in the two left-hand boxes, those without the disease in the two right-hand boxes. Patients testing positive (with the monospot test) are in the upper two boxes, those testing negative in the lower two boxes. The boxes are identified from the upper left as a, b, c, and d. Box a contains those patients who have the disease and who test positive (true positives). Box b contains those without the disease who test positive (false positives). Box d contains those without the disease who test negative (true negatives). Box c contains those with the disease who test negative (false negatives).

With the help of the table, we can now look at the meaning of the three indices.

Sensitivity

Sensitivity is the proportion of patients with the disease who have a positive test result, which has been called "positivity in disease" (Galen and Gambino, 1975). In Box 9.1, boxes $a + c$ give us those patients with the disease, and box a gives us those with the disease who test positive.

Some attributes of sensitivity are especially important for family physicians. A highly sensitive test is very good for ruling out hypotheses. If we have a test that is 100% sensitive and the patient tests negative, we can say with confidence that the patient does not have the disease. Because the test is 100% sensitive, we know that there are no false negatives. A positive test, however, is not so helpful, because we do not know whether it is a true or false positive. If a test is 100% sensitive it will certainly not be 100% specific, and there will be some false positives. Let us consider some examples.

In a study of headache in family practice, we found that tenderness on pressure over the sinuses was 100% sensitive for sinusitis. Absence of tenderness ruled out sinusitis. Presence of tenderness, however, was of little value because so many patients without sinusitis tested positive. In headache patients over the age of 50, an erythrocyte sedimentation rate of greater than 50 mm in 1 hour was 100% sensitive for cranial arteritis. This is very tentative because the disease is rare and there was only one case among the 272 patients in the study. There was also only one false positive, a patient who turned out to have pernicious anemia. Our study supported a clinical impression that the test is very useful for ruling out cranial arteritis.

As we have seen, sensitivity varies with the stage of the disease. Failure to understand this can lead to difficulties for the newcomer to family medicine (Case 9.4).

CASE 9.4

A second-year resident saw a 12-year-old boy in the office during his morning session. The boy had complained of continuous central abdominal pain for several hours. On examination, there was no abdominal tenderness and the temperature was normal. Because there was some frequency of micturition, the resident diagnosed a urinary infection. That same evening, the mother called the doctor on duty because the pain was worse and the boy was vomiting. Examination of the abdomen showed tenderness and muscular rigidity in all areas. A perforated appendix was diagnosed and the boy made a full recovery after emergency surgery.

The pitfall here was that abdominal tenderness and pyrexia, although sensitive signs in the later stages of appendicitis, are not 100% sensitive in the early stages. The family physician cannot, therefore, rely on these for ruling out appendicitis. In this case, the history of continuous abdominal pain should have been sufficient to require re-examination of the patient within 4 hours. An additional error was to make urinary infection a top-ranking hypothesis, because it is uncommon in males of this age and is not usually associated with continuous abdominal pain.

There are many examples of this variation of sensitivity with the evolution of a disease: the chest X-ray in pneumonia, lung cancer, and pulmonary embolus; the ECG in myocardial infarction; and splenic enlargement in infectious mononucleosis, to mention some of them. Few are well documented; textbooks are not written about the early stages of illness.

Specificity

Specificity is the proportion of patients without the disease who have a negative test result. This is sometimes referred to as "negativity in health" (Galen and Gambino, 1975), but note that absence of the disease in question is not synonymous with health. The patient may have some other disease. In Box 9.1, boxes b and d give us those patients without the disease, and box d gives us those without the disease who test negative. Specificity, therefore, expressed as a percentage is therefore

$$\frac{b}{b+d} \times 100$$

Another way of putting this would be

$$\frac{\text{True negatives (TN)}}{\text{True negatives (TN) + False positives (FP)}}$$

In Box 9.1, the specificity of the monospot test is

$$\frac{911}{69+911} \times 100 = 93\%$$

A highly specific test is very good for ruling in hypotheses. If a test is 100% specific and the patient tests positive, we can say with certainty that the patient has the disease. Because the test is 100% specific, we know that there are no false positives. The test is diagnostic. A negative test, however, is less helpful, because we do not know whether it is a true or false negative. If a test is 100% specific, it will almost certainly not be 100% sensitive.

Predictive Value

As we have seen, sensitivity tells us nothing about the false positives, and specificity tells us nothing about the false negatives. Yet it is important for us to know about them. The trouble with false positives and false negatives is that both carry penalties for the patient. A false positive can be hazardous in two ways: by imposing a disease label on a healthy person and by exposing him or her to risky investigations and therapies. A false negative carries a penalty because it misses the diagnosis in a sick patient. Thus, we need a measure that tells us about the false positives and negatives. The predictive value does this.

The positive predictive value is the proportion of positive test results that are true positives:

$$PV^+ = \frac{TP}{TP + FP} \times 100$$

The negative predictive value is the proportion of negative test results that are true negatives:

$$PV^- = \frac{TN}{TN + FN} \times 100$$

The denominator in each case is the number of positive or negative test results, rather than the number of patients with or without the disease. In Box 9.1, the positive predictive value is

$$\frac{a}{a+b}$$

the negative predictive value is

$$\frac{d}{c+b}$$

Synonyms for positive predictive value are the conditional probability of a positive test result, and the post-test probability of disease following a positive result. Synonyms for negative predictive value are the conditional probability of a negative test result, and the post-test probability of no disease following a negative result.

In Box 9.1, the predictive value positive of the monospot test is

$$\frac{17}{17+69} \times 100 = 19.7\%$$

Box 9.2
SENSITIVITY, SPECIFICITY, AND PREDICTIVE VALUE ON THE MONOSPOT TEST FOR INFECTIOUS MONONUCLEOSIS (IM) IN PATIENTS WITH SORE THROAT (PREVALENCE OF IM IN PATIENTS WITH SORE THROAT = 100/1000)

Infectious Mononucleosis
  Monospot Test

	Present		Absent	
Positive	86	a	b	63
Negative	14	c	d	837

$$\text{Sensitivity} = \frac{a}{a+c} \times 100 = \frac{86}{86+14} \times 100 = 86\%$$

$$\text{Specificity} = \frac{d}{b+d} \times 100 = \frac{837}{63+837} \times 100 = 93\%$$

$$\text{Predictive Value Positive} = \frac{a}{a+b} \times 100 = \frac{86}{86+63} \times 100 = 58\%$$

The negative predictive value of the monospot test is

$$\frac{911}{3+911} \times 100 = 99\%$$

The predictive value is a key index, for it tells us the power of a test to change the probability that the patient has the disease in question. There is, however, something very important to bear in mind. We have already mentioned it: *the predictive value varies with the prevalence of the disease.* Let us see how this works in the case of the monospot test. In Box 9.1, the prevalence of mononucleosis in patients with sore throat is 2%. In Box 9.2, the prevalence is 10%. This could be the difference between a family practice and a student health service practice. The effect of this is to increase the predictive value positive to 58%, while the sensitivity and specificity remain virtually the same. The reason is that as the prevalence increases, the proportion of people with the disease increases and the number of false positives decreases.

As we have seen, the variation of predictive value with prevalence can mean that a routine test that may be indicated in a specialty clinic may be contraindicated in family practice.

Having said that predictive value varies with prevalence, we must go on to say that there is one exception. If the sensitivity of a test is 100%, the predictive value of a negative test does not vary with prevalence. There are no false negatives, and the predictive value negative is also 100%. Conversely, if the specificity of a test is 100%, the predictive value of a positive test does not vary with prevalence. There are no false positives, and the predictive value of a positive test is also 100%. Unfortunately, there are not many tests that reach 100% for either sensitivity or specificity. Those that we have we treasure for their capacity to rule out or to rule in a diagnosis.

For the more common tests with sensitivity and specificity of between 80% and 95%, the variation with prevalence is important. Table 9.2 shows how predictive value changes with prevalence for a test that has 95% sensitivity and specificity. As prevalence falls, positive predictive value falls, and negative predictive value rises. Note that a test has greater power to change the pretest or prior probability in the middle ranges of prevalence (40%–60%).

When we get to prevalence rates of 95% and 5%, the test does not help us much. Whether or not this makes the test justifiable depends on the payoff of the diagnosis and the risk of the test. A disease may be so devastating if undiagnosed, and so amenable to treatment, that we do the test even though the disease has a very low prevalence. The test for phenylketonuria is an example of this.

A reminder is in order here. Remember that our definition of test includes elements of the history, examination, and investigation. The experienced clinician selects questions and items of physical examination for their capacity

Table 9.2. THE EFFECT OF PREVALENCE ON THE PREDICTIVE VALUE OF AN EXCELLENT SIGN, SYMPTOM, OR LABORATORY TEST

Prevalence (Pretest likelihood or prior probability of disease)	99%	95%	90%	80%	70%	60%	50%	40%	30%	20%	10%	5%	1%	0.5%	0.1%
Predictive value of a positive test (Posterior probability of disease following a positive test result)	99.9%	99.7%	99.4%	99%	98%	97%	95%	93%	89%	83%	68%	50%	16%	9%	2%
Predictive value of a negative test (Posterior probability of *no disease* following a negative test result)	16%	50%	68%	83%	89%	93%	95%	97%	98%	99%	99.4%	99.7%	99.9%	99.97%	99.99%
(Posterior probability of disease following a negative test result)	84%	50%	32%	17%	11%	7%	5%	3%	2%	1%	0.6%	0.3%	0.1%	0.03%	0.01%

Both sensitivity and specificity equal 95% in every case.
From Sackett et al., *Clinical Epidemiology: A Basic Science for Clinical Medicine*, Little Brown and Co., Copyright 1985. Reprinted by permission.

to change the prior probability. Even before the clinician starts, the patient's presenting symptoms have changed the prior probability in some way.

Despite the panoply of investigations available to us, the history and physical examination—in family practice, especially the history—are still the most effective ways of increasing the probability. Let us see how this works in the case of a patient with chest pain.

Suppose we have a middle-aged man who presents with a typical history of angina of effort: tight substernal pain coming on after a fixed amount of exertion and relieved within 5 minutes by rest. The probability of coronary disease, given these symptoms (conditional probability), is about 90% (Diamond et al., 1979). By taking the history alone, we have raised the probability from the prevalence of coronary disease in males of his age group in our practice (about 5%) to 90%. Now, will an exercise ECG help us? The predictive value positive at this prevalence rate is 98%, a small increase on the previous figure; the predictive value negative is 20%; that is, even if the test is negative there is still an 80% probability of coronary disease. The sensitivity of the test is 60%, the specificity 91%.[4] Let us apply the acid test for an investigation: Will it change our approach to the patient, whatever the result? In this case the answer is "no." If the test is positive, we will still be certain of our diagnosis; but we were already certain. If the test is negative, it will not make any difference, because we will still go by our clinical assessment; with a 60% sensitivity, the rule-out value of the test is low.

Now suppose we have a 40-year-old man with vague left-sided chest pain, unrelated to exercise, but worse on some movements of the chest wall. The history is suggestive of intercostal muscle pain and has no features to indicate coronary disease, although the patient is worried about his heart. The probability of coronary disease in this patient is about the same as any other male of his age in the practice population—about 5%. The predictive value positive of an exercise ECG at this prevalence rate is only 26%. The predictive value negative is 98%, so only 2% of the negatives will be false negatives. Will an exercise ECG help us? A negative result will reinforce our opinion that the patient does not have coronary disease. A positive test will not help us, because 74% of positives will be false positives. In fact, it will probably do harm because it will make it more difficult to reassure the patient that he does not have coronary disease—a big price to pay for a marginal benefit. The physician will do better to have confidence in his or her own clinical judgment.

Now suppose we have a middle-aged man with attacks of substernal pain for several months, occurring at rest and lasting from a few minutes to half an hour, sometimes related to exertion but not relieved by rest, with no tendency to worsening since the onset. The pretest probability of coronary disease in a patient with this history is about 50%. At this prevalence rate, the predictive value positive of the test is 87%—a big increase in the probability of coronary disease. The predictive value negative is 69%, so 31% of negatives will be false negatives, a reduction of 19% in the pretest probability. If positive, the test does help to clarify the management options. The physician will feel justified in treating as ischemic heart disease with appropriate drugs and reduction of risk factors, and referral for further investigation if there is a poor response or if the pain progresses. If negative, the test is less helpful.

In all these patients, the history alone has been enormously effective in assessing the probability of coronary disease. It has provided the family physician with virtually all that is needed for making good management decisions, and the exercise ECG has very little to add.

Before leaving the question of how to select tests, mention must be made of two other tools for helping us to make choices: likelihood ratios and decision analysis. As a tool for helping us with decisions about individual patients, decision analysis has little application in family practice. It comes in useful mainly in developing optimal strategies for complex clinical conditions.[5] Sackett, Haynes, and Tugwell (1985) define decision analysis as "a method of describing complex clinical problems in an explicit fashion, identifying the available courses of action (both diagnosis and management), assessing the probability and value (or utility) of all possible outcomes, and then making a simple calculation to select the optimal course of action." For a description of how it works, see Sackett, Haynes, and Tugwell (1985).

Likelihood Ratios

Likelihood ratios are another way of expressing how good a test is for increasing the probability of a diagnosis. The calculation of the ratios uses indices with which we are already familiar: sensitivity and specificity. The likelihood ratio for a positive result is the odds that a test will be positive in a patient with the disease, in contrast to a patient without the disease. The likelihood ratio for a negative result is the odds that a test will be negative in a patient with the disease, contrasted with a patient without the disease.

The first figure in the likelihood ratio positive (positivity in disease) is the sensitivity of the test. The second figure (positivity in nondisease) is 100 minus the specificity (expressed as a percentage). For example, the likelihood ratio of a positive monospot in infectious mononucleosis (from Box 9.1) is

$$\frac{a}{a+c} \times 100/100 - \left(\frac{d}{b+d} \times 100 \right)$$

That is,

$$85/7 = 12:1$$

The odds of a patient with a positive test result having the disease are 12 to 1. By multiplying the ratio with the pretest odds, we can arrive at the post-test odds for the diagnosis. The pretest odds are calculated as pretest probability/ 1 – pretest probability. Pretest probability is calculated as a + c/a + b + c + d. For our example in Box 9.1, pretest probability = 20/1000, or 0.02. Hence, the pretest odds are 0.02/1 – 0.02, or 0.02. The pretest odds on a patient having infectious mononucleosis were 1:50, or 0.02:1. The post-test odds with a positive test are therefore 0.02:12, or 0.24:1. If we prefer to think in probabilities, odds can be converted to probabilities, and vice versa. To convert odds to probability, we divide it by itself plus one. The post-test odds on infectious mononucleosis becomes a post-test probability of

$$\frac{0.24}{0.24+1} = 0.19 \text{ or } 19\%$$

To convert probabilities to odds, we divide the probability by its complement (one minus itself). The post-test probability of 19% becomes a post-test odds of

$$\frac{0.19}{1-0.19} = \frac{0.19}{0.81} = 0.23$$

In this example, we have treated the test as if the result will be either positive or negative, rather than a continuous variable. It is also possible to express likelihood ratios for different levels of a test result that varies over a range. For the serum uric acid, for example, we can express the likelihood ratio for gout at 7.0, 8.0, and 9.0 mg/100 mL.

Because likelihood ratios are calculated from sensitivity and specificity data, they do not vary with the prevalence of the disease. Like sensitivity and specificity, however, they do vary with the stage of the disease.

As time goes on, information about the likelihood ratios and predictive values of tests have become increasingly available.[5] As family physicians, we should not only get to know these indices for the symptoms, signs, and tests we use ourselves, but also become accustomed to asking our consultants for the likelihood ratios or predictive values of tests they recommend to us. As our patients become more informed, we may also find that they begin to ask these questions themselves.

In testing a hypothesis, the clinician seeks both positive and negative evidence. He or she seeks not only to support it but also to refute it, to rule it in, and to rule it out. Suppose that the first two hypotheses in a patient with weight loss are thyrotoxicosis and diabetes. Suppose that the search has yielded evidence in support of thyrotoxicosis. The clinician will then proceed with tests such as urine and blood glucose, which should be negative if the first hypothesis is correct (unless both conditions are present). Studies of problem-solving have shown that clinicians, like problem-solvers in other fields, show a marked preference for positive over negative evidence. They would much rather try to support their hypothesis than to refute it. This is an experimental confirmation of an observation made centuries ago by Francis Bacon: "It is the peculiar and perpetual error of the human intellect to be more moved and excited by affirmatives than by negatives." (Bacon, 1620, XLVI). The testing of hypotheses raises the difficult question of when the directed search should be ended. When have we collected enough evidence? What is the appropriate level of probability?

The Last Part of the Search

This brings us face to face with the problem of uncertainty and with the potential conflict between precision on the one hand and the patient's well-being on the other. Uncertainty is inherent in medicine. The data we collect are of uncertain value; the observations we make and the tests we perform are subject to error; our diagnoses are probabilistic; both the outcome of the patient's illness and the results of treatment are to varying degrees unknown. The main purpose of our search is to reduce uncertainty. The problem comes when we have to balance the pursuit of greater precision against the risk of further testing. In modern times, precision in medicine has been the overriding value. It is of course a great good and a worthy objective. But greater precision does not necessarily reduce uncertainty. The quest for precision can become mindless, as in the inexorable search for a diagnosis in a patient who is already recovering from an illness. The quest for precision can become a false trail when the true need is to gain a better understanding of the patient.

Until recently, an excessive pursuit of precision did not carry many risks. Now the technology of investigation has advanced so rapidly as to create many hazards, not to speak of enormous expense. Not the least of the hazards is that of finding a spurious abnormality, with all the attendant risks of inappropriate treatment.

Sometimes a test does not carry a hazard by itself, but rather because it may unleash a succession of investigations, the so-called cascade effect (Mold and Stein, 1986). The physician may feel that he or she can maintain control, but this is sometimes easier said than done. The process can become inexorable (Case 9.5).

CASE 9.5

A 79-year-old man was known to have had liver metastases from a carcinoma of the colon for 12 months. He was also known to have gallstones. He eventually developed obstructive jaundice, which was thought to be caused by the tumor. Because he continued to be quite active, it was suggested to him that he should have an ultrasound to try to rule out a stone in the common duct. The result was equivocal, and the radiologist reported that the issue could only be resolved by a transcutaneous cholangiogram, or an endoscopic cholangiogram.

This was put to the patient with the recommendation that no further tests be done. However, he requested a surgeon's opinion and this led to an endoscopic cholangiogram. He found the procedure extremely unpleasant. The X-ray showed multiple intrahepatic obstructions. One of these was bypassed by a tube that drained some bile through the nasogastric tube. He requested that the tube be removed the following day. The same day, he developed septic shock and died within 72 hours.

The Endpoint in Family Practice

Traditionally, the endpoint of the search has been a diagnosis. In family practice, however, this is not always realistic. For reasons already discussed, many of the illnesses seen in family practice do not have a diagnosis in the strict sense of the term.

The illness may be at too early a stage for definitive diagnosis; it may clear spontaneously before diagnosis is possible; or it may be so interwoven with the personal life of the patient as to defy categorization.

In all patients, however, decisions have to be made, even if no diagnosis is possible. It is more helpful, therefore, to describe the endpoint in terms of a treatment decision. The endpoint of the search on any particular occasion is the point at which enough information is available for an informed decision to be made without avoidable risk to the patient.

It is important to understand that endpoints are often different in family practice than in referral specialties. A consultant seeing a referred patient will probably feel the need to make a definitive diagnosis before referring the patient back to his or her own physician. A family physician is not under the same constraint. The continuing relationship with patients means that all problems do not have to be solved right away. Because the relationship itself has no formal endpoint, the search can be discontinued and resumed according to need. In this sense, there is no final endpoint; the family physician should always be ready to revise the hypothesis if new evidence becomes available.

Family physicians, because of their role, make two types of decisions that do not arise as often in other branches of medicine:

1. The decision to wait. In making this decision, the physician is using the evolution of the illness over time as a test of the hypothesis. It is obviously inherent in this decision that no extra risk should be incurred by waiting. The use of time to validate hypotheses in this way can make many investigations redundant. One example of this decision is the eliminative diagnosis referred to earlier, in which the physician decides that the illness is transient and minor, then waits for the hypothesis to be verified.
2. The decision to refer. The endpoint of a search may be the decision to consult with or refer to another physician. This decision may have to be made before a definitive diagnosis is arrived at, for example, with a severely ill baby or a patient with an acute abdomen. It is clear that the objective of the family physician in these cases is different from that of the specialist. The family physician has fulfilled his or her obligation if the referral was made in time for the patient to receive effective treatment. The physician has failed to fulfill his or her obligation if the outcome of the illness was worsened by delaying referral in an effort to provide a more definitive diagnosis.[6]

The Routine Search

This comprises the routine systems inquiry and physical examination. The chief aims of the routine part of the search are to prompt alternative hypotheses by bringing to light cues that have not emerged in the directed part of the search, to collect baseline and background data on the patient, and to screen for symptomless conditions such as hypertension.

The routine search is sometimes referred to as a complete history and physical. This is a misnomer, for even the routine search is a selection from a much larger number of possible tests. As in the directed search, the tests are selected for their usefulness in achieving the objective. Internists would probably include ophthalmoscopy in their routine but not laryngoscopy—for the very good reason that ophthalmoscopy is more useful in generating new cues in patients seen by internists. For similar reasons, otolaryngologists would probably make the opposite choice. For four reasons, the family physician tends to make different use of routines than some other clinicians. First, because the patient is usually well known to the family physician, he or she may already have all the baseline data needed. Second, in minor and transient disorders, little in the way of a routine search is required. Third, because the family physician deals with such a wide range of clinical problems, from minor to life-threatening, no single routine is appropriate for every patient. He or she therefore develops different routines for different problems: one for sore throat, one for fatigue, one for dyspepsia, and so on. Finally, the affective component is so important that some question about feelings is routine unless covered earlier in the process.

THE SEARCH FOR COMMON GROUND

Common ground between doctor and patient about the definition of the problem, the goals of treatment, and the care plan is a key element in the patient-centered clinical method. The search for common ground is a process of clarifying the issues, encouraging the patient's questions, and seeking his or her agreement with the plan. The whole consultation is an exchange of meanings between patient and doctor, culminating in an interpretation of the illness that is a joint creation of doctor and patient. The contribution of the patient will vary with the nature of the problem and the patient's expectations. In family practice, the process often will not have led to a high degree of certainty. Nevertheless, collaborative decisions have to be made, even if the decision is to wait.

THE CARE PLAN AND THERAPY

We make a distinction here between a care plan and therapy. A care plan may or may not include therapy. Even if, at the end of a consultation, there is no specific therapeutic plan, it is still necessary to have a care plan, including arrangements for follow-up, further investigation, and reporting back. It is misleading to think of therapy only in terms of decision-making. Therapy includes decision-making but much more. Therapy that heals requires a deep involvement of the physician and a close attention to all the patient's needs and as much common ground as can be attained. The whole consultation is potentially therapeutic (Case 9.6).

CASE 9.6

A married woman in her mid-forties, a professional pianist and accompanist, was struck with a severe constricting chest pain while playing the piano. She was taken directly to the hospital and discharged a few days later with a diagnosis of angina. She said later that she left the hospital with the feeling that a sword of Damocles was hanging over her. She returned to work with some trepidation and had a recurrence of severe pain. This time she had angiograms, followed by coronary bypass surgery. From that day onward, she referred to this as her "open heart operation."

She made a good recovery and was discharged home 2 weeks later. During this time each member of the family—patient, husband, and son—kept his or her own counsel, each thinking that one or both of the others knew something he or she did not know. No one addressed this problem, and each withdrew into his or her own way of dealing with the crisis. The patient changed from being a talkative, rather exuberant woman to being quiet and depressed. She looked fragile and lost weight. Her husband and son saw this as a portent of a tragic outcome, and neither of them knew what to do. When the family were together, the subject was avoided. In the 3 months after the patient's discharge, she had frequent chest pain. Any attempt to play the piano resulted in pain. She paid frequent visits to her physician, who at each visit did an ECG, reassured her that it was all right, and reminded her to be careful. She was given quinidine, which made her think of herself as in danger of heart irregularities. The drug also gave her diarrhea and abdominal distress. Antidepressives and benzodiazepines were prescribed but did not help. She was advised also to give up her attempts to play the piano.

At this point, she came under the care of another physician, introduced by a mutual friend who was concerned for her life and health. She was depressed, in poor physical condition, and having frequent pain. She said that she wanted to feel better but was not interested in a long life if its quality could not be improved. Her inability to play the piano was a great loss to her and she did not know whether she wanted to live without her music.

In the course of several visits over the next few weeks, the following needs were identified and addressed: (1) The need for a definitive cardiac assessment. A cardiologist was consulted and gave her an excellent prognosis, with assurance that her chest pain was not cardiac. It was agreed that he would see her once a year for reassessment, but that apart from this, no further ECGs would be done. (2) The need to reduce and discontinue all medications, because they were not helping. This was done over the course of 2 months. (3) The need for physical rehabilitation. A physiotherapist experienced with cardiac patients was found. The patient embarked on a program of relaxation, pain control, and muscle strengthening. (4) Her need to play the piano. She was encouraged to sit at her piano and run her fingers over the keys. At first she could tolerate only a few minutes of this, but as her muscular strength increased, she was able to play for increasing periods. She was angry and frustrated with her playing at first, but was determined to play as well as ever. (5) Her need to understand how all this came to happen to her. This took weekly visits over many months. (6) Her family also had the need to understand what had happened, especially to appreciate the effects on the patient of their withdrawal and silence.

Within a year, the patient had recovered. She was free from pain, off all medication, and playing the piano for 2 to 3 hours a day. She had become her normal talkative self again.

No single individual would have been able to meet all this patient's needs. Each had to play his or her part: the family physician, the cardiologist, the physiotherapist, and the family. More than this, each needed to understand how his or her part fitted with the others. They had to work as an orchestra, rather than a number of soloists. The family physician was the conductor of the orchestra but also provided a *sine qua non* of the therapy: a belief in the patient's eventual recovery. The family physician helped the patient to understand her illness and to believe in recovery. She also selected a cardiologist and a physiotherapist who were appropriate for the patient's needs. If either had been ill-chosen, the therapy might have failed.

Much of diagnosis is a categorizing, generalizing process. A collaborative care plan is a synthesizing, individualizing process. The approach to care is probably more individualized in family practice than in any other field of medicine. It has much in common with the approach described by occupational therapists (Mattingly and Fleming, 1994). Obviously, the more precisely defined the problem, the less scope for variation in treatment. If a patient has pernicious anemia, the treatment in all cases is vitamin B_{12}. Even in this case, however, there may be aspects of management that, if neglected, can lead to failure of treatment. How likely is the patient to comply, for example? What is to be done to ensure that the patient is followed up? Few problems in family practice are as easy to define as pernicious anemia.

The complexity of problems, the frequent difficulty in achieving diagnostic precision, and the close personal knowledge of patients all combine to make therapy the most challenging and the most rewarding part of family practice. Gayle Stephens (1975) has called it "the quintessential skill of clinical practice and the ground of what family physicians know that is unique."

In a study of decision-making in general practice, Essex (1985) identified 10 categories of factors affecting decisions:

- Health problem (urgency, seriousness, natural history, etc.)
- Patient (expectations, culture, compliance, etc.)
- Family (impact on, requests from, etc.)
- Other people (person accompanying patient, effect of problem on others, etc.)
- Doctor (communication difficulties, experience with problem, knowledge/ignorance, mental state, workload, uncertainty, etc.)
- Investigations (indications, reliability, results)
- Resources (availability, constraints)
- Time factors
- Ethical and medicolegal factors
- Management (indications and contraindications, drug side effects and interactions, risks and benefits of therapy, etc.).

In a qualitative study using semi-structured interviews with general practitioners, Jones and Morrell (1995) found that the doctors frequently used personal background knowledge of patients in decision-making. Four areas of knowledge were described: patient's coping abilities; social supports and stressors, especially in the family; social circumstances; and the doctors' feelings about the patients. Jones interviewed doctors about patients they had seen the same day, with the patients' records to assist their recall. The knowledge used was mainly of the tacit kind (Polanyi, 1962) and clearly had an affective component.

The result of all these interacting factors is that two patients with the same condition may be treated quite differently. Consider the example of two mothers phoning in the early hours of the morning about a sick child. One is well known to you, has good coping skills but tends to be overanxious, and is able to give a good clinical description of the child, from which it appears that there are no indications of serious illness. The other is an immigrant who is not well known to you, has difficulty with the language, gives equivocal answers to your questions, and leaves you uncertain about the child's level of consciousness. The decision will probably be to see the second child at once and to reassure the mother of the first, with arrangements to see the child later. Patients with the same kind of acute sore throat may be treated differently if one is a student with an exam the next day, one a married office worker with no children, and another a single mother on welfare with no transport who has three young children.

As we have already seen, family physicians in some cases proceed directly from assessment to treatment, without going through a stage of specific diagnosis. The need for this is dictated by the conditions of family practice, with its early stages of disease, undifferentiated illness, and high level of uncertainty.

It is in arriving at a collaborative care plan with the patient that the family physician has the greatest scope for creativity. How a patient's problem is addressed depends on how it is perceived. Failure to understand the context of a problem will limit the range of decision alternatives. It is in this area that family medicine demands that a physician be skilled at synthesis rather than analysis. Case 9.7 illustrates the relationship between perception of the problem and choice of management.

The approach preferred by the physician may not be in accordance with the patient's expectations; it may even be in conflict with the patient's wishes. This is a challenge to the physician's skill in finding common ground. Therapy that the patient does not agree with is very unlikely to be beneficial. If the clinical method has been patient-centered, a search for common ground should have preceded treatment decisions.

CASE 9.7

A 19-year-old woman injured her knee while playing baseball and was admitted to the hospital for surgery. When seen for follow-up by Dr. A, she showed weakness and muscle wasting in the leg and complained of a number of general symptoms (fatigue, sweating, and pain in the neck). When Dr. A suggested that she was not doing her exercises, she became hostile and angry. Eventually she saw another doctor (Dr. B), who found her with severe muscle wasting in the leg and still complaining of the same general symptoms. After excluding some physical causes of her symptoms, Dr. B invited her to talk about the impact of her injury on her life. It turned out that the injury, by forcing her to cease her athletic pursuits, had, at a critical stage in her life, removed the main basis of her self-esteem. Given some insight into the problem, and the opportunity to discuss it with the doctor, she made a gradual recovery from her illness and returned to full activity.

Dr. A saw a hostile and uncooperative patient with an injured knee; Dr. B saw a patient with an injured knee and a life crisis.

EXTRANEOUS FACTORS IN CLINICAL DECISION-MAKING

It is important to recognize, however, that factors outside the clinical situation may have a powerful influence on the process. Some of these factors are as follows.

Clinical Practice Guidelines (CPGs). One product of the evidence-based medicine movement has been a proliferation of CPGs that frequently target family practitioners. Increasingly, measures of practice quality use adherence to guidelines as one metric. Evidence-based guidelines are based on studies involving large numbers of patients who may or may not be similar to one's practice population, casting doubt on their applicability. Nevertheless, they have a strong influence on decision-making in family practice, more so when tied to remuneration mechanisms.

Institutional. In deciding on a search strategy, a physician may be heavily influenced by the rules of the institution. With the growth of managed care, there is an increasing tendency to standardize care. The clinical guidelines published by expert committees may become institutional rules rather than general statements requiring interpretation for individual patients.

Patients' expectations. As a result of reading medical articles in the press, or of hearsay, or of a need to take action in their care or need to exercise some control over their care, patients may ask questions about or request tests that the physician may find difficult to resist, even though there is no logical justification for them.

Fear of litigation. The prevalence of malpractice suits has had a powerful influence on the search strategies of physicians, the effect being to encourage defensive medicine.

Physician factors. Another influence on the diagnostic process is the physician's own personality, feelings, and experience. Physicians who feel insecure or who cannot tolerate uncertainty tend to carry out more tests than those who feel secure and tolerate uncertainty well. A physician's strategy may be influenced by feelings of anxiety about a particular patient or type of problem. If the physician feels he or she has made past errors with a patient, or with a particular problem, for example, he or she may tend to be over-meticulous in investigations or especially liable to refer the patient to a specialist.

The time factor. All physicians have to work within time constraints. Because workload is so unpredictable, this is particularly the case in primary medical practice.

IDENTIFICATION OF ERRORS

As mentioned earlier, one of the reasons for knowing the theory of clinical decision-making is that it enables the clinician to identify errors and thus to enhance his or her skills. Errors can be classified according to the level at which they occur: cues, hypotheses, search, or management. Some examples are given in the following.

Cue Blindness (Cutoffs)

This describes a situation in which the clinician fails to respond to cues presented by the patient. We will give three examples, two from observation of trainees, one from my (IRMcW's) own practice.

A resident saw a number of patients in one morning session, all with malaise, fever, and aches and pains. They all appeared to be suffering from a mild epidemic virus infection. One of them, however, when describing his symptoms, said " . . . and my water is like tea." The resident did not respond to this cue but, after prompting, obtained a urine specimen that was strongly positive for bile.

A resident was about to see a 19-year-old unmarried woman with a sore on her lip. When asked about what question was in his mind, he said, "Why has she come with this minor problem?" When the resident opened the interview by saying "How are you?" the patient replied "Okay, I guess." In the local idiom, this actually means not okay. The resident did not respond to this cue and went on to examine the lesion—a herpes simplex infection. He then asked her about her expectations, to which she replied: "I want to get rid of it—fast." The resident assured her that it would soon go away and did not require any treatment. However, the patient did not look pleased as she left the room, and the resident admitted to feeling dissatisfied with the interview. By cutting off two cues to her feelings, he had missed the opportunity of learning about her fears. Because his reassurance was not based on knowledge, it was ineffective.

The patient from my own practice (IRMcW) was a 65-year-old man with a fever of unknown origin and a very high erythrocyte sedimentation rate. Although his temperature was swinging between normal and 103°F, he was not ill enough to suggest an infection. All investigations for infection, auto-immune disease, and malignancy were negative, and an internist I consulted could not suggest a diagnosis. Some time after the onset of the illness, the patient mentioned that he was getting headaches, to which I did not pay much attention, regarding them as a result of his fever. Eventually, I consulted a second internist, who immediately focused on the headaches as a significant cue. He diagnosed cranial arteritis, and the patient responded dramatically to prednisone. This is an example of a common pitfall—the cutting off of a cue that does not appear until later in the course of the illness. It is also relevant that the second consultant had seen many cases of cranial arteritis and had published one of the largest series in the literature.

Another reason for cutting off cues is the mental set of the clinician. The following story was told by a resident about a clinician he was working with. The patient suffered from anterior chest pain, and the clinician was taking a history with a diagnosis of ischemic heart disease in mind. Suddenly the patient interjected, "and I feel like crying all the time." The clinician failed to respond to this cue and continued to ask questions about his pain. The eventual diagnosis was depression. In this case, the clinician had a "set" on a certain line of inquiry, which blinded him to the most valuable cue of all.

Premature Convergence on a Hypothesis

In the early stages of hypothesis formation, it is important for the clinician's thinking to be lateral and divergent, considering many possible explanations for the patient's symptoms. One common error at this level is premature convergence on a hypothesis of viral infection in a patient with a mild febrile illness. This leads to failure to test such alternative hypotheses as urinary infection.

Errors in the Search

Two opposite errors are common in the search strategy. The first is redundancy. In this case, investigations are continued far beyond the point necessary for making an informed decision. Over-investigation is perhaps the most common error in medicine today. Sometimes it is due to the inexorable search for a diagnosis in a patient who is already recovering from the illness. Another example of this error, often found early in the family medicine residency, is the use of investigations when clinical observation would provide a better search strategy. For many illnesses encountered in family practice, such as the pre-eruptive pain of herpes zoster, clinical observation is the only way of making the diagnosis.

A second common error is inadequate testing. Sometimes very simple procedures will increase the validity of a diagnosis without additional risk or expense: an erythrocyte sedimentation rate in a patient with fatigue and depression, a rectal examination in a patient with abdominal pain, a urine analysis in a patient with fever. Yet these opportunities for validation are often not taken if the clinician feels that he or she has good positive evidence for a hypothesis. This is an example of the well-known preference of all problem-solvers for positive rather than negative evidence.

A third type of error, described earlier, is the premature ruling out of an important diagnosis because of reliance on a test with low sensitivity in the early stages of illness.

Management Errors

A common fault in management is failure to consider some of the important variables that should enter into the decision, such as the risks of treatment or the ethical issues. Another is the failure to consider the effect of management on the ecology of the family, as in Case 9.8.

The doctor's chief error here was in not foreseeing that his management strategy would put an intolerable strain on a precariously balanced system. The strain produced acute anxiety, with psychogenic diarrhea and wasting. Moreover, complete bed rest was probably not good treatment for back pain in an 87-year-old. Even if it had been correct, it could only have been carried out by mobilizing a home support system. If the patient-centered method had been followed, the management plan would not have been implemented without seeking the response of the patient and her husband. Even if they had agreed, an exploration of the patient's feelings at a follow-up visit would have disclosed her anxiety and made clear the harmful consequences of the therapy.

CASE 9.8

An 87-year-old woman was seen at home by her family physician for acute low back pain. Apart from loss of central vision due to macular degeneration, she was in good health for her age. She and her 89-year-old husband were living independently and just managing to cope with the daily household tasks. The doctor ordered 2 weeks of complete bed rest and, because he arranged for no home help, the whole burden of care fell on the shoulders of the husband.

Because the patient's husband was unfamiliar with the household tasks he was assuming, he had to ask his wife repeated questions about them and was unable to understand her answers from the bed because of his deafness. This produced great anxiety and feeling of helplessness in his wife, which was exacerbated by her blindness.

While resting in bed, the patient developed frequent loose stools and began to lose weight rapidly. Carcinoma of the colon was suspected, and she was admitted to the hospital for investigation, which proved to be negative. At this point, her daughter arrived from a distance and stayed for 6 weeks. Under her daughter's care, the patient gradually recovered. The old couple lived on into their nineties in good health.

NOTES

1. See Chapter 6, p. . <AU: in notes 1 and 2, if page number is desired, it will need to be added in page proofs.>
2. See Chapter 6, p. .
3. Used with permission of M. Stewart, Principal Investigator of the project Communicating with Breast Cancer Patients, Centre for Studies in Family Medicine. See related paper, Stewart M, et al. (2007).
4. We have based this example on cases described in Sackett DL, Haynes RB, Tugwell P, *Clinical Epidemiology: A Basic Science for Clinical Medicine* (Boston, MA: Little, Brown, 1985).
5. An excellent resource for this information may be found at essential evidence plus (http://www.essentialevidenceplus.com/). <AU: There are two callouts for note 5 in the text; please verify which is correct and delete incorrect callout.>
6. See Chapter 22 for a more extensive discussion of referral.

REFERENCES

Anspach RR. 1988. Notes on the sociology of medical discourse: The language of case presentation. *Journal of Health and Social Behavior* 29:357–375.
Aronowitz RA. 2001. When do symptoms become a disease? *Annals of Internal Medicine* 134:803–808.
Bacon F. 1620. *Norvum Organon*.

Balint M. 1964. *The Doctor, His Patient and the Illness.* London: Pitman Medical.

Beckman HB, Frankel RM. 1984. The effect of physician behavior on the collection of data. *Annals of Internal Medicine* 101:692.

Borkan J, Reis S, Steinmetz D, Medalie J. 1999. *Patients and Doctors: Life-Changing Stories from Primary Care.* Madison: The University of Wisconsin Press.

Brown J, Stewart M, McCracken EC, et al. 1986. The patient-centered clinical method. II: Definition and application. *Family Practice* 3:75.

Brown JB, Stewart MA, Ryan B. 2001. Assessing communication between patients and physicians: The Measure of Patient-Centered Communication (MPCC). Paper #95–2 (2e) Working Paper Series. London, ON: Centre for Studies in Family Medicine, The University of Western Ontario.

Brown J, Stewart M, Weston W. 2002. *Challenges and Solutions in Patient-Centered Care: A Case Book.* Oxford: Radcliffe Medical Press.

Campbell K, Wulf Silver R, Hoch JS, Osbyte T, Stewart M, Barnsley J, et al. 2005. Re-utilization outcomes and costs of minor acute illness treated at family physican offices, walk-in clinics, and emergency departments. *Canadian Family Physician* 51:82–83.

Cannon WB. 1890. The case method of teaching systematic medicine. *Boston Medical Surgery Journal* 142:31–36.

Charon R. 1986. To render the lives of patients. *Literature and Medicine* 5:58–74.

Charon R. 2001. The patient–physician relationship. Narrative medicine: A model for empathy, reflection, profession, and trust. *Journal of the American Medical Association* 286(15):1897–1902.

Crombie DL. 1963. Diagnostic methods. *Practitioner* 91:539.

Crookshank FG. 1926. The theory of diagnosis. *Lancet* 2:939.

Diamond GA, Forrester JS, Hirsch M, et al. 1979. Application of conditional probability analysis to the clinical diagnosis of coronary heart disease. *New England Journal of Medicine* 300:1350.

Donnelly WJ. 1989. Righting the medical record: Transforming chronicle into story. *Soundings* 72(1):127–136.

Dwamena F, Holmes-Rovner M, Gaulden CM, Jorgenson S, Sadigh G, Sikorskii A, Lewis S, Smith RC, Coffey J, Olomu A. 2012. Interventions for providers to promote a patient-centred approach to clinical consultatons. *Cochrane Database Systematic Review* (12): CD003267.

Engel GL. 1977. The need for a new medical model: A challenge for biomedicine. *Science* 196:129.

Engel GL. 1980. The clinical application of the biopsychosocial model. *American Journal of Psychiatry* 137:535.

Essex BJ. 1985. Decision analysis in general practice. In: Sheldon M, Brooke J, Rector A, eds., *Decision-Making in General Practice.* London: Macmillan.

Fabrega H. 1974. *Disease and Social Behavior.* Cambridge, MA: MIT Press.

Feinstein AR. 1967. *Clinical Judgment.* Baltimore, MD: Williams and Wilkins.

Freeman TR. 2014. The case report as a teaching tool for patient-centered care. In: Stewart M, Brown JB, Weston WW, McWhinney IR, McWilliam CL, Freeman TR, eds., *Patient-centered Medicine: Transforming the Clinical Method*, 3rd ed. Oxford: Radcliffe Medical Press.

Galen RS, Gambino SR. 1975. *Beyond Normality: The Predictive Value and Efficiency of Medical Diagnoses.* New York: John Wiley.

Gatrell AC, Elliott SJ. 2009. *Geographies of Health: An Introduction.* Chichester, West Sussex, UK: Wiley-Blackwell.

Ge B, Stewart M. 2006. Comparison of clinical communication patterns of internists in outpatient departments of teaching hospitals and general practitioners in community-based clinics in Beijing. Submitted in partial fulfillment of requirements for the degree of Master of Clinical Science, Western University, London, Ontario.

Gombrich EH. 1960. *Art and Illusion: A Study in the Psychology of Pictorial Representation.* Princeton, NJ: Princeton University Press.

Greenhalgh T, Hurwitz B. 1998. *Narrative Based Medicine: Dialogue and Discourse in Clinical Practice.* London: BMJ Books.

Griffin SJ, Kinmonth AL, Veltman MWM, Gillard S, Grant J, Stewart M. 2004. Effect on health-related outcomes of interventions to alter the interaction between patients and practitioners: A systematic review of trials. *Annals of Family Medicine* 5(2):595–608.

Henbest RJ, Fehrsen GS. 1992. Patient-centredness: Is it applicable outside the West? Its measurement and effect on outcomes. *Family Practice* 9(3):311–317.

Howie JGR. 1973. A new look at respiratory illness in general practice: A reclassification of respiratory illness based on antibiotic prescribing. *Journal of the Royal College of General Practitioners* 23:895.

Jones J, Morrell D. 1995. General practitioners' background knowledge of their patients. *Family Practice* 12(1):49.

Kleinman A, Eisenberg J, Good B. 1978. Culture, illness and care: Clinical lessons from anthropologic and cross-cultural research. *Annals of Internal Medicine* 88:251.

Levenstein JH, McCracken EC, McWhinney IR, et al. 1986. The patient-centered clinical method. I: A model for the doctor–patient interaction in family medicine. *Family Practice* 3:24.

Little P, Everitt H, Williamson I, Warner G, Moore M, Gould C, et al. 2001a. Observational study of effect of patient centredness and positive approach on outcomes of general practice consultations. *British Medical Journal* 323:908–911.

Little P, Everitt H, Williamson I, et al. 2001b. Preferences of patients for patient-centred approach to consultation in primary care: observational study. *British Medical Journal* 322(7284): 468–472.

Lussier M-T, Richard C. 2008. Because one shoe doesn't fit all: A repertoire of doctor-patient relationships. *Can Fam Physician* 54(8):1089–1092.

Mair A. 1973. *Sir James Mackenzie, M.D., General Practitioner, 1853–1925.* Edinburgh: Churchill Livingstone.

Marinker M. 1983. Communication in general practice. In: Pendleton D, Hasler J, eds., *Doctor–Patient Communication.* London: Academic Press.

Mattingly C, Fleming MH. 1994. *Clinical Reasoning: Forms of Inquiry in a Therapeutic Practice.* Philadelphia: F. A. Davis.

Miller WL. 1992. Routine, ceremony or drama: An exploratory field study of the primary care clinical encounter. *Journal of Family Practice* 34(3):289.

Mold JW, Stein HF. 1986. The cascade effect in the clinical care of patients. *New England Journal of Medicine* 314:512.

Moorehead R. 1999. Sir James Mackenzie (1853–1925): views on general practice education and research. *J Royal Soc Medicine* 92:38–43.

Moral RR, Almo MM, Jurado MA, de Torres LP. 2001. Effectiveness of a learner-centred training programme for primary care physicians in using a patient-centred consultation style. *Family Practice* 18:1:60–63.

Polanyi M. 1962. *Personal Knowledge.* Chicago: University of Chicago Press.

Rudebeck CE. 1992. General practice and the dialogue of clinical practice. *Scandinavian Journal of Primary Health Care*, 10:7–87 Supplement 1.

Sackett DL, Haynes RB, Tugwell P. 1985. *Clinical Epidemiology: A Basic Science for Clinical Medicine*. Boston, MA: Little, Brown.

Stephens GG. 1975. The intellectual basis of family practice. *Journal of Family Practice* 2:423.

Stewart M, Brown JB, Donner A, McWhinney IR, Oates J, Weston WW, et al. 2000. The impact of patient-centered care on outcomes. *Journal of Family Practice* 49(9):796–804.

Stewart M, Brown JB, Hammerton J, Donner A, Gavin A, Holliday RL, et al. 2007. Improving communication between doctors and breast cancer patients. *Annals of Family Medicine* September/October; 5(5):387–394.

Stewart M, Brown JB, Weston WW, McWhinney IR, McWilliam CL, Freeman TR. 2014. *Patient-Centered Medicine: Transforming the Clinical Method*, 3rd ed. Oxford, UK: Radcliffe Medical Press Ltd.

Stewart M, Ryan B, Bodea C. 2011. Is patient-centred care associated with lower diagnostic costs? *Healthcare Policy* 6(4):27–31.

Stewart MA, McWhinney IR, Buck CW. 1979. The doctor–patient relationship and its effect upon outcome. *Journal of the Royal College of General Practitioners* 29:77.

Tait I. 1979. The history and function of clinical records. M.D. thesis, University of Cambridge.

Weed LL. 1969. *Medical Records, Medical Education, and Patient Care*. Chicago: Year Book Medical Publishers.

Winker MA. 2006. Clinical crossroads: Expanding the horizons. *Journal of the American Medical Associaton* 295(24):2888–2889.

CHAPTER 10

༄

The Enhancement of Health
and the Prevention of Disease

Family physicians are in an unrivaled position for helping their patients to maintain and improve their health. They see each of their patients, on the average, three or four times a year. Many of these visits are for self-limiting problems in healthy people. They provide, therefore, an excellent opportunity for health counseling and the early detection of disease. Because of their personal knowledge of patients and their families, family physicians may be aware of resources, both inner and outer, that are important for the maintenance or recovery of health. In secondary prevention, they can take responsibility for the whole process, from case finding through investigation to the approach to the problem.

WHAT IS HEALTH?

The meaning of health has always proved to be elusive. According to the Constitution of the World Health Organization, health is "a state of complete physical, mental and social well-being and is not merely the absence of disease or infirmity." For the great majority of people this represents an impossible ideal. In the words of René Dubos (1980, p. 349), "positive health is not even a concept of the ideal to be striven for hopefully. Rather it is only a mirage, because man in the real world must face the physical, biological and social forces of his environment, which are forever changing, usually in an unpredictable manner and frequently with dangerous consequences." In the words of Gordon (1958, p. 638),

> The "positiveness" of health does not lie in the state, but in the struggle—the
> effort to reach a goal which in its perfection is unattainable. . . . the words health

and disease are meaningful only when defined in terms of a given person functioning in a given physical and social environment. The nearest approach to health is a physical and mental state fairly free of discomfort and pain, which permits the person concerned to function effectively and as long as possible in the environment where chance or choice has placed him.

Health and "normality" always have to be defined in terms of a particular person or group in a particular environment. Inquiring of the patient what the meaning of health is to him or her in particular often reveals the unique nature of the concept to that person. To an elderly woman who is caretaker for her husband, keeping her osteoarthritic knees relatively pain free is her definition of health, while to a young woman being able to compete in a marathon signifies good health. The person's values must be taken into account. Health is a value, and to some it may not be the highest value. It is sometimes sacrificed in the service of others. It is sometimes squandered in the pursuit of pleasure, fame, or fortune.

Value judgments also enter into physicians' concepts of health, especially when they concern human behavior. In accepting unthinkingly the norms of his or her own class and culture, the physician may not even realize that a value judgment is being made. It is important, therefore, to be clear about what *normal* means.

THE MEANING OF NORMAL

To identify individuals at high risk requires an understanding of the meaning of *normal*. In the history of medicine, few errors have led to so much harm as the failure to be precise about the meaning of the term. Although present when the physician is assessing and treating illness, the risk of harm is especially great in preventive medicine, for here the physician is identifying abnormalities in patients who have not come for treatment of symptoms or who have come with symptoms that bear no relation to the identified abnormality. Identification of the abnormality may then lead to treatment that has risks and costs. At the very least the patient will have an anxiety he or she did not have before.

To think clearly about normality, the physician must have an appreciation of human variability. Two types of variability are found in humans, the first of which is *individual variation*. In a given person, physiological values vary widely from minute to minute, hour to hour, day to day, week to week, and so on. These variations are manifestations of the adaptability of the organism to environmental change. Variations occur within a certain range compatible with life. Variations outside this range, if sustained, lead to pathological change and perhaps death of the organism.

The other kind is *variation between individuals*. Physiological values vary between one individual and another. If a value is plotted in a population, the result is a distribution curve with most members of the population having values about the middle of the range and smaller numbers at the two extremes. This type of variation is partly genetic but also partly the result of adaptation of individuals to different environments.

Variations resulting from adaptation are particularly noticeable when two populations from different environments are compared. The distribution of blood pressure and blood cholesterol in certain African tribes is quite different from their distribution in North Americans. The intestinal mucosa of an average Thai peasant has the same appearance as the mucosa of a North American with sprue (celiac disease). What we have said about physiological variables is equally true of cultural and behavioral variables. There are vast differences in what is considered normal behavior between different cultures and between subcultures and social classes of the same society. A degree of aggressiveness that is normal in the white North American may be considered pathological in a Pueblo Indian. A European who complained of being under a spell would be considered delusional; a rural African might be providing an explanation of symptoms consistent with his or her view of the world.

The history of medicine is full of examples of unnecessary suffering imposed on patients because they have been erroneously classified as abnormal. Some dubious practices—the wholesale removal of large tonsils, for example, was in vogue until after the mid-twentieth century. One that is of particular interest to family physicians is the practice, common in the late nineteenth century, of keeping young people with sinus arrhythmia in bed for months on end. This particular error was rectified by James Mackenzie, the British physician who showed the harmlessness of sinus arrhythmia by following a group of patients for 15 years.

John Ryle (1948) wrote,

> Each new instrument has left a trail of faulty diagnoses in its wake. The stethoscope, through misinterpretation of natural sounds or innocent murmurs, at one time created its thousands of cardiac invalids. The sphygmomanometer—through unfamiliarity with normal ranges and fluctuations of blood pressure—has created blood pressure invalids in a similar fashion. The gastroscopist who did not sufficiently recognize that the gastric mucosa, like the face, was responsive to normal stimuli, at first, exaggerated the importance of gastritis. Many laboratory methods have also been liable to misinterpretation through failure to study the limits of variability which are observable in health (p. 69).

Mitral valve prolapse (MVP) provides a more recent example. Prolapse of the posterior leaflet of the mitral valve was first recognized during angiography and a relationship with late systolic click and murmur was noted. The development of echocardiography aided recognition of the condition and it became a common finding in patients without abnormal clinical features. As availability of this technology increased, recognition of MVP became more common. Soon the finding of MVP by echocardiography was being taken as an explanation for a whole range of signs and symptoms, including atypical chest pain, arrhythmias, syncope, dyspnea, panic and anxiety, numbness or tingling, effort syndrome, and skeletal abnormalities. MVP syndrome became a popular and overused diagnosis.

In 1983, the results of a study of the Framingham population became known. Echocardiography was done on 4967 people, 5% of whom had MVP. In women, the prevalence declined from 17% in their twenties to 1% in their eighties. In men the prevalence remained between 2% and 4% in all age groups. A systolic click or murmur was found in only five people out of the 208 with echocardiographic MVP. Symptoms of chest pain, dyspnea, and syncope were no more common in the 208 with echocardiographic prolapse than in those without. Only half the people with systolic clicks have echocardiographic prolapse. Subsequent studies have demonstrated a much lower prevalence of MVP with values typically in the range of less than 1% up to 2.4%. In a study of 24,265 (12,926 females and 11,339 males) echocardiograms carried out for clinical reasons, the prevalence of MVP was found to be only 0.4% in women and 0.7% in men (Hepner, Ahmadi-Kashani, and Movahed, 2007). In a study of the offspring cohort of the Framingham Heart Study, the prevalence of MVP was 2.4%, with 1.3% showing classic prolapse and 1.1% nonclassic prolapse. Complications such as heart failure, atrial fibrillation, cerebrovasular disease, and syncope were no more common in those with prolapse than in those without. Also, the frequencies of chest pain, dyspnea, and electrocardiographic abnormalities were the same in those with and without prolapse (Freed et al., 2002). It thus appears that non-classic MVP, found only on echocardiography, is, like sinus arrhythmia, a variant of normal. Confirmation of this will await the follow-up of this cohort of people. This normal variant can now be distinguished from the MVP with mitral regurgitation found in those over 50 years of age.

How have these examples happened? Several recurring errors can be identified.

1. The distinction between normality and abnormality is regarded as an either/or question. A person is either hypertensive or not hypertensive, diabetic or not diabetic, developmentally delayed or not developmentally delayed. This kind of thinking flies in the face of the truth. Variables such as blood pressure and blood cholesterol are continuously distributed in the population. They are also continuously related to mortality and other undesirable outcomes. It is difficult to identify a point at which blood pressure suddenly becomes associated with an increased risk of dying. A person with a diastolic blood pressure of 100 mm Hg has a greater risk of dying than one with a diastolic blood pressure of 90 mmHg, one with 90 mmHg has

a greater risk than one with 80 mmHg, one with 80 mmHg a greater risk than one with 70 mmHg. Statements about the normality or abnormality of a continuously distributed variable are meaningless unless they are combined with a quantitative statement about the implications of the result. The implications will obviously depend on a number of other variables, including age, sex, existence of other diseases, and environment.

2. The term *normal* is confused with *average*. This is exemplified by the practice of plotting the results of a test in a representative population and arbitrarily defining as abnormal all results that lie outside two standard deviations from the mean. A moment's thought is enough to demonstrate the inadequacy of this concept in clinical medicine. Conditions such as abnormally low blood pressure and abnormally high intelligence are quite compatible with excellent health. Some conditions that are average are unhealthy—dental caries before fluoridation, for example. A condition may be accepted as healthy in one population because it is average, even though in another population the distribution of the variable may be quite different. We may question, therefore, whether the "normal blood pressure" in North America should be considered normal when compared with the level attained in other communities. Values within the normal range cannot be taken as an indication of health, nor can values outside this range be taken as an indication of disease. The fallacy in this approach is graphically illustrated by the probability of finding an abnormal result when multiple tests are done (Table 10.1). If enough tests are done, almost everybody is "abnormal." This had led Edmond Murphy (1976) to define (in jest) a normal person as "one who has been insufficiently investigated." There are several ways of

Table 10.1. PROBABILITY OF OBTAINING
AN ABNORMAL RESULT WHEN MULTIPLE
TESTS ARE DONE

Number of Independent Tests	Percentage of Times an Abnormal Result Is Found
1	5
2	10
4	19
6	26
10	40
20	64
50	92
90	99

Reprinted with permission from Galen RS, Gambino SR. 1975. *Beyond Normality: The Predictive Value and Efficiency of Medical Diagnoses.* New York: John Wiley.

guarding against this error. One is to report data in percentiles, as in the percentile growth charts we use to assess the development of infants and children. The percentile chart tells us how unusual the data for an individual child are in terms of the reference population that was used to compile the chart. The percentile chart is a very useful tool for clinicians, provided they do not equate deviation with disease and average growth with normality. The chart must obviously be used in conjunction with other criteria: the child's general health, other manifestations of disease, and whether or not the deviation is also a deviation in the child's own growth curve. Another way of avoiding this error is to use referent values rather than the normal range as our criteria. The referent value relates the result of a test to its predictive value for a particular disease. Referent values for a particular test in a particular disease will vary with age, sex, and other population characteristics. The use of referent values is illustrated by Table 10.2. This tells us that 82% of subjects with a serum uric acid level of 9 mg/dL or higher subsequently develop gout.

3. The criteria of abnormality for a new test may be arrived at by testing an unrepresentative sample of the population, such as people admitted to hospital or attending a particular clinic. After a time, a random sample of the population is tested and the criteria are corrected. When data are collected to establish the normal range for any variable, great care has to be taken to ensure that the sample chosen is truly representative of the whole population.

4. Physicians reflect the cultural norms of their own society and social class and they may, therefore, classify as abnormal or unhealthy some behaviors that are only unfashionable or unpopular. Sexual behavior is especially likely to be treated in this way. It is not long since masturbation was classified as a disease and treated with severe measures. In the present moral climate, sexual activity is unlikely to be classified as abnormal, but the

Table 10.2. REFERENT VALUES FOR SERUM
URIC ACID (USUAL RANGE 3–6 MG/DL)

Referent Value	Diagnosis	Predictive Value (%)
7.0	Gout	21
8.0	Gout	35
9.0	Gout	82

Reprinted with permission from Galen RS, Gambino SR. 1975. *Beyond Normality: The Predictive Value and Efficiency of Medical Diagnoses.* New York: John Wiley.

opposite error has taken its place. By unintentional and unconscious signals, physicians can convey to patients that they consider them abnormal for not being sexually active.

What are the implications of these observations for the family physician?

1. In judging the significance of a finding, it is important to ascertain that the result is not one extreme of an individual variation. A good example of this is the tendency of blood pressure to be higher at the first than at subsequent readings—hence the need to establish the patient's normal range of variation before embarking on treatment for hypertension.
2. In using percentile charts as the criterion for normality (in developmental assessment, for example), the physician should bear in mind the meaning of "normal" and "abnormal" results.
3. In judging the abnormality of a result, rather than using the statistical average or normal range as a standard, the physician should, where it is available, use the reference value.
4. Because of the long-term relationship with patients, the family physician is in a good position for obtaining baseline values from patients. This enables the physician to compare subsequent readings on the same patient with this baseline value—a potentially much more useful comparison than that with a "normal range." For example, if the physician knows that a woman's usual systolic blood pressure is 100 mmHg, the fact that her blood pressure at 28 weeks of pregnancy is 120 mmHg will warn of the possibility of preeclampsia, even though her reading is well within the normal range.
5. Because they care for more or less unselected populations, family physicians are in an excellent position to determine the range of normality for many kinds of variables. This is one of the most useful kinds of research a family physician can undertake.
6. Family physicians should be constantly aware, when dealing with family and personal problems, that it is very easy to convey value judgments without knowing that they are doing so.

SALUTOGENESIS

The concept of *salutogenesis* switches our perspective from the causes of disease to the maintenance and improvement of health. It recognizes that stressors are universal and omnipresent, but not necessarily pathological. Their pathogenicity depends on the character of the stressor and the resources available to the individual. Research is focused on the sources of successful resistance. Antonovsky (1987) attributes successful resistance to a sense of coherence (SOC) that has three core components:

1. *Comprehensibility*. Stressors, either internal or external, should make cognitive sense to the person.
2. *Manageability*. To cope with the stressors, resources should be available either to the person or his or her supporters.
3. *Meaningfulness*. The person should feel that the experience is congruent with his or her beliefs and values.

The SOC is an expression of the fit between an individual and his or her social environment. The person must feel that he or she is valued and rewarded at home, at work, and in other social contexts. The inner and outer resources are mutually interactive. Inner self-confidence is increased by a sense of belonging, and the increased confidence leads to stronger social integration. A strong supportive network may balance weaker inner resources, and vice versa. Helping patients arrive at a meaningful (to them) understanding of their symptoms sustains the SOC and is an essential part of the physician's task.

Siegrist (1993) emphasizes the importance of the emotions in an individual's response to experience. The response is not cognitive alone. The affective response to stressful experience often bypasses or overrides the cognitive. The devastating effect of unemployment, for example, can lower a person's feeling of self-worth, reduce the sense of belonging, and cut him or her off from a major source of social approval. Unemployment is associated with high rates of illness and increased death rates.

SELF-ASSESSED HEALTH AND MORTALITY

The association between self-assessed health and mortality was first reported in an analysis of the Manitoba Longitudinal Study on Aging (Mossey and Shapiro, 1982). The self-assessments were given in response to the question "For your age, in general, would you say your health is excellent, good, fair, poor, or bad?" The answers proved to be better predictors of survival during the follow-up period than the extensive data on respondents' health from the Manitoba Health Insurance Plan. The data recorded diagnoses and utilization of medical services. Respondents with poorer subjective health status experienced greater mortality throughout the 7 years of the study. The finding has since been replicated in five other studies (Idler, 1992). How can we explain this surprising fact? Respondents may have been intuitively aware of their bodily state in a way that was not reflected in the objective evidence of health status. Alternatively, their assessment may have reflected a sense of coherence, or lack of it, which exerted an independent effect on their subsequent health. Self-assessment of health covaries with education, marital status, and income. For any given level of objective health status, those who have less education, lower income, and who are unmarried have poorer self-assessments of health.

The implication for family physicians is that what people say about their health should be taken seriously, even if it contradicts other evidence. Hollnagel and Malterud (1995) have drawn attention to the lack of research on patients' healing potentials in general practice and on the lack of any system for recording patients' resources in primary care classifcation systems. Giving people confidence and supporting them in a sense of control is associated with better health and improved function. Sobel (1995, p. 243) says, "There is a biology of self-confidence." Giving patients prescriptions for lifestyle and behavior changes that are difficult to achieve may only increase their sense of failure. A sense of being in control gives patients the confidence to set their own goals. Achieving the goals, even if they are limited, further increases the feeling of confidence. For example, Lorig, Mazonson, and Holman (1993) reported that the best predictor of improvement by participants in an arthritis self-management course was the patients' self-assessment of how likely they were to improve.

GENERAL PRINCIPLES

By convention, preventive practice has been divided into four categories:

1. Primary prevention increases a person's ability to remain free of disease.
2. Secondary prevention is the early detection of disease—or precursors of disease—so that treatment can be started before irreversible damage has occurred.
3. Tertiary prevention is the management of established disease so as to minimize disability.
4. Quaternary prevention refers to rehabilitation of those with disease.

All these refer to preventive services for individuals. Measures to maintain health are also applied to communities and populations. They may involve clean water, food inspection, sanitation, waste disposal, pollution control, accident prevention, or social services that relieve poverty, protect children, and improve access to health care. Even though in many societies a dependable infrastructure can be relied on for the basic protection of public health, family doctors rooted in their communities may encounter hazards to public health at any time through the experience of their patients. An outbreak of food poisoning in an institution may point to poor food hygiene. A local cluster of cases may raise suspicions of environmental pollution, as in the case of the Love Canal (see Chapter 2). In some communities, the health problems may require an approach at both individual and population levels. For family doctors in many Native North American communities, the epidemic of diabetes calls for work at the community level as well as the care of individual patients. The same applies in the central areas of large cities, where individual prevention may be vitiated by social breakdown. In poor countries, the lack of infrastructure may render individual prevention ineffective. For example, a reliable supply of electricity is necessary for the refrigeration of vaccines.

PROMOTION OF HEALTH VERSUS PREVENTION OF DISEASE

The categorization of preventive activities into primary, secondary, tertiary, and quaternary was intended to apply to specific diseases. Some would add to this list a category termed *primordial prevention* or *prevention of risk factors*. This is better known as health promotion. The 1986 Ottawa Charter for Health Promotion (WHO, 1986) focused attention on fundamental determinants of health such as food, shelter, education, and safety that contribute to an environment that supports health and enables people to preserve their health. Health promotion is the development of a person's general resistance resources (GRR) (Antonovsky, 1979). Health is attained through a healthy environment, balanced diet, and physical fitness, as well as the fostering of coping skills, self-confidence, and self-control. Antonovsky has described this approach as "salutogenesis."

THE HEALTH ENHANCEMENT CONTINUUM

The enhancement of health covers a spectrum from environmental and social policies at one end to good clinical practice at the other (Table 10.3). The environmental determinants of health create the conditions for enhancement of health at the personal level. Although family physicians in industrialized countries do not usually have primary responsibility for environmental health, they can often identify local health problems in the course of their work. In poorer countries where public health services cannot as readily be taken for granted, family physicians may have a more direct responsibility for this aspect of health.

Social class is one of the strongest predictors of health and disease. Even in countries with universal access to health services and an effective social safety net, lower income and social status are associated with poorer health. The association has not been fully explained. It is likely that social status is a surrogate for several determinants of health, such as nutrition, housing, quality of environment, education, work satisfaction, control over one's life, and attitudes toward prevention.

Table 10.3. THE HEALTH ENHANCEMENT CONTINUUM

Environmental and Social Policies	Assessment of General Resistance Resources (GRR)	Enhancement of GRR	Risk Assessment	Risk Reduction	Presymtomatic Diagnosis	Early Diagnosis	Rehabilitation to Enhance Recovery	Care and Support of Patients with Chronic Disease and Their Families to Maintain Function and Reduce Complications
Housing	Self-assessed health status	Support	Smoking-related diseases	Smoking cessation	Screening and case finding	Prevention of complications by early diagnosis of serious treatable disease e.g., meningitis cranial arteritis myocardial infarction major depression	E.g., industrial injuries	E.g., Diabetes
Electric power	Confidence	Health education and counselling	Substance abuse	Reduction of alcohol intake	Hypertension		Stroke	Hypertension
Clean air	Coping ability	(e.g., nutrition, exercise sexuality, accident)	Coronary heart disease	Reduction of serum cholesterol	Cervical cancer		Accidents	Breast cancer
Clean water	Social support	Immunization	Family violence	Nutrition education	Breast cancer		Musculo skeletal disorders	Multiple sclerosis
Parks and recreation	Family function	Family planning	Accidents in aged	Accident prevention				COPD
Nutrition education	Work satisfaction	Prenatal care	STD	Referral to social services counseling				Chronic arthritis
Food inspection	Exercise	Child care	Teenage pregnancy					Schizophrenia
Occupational health and safety	Immunization status							Chronic depression
Insect control	Income security							Alzheimer's disease
Accident prevention	Knowledge of hygiene							
Child support and protection								
Access to health services								
Unemployment insurance								
Health education								
Social stability and law enforcement								

The next part of the spectrum concerns the identification of strengths and the enhancement of general resistance resources in individuals, followed by risk assessment and reduction. Prevention merges with clinical diagnosis and management in presymptomatic and early diagnosis, management, and rehabilitation. Measures for the enhancement of health are not limited to one part of the spectrum. General resistance resources (GRR), for example, are important both in the maintenance of health and in the recovery from disease. Assessment of GRR is an aspect of patient-centered medicine.

Identification of risk factors may be followed either by treatment (e.g., for hypertension) or by counseling in behavior change (e.g., for smoking). Because this involves either treatment of people without identifed disease or interference in a person's way of life, it is only justified when supported by strong evidence.

Health education is the provision of information, advice, and sometimes training in activities that can promote health. There are numerous examples: prenatal classes, preparation for parenthood, family planning, prevention of accidents in children, advice on seat belts and crash helmets, prevention of falls in the elderly, and information for travelers. Education for new experiences such as childbirth and parenthood is based on the principle that coping ability is enhanced by preparation. Health education is an activity for the whole healthcare team, including nurses, occupational therapists, physiotherapists, and nutritionists. Brochures, books, and the Internet can be valuable resources. Health education can also play a part in tertiary prevention. Counseling before surgery can reduce postoperative pain and time in the hospital. Video presentations can help patients to make choices between alternative therapies—for example, when facing a decision about prostatectomy.

A screening procedure is one that is applied to an unselected population to identify those members who are either diseased or at risk for a disease. For example, the population of a factory or a town may be screened for hypertension. In case finding, a person is identifed as diseased or at risk by the physician responsible for his or her health care. For example, a patient may be identified as hypertensive while attending for skin infection. It will be clear that case finding, rather than screening, is the method used in family practice. The family physician is responsible for the identification of the abnormality, its investigation and treatment, and follow-up.

HUMAN BEHAVIORAL COUNSELING

Human behavioral patterns have been identified as contributing as much as 40% of causes for premature death (Schroeder, 2007) and it is here that behavioral counseling techniques are intended to have an impact. The US Preventive Services Task Force (USPSTF) defines behavioral counseling interventions as preventive services that are designed to assist individuals to engage in healthy behaviors and limit unhealthy ones (Curry, Grossman, Whitlock, et al., 2014). Such interventions range from individual and marital therapy to group educational visits, smoking cessation counseling, regular exercise healthy diets, and others. Family physicians can assist patients not only on an individual basis in their practices, but also by supporting community, public health, and policy initiatives that support healthy living environments.

Motivational interviewing techniques are useful in family practice by taking into account that patients make significant changes in lifestyle in stages. These stages consist of pre-contemplation (no particular thoughts or intent to change), contemplation (thinking about making changes), preparation (getting ready to make changes), action (changes in behavior are made), and maintenance (changes achieved are consolidated and measures taken to prevent relapse) (Prochaska, 1979). Health promotion interventions are tailored to the particular stage of the patient. In the pre-contemplation phase, it may consist of increasing a person's awareness of the problem and providing education about known consequences of it. If a patient is in the contemplation phase, the physician encourages discussion about the patient's perception of the pros and cons of undertaking the needed change and validates the reasons for it. When a patient is in the preparation stage and has made a commitment to it, the intervention consists of supporting self-efficacy, identifying and assisting problem-solving, and encouraging small initial steps. Once a major change has been made, it is important to provide supportive follow-up and to discuss coping strategies for relapse. This last step is important since, in its absence, an individual will tend to view any relapse as a failure and reason to give up, rather than an expected event that can be made into a positive step.

By tailoring a health promotion or preventive intervention to the stages of change, the practitioner's and patient's time and the effectiveness of the intervention are made optimal. This approach has been shown to be useful in smoking cessation and other addiction counseling, and making lifestyle changes, including diet and exercise (Burke, Arkowitz, and Menchola, 2003). Motivational interviewing techniques have been shown to be adaptable in family practice and to improve communication in a variety of lifestyle-related issues (Soderlund, Madson, and Rubak, 2011).

THE EVALUATION OF SCREENING AND CASE FINDING

To justify the application of a screening or case-finding procedure, the following conditions should be fulfilled:

1. The disease in question should be a serious health problem.
2. There should be a pre-symptomatic phase during which treatment can change the course of the disease more successfully than in the symptomatic phase.

3. The screening procedure and the ensuing treatment should be acceptable to the public.
4. The screening procedure should have acceptable sensitivity and specificity.
5. The screening procedure and ensuing treatment should be cost-effective.

Severe hypertension fills these criteria because if untreated, it is associated with a higher mortality rate from stroke and heart disease; because the detection procedure has high specificity and sensitivity; and because treatment before end organ damage has occurred has been shown by randomized trial to increase survival. On the other hand, prostate-specific antigen fails by these criteria as a screening test for prostate cancer because of relatively low sensitivity (63%–83%)[2] and specificity (90%). Sensitivity decreases with increasing age, and in cases of benign prostatic hypertrophy, controversy exists over whether early prostatectomy increases survival (Fradet, 2007; Labrecque, Legare, and Cauchon, 2007), and there are recognized complications of biopsy from screening due to false positive results. Moreover, there is no evidence from randomized controlled trials that prostatectomy for early carcinoma increases survival.

The efficacy of screening is sometimes accepted on evidence that fails to take account of certain pitfalls. First, patients who volunteer for screening programs are often those who are destined for favorable outcomes for other reasons. Second, the increased survival demonstrated as a result of screening may be only the longer time the disease is known to exist (lead time bias). And third, screening programs will tend to identify slowly progressive variants of disease since these are more likely to have a long pre-symptomatic phase. For example, a very malignant carcinoma is unlikely to be identifed by screening because it is likely to cause symptoms early in the course of the disease. For all these reasons, the best evidence on which to base a screening procedure is that obtained by a randomized, controlled trial, with mortality, rather than duration of survival, as the endpoint. The increasing availability of screening tests has made it essential that decisions on screening should be made only after rigorous and critical examination of the evidence. As we will see in the next section, this is often not the case.

SCREENING-HISTORICAL ANTECEDENTS: PARTIAL PATIENTS

Armstrong (1995) drew attention to the emergence of what he designated "surveillance medicine" in the twentieth century. Historically, the "medical gaze" shifted from bedside medicine, in which illness and symptoms were the same, to hospital medicine in the late eighteenth century with the establishment of the hospital system in Paris. In hospital medicine, symptoms and signs were linked to underlying pathology whose existence could be inferred. The clinical-pathological correlation became the focus of work in biomedicine. Linking the pathological lesion and causal agent seemed to put medicine on an objective footing. With the advances in technology and biological understanding, biomedicine has made great advances in treating illnesses in individuals, but perhaps has had less impact on population health.

Beginning with concerns about the health of children and eventually concerns about the health of the population as a whole, twentieth century socio-medical surveys were instrumental in developing the idea that illness and disease existed in a continuum that included a premorbid state, prior to the development of signs and symptoms. The "medical gaze" shifted from the body of the patient with signs and symptoms to the community and to lifestyle. The community became the "space" of illness.

As an "epidemiological transition" from infectious diseases to non-communicable chronic diseases occurred, the idea of a specific causal agent gave way to a multifactorial model. Techniques of statistical probability reinforced the notion of a "quantitative gradation" of ill health. "Thus individuals at high risk came to be interpreted as having a latent medical condition, even though there was only a probability that they would ever develop symptoms or pathological change" (Greaves, 2004, p. 116). It was no longer necessary for individuals to feel ill and seek medical attention to become patients. They could be identified through testing to have risk factors and be deemed medically abnormal. The individual's subjective experience became unnecessary to making a diagnosis.

Building on this concept of "surveillance medicine," David Greaves (2004) develops the notion of "partial patients." Such individuals represent a social category of individuals who do not feel themselves to be ill or disabled, but have been medically informed that they may have or may be at risk for having a disease. There are two major types of partial patients: those who are identified from screening or preventive medicine practices (e.g., raised serum cholesterol, hypertension, genetic family history of Huntington's disease) and those who have a recognized medical condition that has caused them to be ill in the past but which is in remission or controlled at present (e.g., controlled diabetes mellitus, stable angina, cancer in remission). It is the first type, those identified from screening or preventive medicine practices, which are principally considered in this chapter.

Greaves sees partial patients as a natural consequence of a biomedical approach. Separating the subjective illness from diagnosis made it conceptually possible to seek out disease in apparently healthy populations. It is necessary for family physicians to recognize that surveillance medicine places on them an onus to ensure that screening practices are of benefit and that the pros and cons of screening tests are adequately conveyed to their patients.

Problems in the Interpretation and Application of Evidence

Even when the evaluation has been conducted by experts in the field, there have been many examples of failure to apply rigorous standards to evidence.[1] Indeed, the involvement of experts carries its own risks, since deep involvement in an issue can generate so much enthusiasm for promoting it that contrary evidence is ignored.

The following are some examples:

Ignoring Contrary Evidence

In the latter half of the twentieth century, research on diet and heart disease focused on saturated fats and failed to take into account other factors such as sugar, even though at the same time there was compelling evidence that sugar intake was an important factor (Sinatra, Leder, and Bowden, 2014). The work of Ansel Keys (Keys, Menotti, Aravanis, et al., 1984) was highly influential in thinking about the rise of cardiovascular disease (CVD) that was then occurring. The diet-heart hypothesis holds that saturated fat in the diet and, in some versions of the hypothesis, dietary cholesterol are major contributors to heart disease. Alternatively, Yudkin (1964) had amassed stronger evidence that dietary carbohydrates, especially refined sugars, were a much stronger contributor. Despite evidence to the contrary showing that saturated fats are not important contributors to CVD, the diet-heart hypothesis has dominated medical thinking and popular culture for many years. Avoiding fats in the diet may have contributed to the increase in dietary carbohydrates that has characterized Western diets and this, in turn, has been linked to the "epidemic" in diabetes. As attention has changed from a focus on dietary fats, other and better supported theories regarding CVD have emerged, such as those concerning inflammation and mitochondrial dysfunction as well as ROS (reactive oxygen species), which is increased by dietary carbohydrates and vegetable oils used in cooking. *Trans*-fatty acids have been shown to be involved in cardiac dysfunction and blood lipid abnormalities causing significant cardiac pathology. So, while saturated fats have been blamed, the real culprits were trans-fatty acids and carbohydrates, including starchy foods such as potatoes and rice, processed cereals, pasta, and bread. It is striking that even as the focus on saturated fats began, there was evidence that dietary carbohydrates were to blame. It has taken over 50 years to overcome this erroneous orthodoxy.

Failing to Take into Account the Impact of False Positive Tests

Tests like Papinicolaou smears, mammograms, and prostate-specific antigen are initial screens which, if positive, require additional tests to confirm the result. When the number of false positive screening tests is high, large numbers of normal people are subjected to these further tests, with their attendant risks, and to the anxiety caused by the process.

For example, a screening test with a sensitivity of 90% and specificity of 96%, if used in a population where the prevalence is 0.6% (not uncommon for some cancers in family practice), the 88% of those who are found to be abnormal will be false positives. This means that if 1000 people are screened, 6 will have the condition and 40 will be falsely labeled as positive and will undergo further testing, which may itself involve some morbidity and even mortality (for more on the risks of screening, see Woolf and Harris, 2012).

The Ritual of Annual Testing

When new screening tests are introduced, there generally follows a period when they are carried out on an annual basis. As knowledge of the impact of the test on population health accumulates and the cost–benefit ratio is adjusted, testing intervals are frequently changed. Pap smears used to be recommended on an annual basis for all women when they became sexually active. More recently, the recommendation has been changed to initiate testing at age 21 and screen every 3 years until age 65. For women 30–65 years of age, screening may be lengthened to every 5 years when cytological screening is combined with testing for human papilloma virus (HPV) (US Preventive Services Task Force, 2012).

The Chimera of Universal Consensus

When all the evidence has been considered, decisions about screening still depend on judgment. There is no single correct answer to questions like the cutoff point between "normal" and "abnormal," the level at which treatment is indicated, or the frequency of testing. The answers vary from one country to another, depending on cultural and economic factors. After reviewing cholesterol guidelines in six countries, Rosser et al. (1993) concluded that policy and guidelines tended to be more influenced by political and economic factors than by evidence of health benefit. The assessments produced by the international Cochrane project will probably be interpreted differently in each national jurisdiction.

Extrapolation Beyond the Group Investigated in the Trial

When a trial has established that a screening test is justified in one age and sex group, there is a tendency to assume that the evidence also justifies the procedure in other groups such as females and the elderly of both sexes. This cannot be taken for granted since biological differences between males and females, and between children, mature adults, and the elderly, make it very likely that different criteria will apply. Most of the early research on cholesterol and heart disease has been conducted on middle-aged men. More than 10,000 men with preexisting coronary disease were enrolled in trials of cholesterol reduction, but only just over 400 women—too few for definitive results (Rich-Edwards, Manson, Hennekens, and Buring, 1995). Only 5800 of more than 30,000 people enrolled in primary prevention trials of cholesterol reduction have been women—not enough to obtain the necessary statistical power. With greater knowledge, it is now recommended that all men over age 35 be screened for lipid abnormalities, but for women screening not begin until age 45 in those at high risk (USPSTF, 2008). Clinical trials may include balanced numbers of both sexes, but may not report the results separately. Trials also tend to recruit people with fewer coexisting diseases than the general population.

The Concept of Risk

It is useful to distinguish between risk and uncertainty. Risk refers to the situation in which it is possible to determine the probability of different outcomes. Uncertainty exists where no such probabilities are possible. It is not uncommon to find uncertainty referred to as risk, thus obscuring a lack of knowledge. The identfication of risk factors has become a major objective of epidemiological research and an increasing number of reports are appearing in major medical journals (Skolbekken, 1995). Much of this research has been criticized for its conceptual confusion (Hayes, 1992) and lack of rigor (Feinstein, 1988). Many studies do not begin with a hypothesis based on clinical observation. The factors to be tested for association with the target disorder are therefore not determined in advance. Instead, large numbers of variables are subjected to statistical manipulations that are easily done with modern computers. When a statistically significant relationship comes out, it may be wrongly interpreted as a causal relationship. Rarely a week passes without one of these findings being reported in the media, raising public anxieties and undermining people's confidence in their ability to lead a healthy life. Reports with major methodological errors have been accepted by leading medical journals. More than 80,000 articles on risk were published between 1987 and 1991 (Skolbekken, 1995).

The identification of a causal factor, such as smoking for lung cancer, usually begins with a clinical observation or a hypothesis based on some logical connection between factor and target disorder. A cohort of patients with the target disorder is assembled with special care to avoid selection bias. A matching group without the target disorder is obtained, again with care to match the groups for all variables that could influence the factor in question. The groups are then compared for the presence of the factor. For any factor that depends on self-reporting, such as diet or smoking, great care must be taken to validate questionnaires and avoid recall bias. Many studies do not follow this procedure. Since there is no hypothesis to guide the formation of a cohort, a convenience cohort, selected for some other purpose, is used. The investigators thus have no control over the way data were collected, either at entry to the study or afterward. To avoid selection bias, it is crucial that the target disorder should be sought with equal thoroughness in groups with and without the disorder, so that "silent" cases in the latter group will not be missed. For example, the apparent association of alcohol and breast cancer could be explained if heavy drinkers were more likely to be diagnosed because of increased medical attention, or if moderate drinkers were of a different social class from abstainers, and more likely to attend for screening.

Even when well-designed studies have shown a causal relationship between factor and target disorder, and randomized trials have shown that modification of the factor can change the outcome, unjustified extrapolations may be made to groups of people not represented in the cohort. Studies of men may be extrapolated to women, or studies of younger people extrapolated to the elderly (McCormick, 1994).

Flawed methodology leads to the accumulation of "risk factors" that are no more than statistical associations between observations. More than 300 risk fac- tors for coronary disease have been identified (Skrabanek and McCormick, 1990). The term *risk factor* covers a number of quite different concepts of risk. It does not distinguish between factors that are causal, such as smoking for lung cancer, and those that are contingent, such as age and sex for coronary heart disease. Nor does it distinguish between factors that are unalterable and those that can be changed. Whether a risk factor is called a disease or a cause of disease is a matter of convention. Blood cholesterol above a critical level is called a risk factor for coronary heart disease. Blood sugar above a critical level is called a disease—diabetes mellitus—even if there are no symptoms. Symptomless carcinoma of the prostate, discovered at transurethral prostatectomy, is called a disease, not a risk factor, even though it may not progress to the stage of symptoms.

Foss and Rothenberg (1987) maintain that risk factors tend to be called *causes* if they fit with the prevailing mechanistic paradigm; behavioral factors are still called *risk factors* even when they have a causal relationship with disease. Skrabanek and McCormick (1990, p. 94) believe that risk factors should be called "risk markers" to emphasize that they are associated with altered probability of developing disease rather than necessarily being causally related.

Epidemiology came of age when the doctrine of specific causation held sway. Infectious diseases provided the model for diseases to be defined in terms of single causal agents, even though multiple factors in host and environment contributed to the web of causation. The factor isolated as the cause was the one "necessary" for a case to be classified as an example of the disease. With the infectious diseases of the nineteenth century, the doctrine worked well. Now, infectious disease is often nosocomial, and the "cause" has to be sought in some change in the host. The doctrine of specific causation does not work well for chronic diseases, which cannot usually be classified in terms of a single necessary cause. Epidemiology has thus becoming a probabilistic science. Identification of factors strongly associated with disease is a valid procedure, provided that they are treated as hypotheses to be tested. If a prospective study shows a causal relationship, then the factor should be classified as a cause. The magnitude of its contribution to the causal web should also be expressed in terms of probability.

The necessity of having a hypothesis should not blind us to the importance of unexpected findings. Many important discoveries have been the unexpected result of research done for some other purpose. The usual course of events is that the finding is confirmed by a study in which the unexpected finding becomes a new hypothesis.

Perception of Risk from Relatives' Knowledge of Their Family Histories

Risk perceptions have been shown to be held by people with a family history of breast cancer, colon cancer, diabetes, and heart disease (Walter and Emery, 2006). Understanding of familial risk may be influential in motivating preventive measures and healthy behavior. Structured models have been developed to integrate different health beliefs and to understand their role in predicting health-related behavior.

Levanthals' Common Sense Model of Self-Regulation of Health and Illness (CSM) (Leventhal et al., 2003) arose from the observation that biomedical symptoms (or identity) represented only one type of perceptual information needed to appraise a health risk situation. Other attributes of threats used in the CSM were as follows (Walter and Emery, 2005):

1. Identity: internal or external sources of information of a relative's illness (e.g., a symptom of information that a relative has a disease)
2. Time scale of the threat (timeline)
3. Potential to affect life expectancy or quality of life
4. Perceived cause of the illness
5. Controllability: the possibility of coping with the illness.

In their study, Walter and Emery used the framework of the CSM to compare and contrast perceptions about family history among primary care patients with a family history of cancer, heart disease, or diabetes.

Participants were recruited from two general practices and the sampling strategy aimed to gain as broad a range as possible of age, gender, educational levels, and degree of family risk. Semi-structured qualitative interviews were conducted by one person (F. M. Walter), mainly in the interviewees' homes, and lasted about an hour. Flexibility allowed for discussion of important issues.

Walter and Emery's study was the first to examine inter-disease variations in perceptions of their family history among a primary care sample. It demonstrates some benefits of obtaining the relevant data in this way. From the scientific point of view, the lengthy interchange between interviewee and investigator allows for accuracy of the data. For the family practitioner, it obtains this important data at first hand and can enter data into the patient's chart (neither of the investigators were members of the two practices). Walter and Emery present their results in comparison with the CSM categories of *consequences and timeline, cause, controllability and relative threats of cancer, heart disease, and diabetes.* In each case, interviewee's comments are quoted verbatim and together with the investigator's findings.

Before the above-mentioned publications, Fiona Walter and her colleagues had published two other papers on the same theme.

Walter and Emery write, "The family history is becoming an increasingly important feature of health promotion and early detection of common chronic diseases in primary care. Previous studies of patients from genetics clinics suggest a divergence between how persons with a family history perceive and understand their risk and the risk provided by health professionals ... what exactly constitutes having a family history of an illness varied among participants. The development of a personal sense of vulnerability to the illness in the family depended not only on the biomedical approach ... but also on an interplay of other factors" (p. 405). These included the emotional impact of witnessing the illness in the family, members' personal relationships in the family, and different beliefs about the contribution to illness of nature and nurture. Family health history may make some diseases more salient to individuals but is often lower than their calculated risk (Acheson, Wang, and Zyzanski, 2010).

Absolute Risk, Relative Risk, and the Number Needed to Treat

The family physician needs some way of applying epidemiological data to individuals and of explaining their implications to patients. The "number needed to treat" is a way of conveying both statistical and clinical significance. It is defined as the number of patients the physician will need to treat to prevent one adverse event. For patients, it is much easier to understand than percentages. We have to remember that many of our patients have difficulty with percentages, even to the extent of reckoning the amount of a waiter's tip.

Research findings are often expressed in terms of the relative risk reduction. This has no bearing, however, on the probability that an individual will acquire the disease. If the absolute risk is very small, the increase in risk, though relatively high, may in fact be very small. The 30% greater risk of lung cancer in passive smokers, compared to other nonsmokers, moves them from a probability of 0.09 per 1000 to 0.12 per 1000 (Skrabanek and McCormick, 1990, pp. 40–41).

The number needed to treat is the reciprocal of the absolute risk reduction (Laupacis, Sackett, and Roberts, 1988). Cook and Sackett (1995) use data from a review of antihypertensive therapy (Collins et al., 1990) as an illustration. Patients with mild hypertension receiving placebo had a 1.5% expectation of a stroke over 5 years, compared with 0.9% in those receiving antihypertensive drugs, giving a risk reduction of 0.015 – 0.009 = 0.006. The reciprocal of this number is about 167, so that 167 patients would need to be treated for 5 years to prevent one stroke. This assumes that the individual patient's baseline risk is the same as the baseline risk of patients in the trial, which may not be the case. If the baseline risk of a patient is higher by a factor f times the risk of patients in the trial, the new number needed to treat is the original number divided by f. If the patient's baseline risk is estimated to be twice the risk of those in the trial, the number needed to treat would be 167/2 or 83.

This could be explained to a patient with the same baseline risk as the trial patients in the following way. "If 100 men like you are followed for 5 years, about two will have a stroke, 98 will not. We do not know whether you are one of the two or one of the 98. If you reduce your blood pressure by taking antihypertensive medication, you can jump to another group. Then out of 100 men like you, one will have a stroke, 99 will not. We still do not know whether you are the one, or one of the 99. Which group do you wish to belong to: those who accept the status quo, or those who take medication?"

CLINICAL GUIDELINES

The sheer volume of evidence now available makes it impossible for any one physician to base his or her practice on his or her own critical review of the literature. To meet this need, institutions, academic bodies, professional groups, and others developed recommendations or guidelines on matters such as diagnostic tests, management of disease, and preventive procedures. The process varies from one group to another. Sometimes the guidelines are developed by a group of experts on the subject in question. The problem with this is that experts develop enthusiasms for their subjects and may be inclined to brush aside critical evidence. Even when dissenting voices are raised, they may find it difficult to gain a hearing. The process is "top down." Recommendations are handed down to practitioners without the opportunity of feedback while the guidelines are being developed. This may set the stage for disputes between practitioners and experts. The situation becomes more complex when members of panels that develop guidelines have financial ties to industry that benefits from the recommendations, thus creating conflicts of interest (Norris, Holmer, Ogden, et al., 2011).

The process designed by the Dutch College of General Practitioners (NHG) is an example of the opposite "bottom up" approach, in which practitioners initiate and participate in the whole process. The aim is to achieve a balance between evidence-based guidelines and guidelines that are feasible in practice (Grol, Thomas, and Roberts, 1995). An independent advisory board of experienced practitioners selects the topic. A working party of four to eight family physicians is appointed, representing a mix of scientific and practical experience. The group analyzes the literature, explores clinical experience, and builds a consensus leading to draft guidelines. Since scientific evidence is often lacking or conflicting, the discussions are often extensive. Only 5% to 10% of guidelines can be based on scientific evidence (Grol, Thomas, and Roberts, 1995).

The draft guidelines are sent for comment to 50 randomly selected general practitioners and to external reviewers, who are usually experts in the subject. After this review, the working party has to defend its guidelines before a critical group of general practitioners with high academic and professional standing. The definitive guidelines are then published in the scientific journal for Dutch family physicians and educational programs are developed. Finally, the impact of the guidelines is assessed by surveys, and updates are provided when new evidence becomes available. About half the members of working groups are general practitioners with academic appointments, some of whom have done research on the subject of the guidelines. The guidelines are reviewed and brought up to date every 3–5 years depending on the emergence of new information. The dissemination of the guidelines is accompanied by educational initiatives. After 10 years they have developed and disseminated over 70 guidelines (Grol, 2001).The Dutch system would only be possible in a country where general practice research and academic general practice are well supported.

Clinical guidelines are a tool that can enhance care for patients, and general agreement on the methods and procedures for their development (Burgers, Cluzeau, et al., 2003) has improved the quality of guidelines. However, there remain some issues (Grol and van Weel, 2009). Not all clinical guidelines adhere to the AGREE Collaborative criteria (http://www.agreetrust.org/), which leads to sometimes wide variation and hence confusion. They frequently are aimed at single disease entities and do not take into account the complexity introduced by multimorbidity. Many clinical guidelines contain many recommendations and do not highlight the most important ones or key targets, making implementation more difficult. Finally, tools to implement them in practice are often lacking. "The limitations and importance of drawing guidelines for highly different circumstances under which practitioners encounter their patients should be acknowledged. This is even more important when financial incentives are linked to evidence-based guidelines" (Grol and van Weel, 2009, p. 438).

With the evolution of managed care, there are fears that guidelines will eventually become mandatory, thus limiting the clinical freedom of physicians to apply them with discretion. There is a fear also that, in legal cases, failure to follow the guidelines may be used as evidence of malpractice.

PREVENTIVE METHODS IN FAMILY PRACTICE

The source of a family doctor's effectiveness is his or her knowledge of the strengths and vulnerabilities of individual patients and their families. Statistical probabilities and authoritative recommendations always have to be applied to an individual. A heavy smoker should be counseled to stop, but what if he is a chronic schizophrenic who derives from smoking one of his few comforts? Amniocentesis should be offered to pregnant women aged 35 or over, or if her risk of having a Down's syndrome child is similar to that of a 35-year-old woman. But what if she is a 33-year-old single mother with poor coping skills and doubts about her ability to raise a Down's syndrome child, or if she is a married woman whose husband is ambivalent about parenthood? Family doctors' knowledge of their patients can enhance their effectiveness in other ways: interventions can be made when patients are most receptive to them, and opportunities can be taken to increase patients' confidence in their health.

For many years one of the mainstays of preventive medicine in family practice was the annual physical examination, at which a history and physical examination were combined with a battery of screening tests. The practice of applying a package of screening tests to a population is also called "multiphasic screening." Experimental evidence available has failed to show that the type of multiphasic screening applied during an annual physical examination has an impact on overall mortality rates (Holland et al., 1977; Dales, Friedman, and Collen, 1979). These studies failed to demonstrate any statistically significant differences in the overall death rates between the treatment and control groups. However, in one study (Dales et al., 1979) mortality from some of the diseases to which screening was directed showed significantly improved rates in the screening group. These findings indicate that screening programs must be evaluated by specific as well as overall mortality.

As a preventive strategy for family practice, the annual physical examination was also open to a number of other objections:

1. It bears little relation to the specific needs of different age groups.
2. Because of the global nature of the complete physical examination, it often includes tests that fail to fulfill the criteria for acceptance of a screening or case-finding procedure—electrocardiography, for example.
3. Annual testing may be no more effective than less frequent testing (see earlier discussion).
4. In most practices, complete physicals are given only to that section of the population who demand it or at least are compliant. If every member of a practice of 2000 patients had a 20-minute annual health examination, it would occupy the physician full-time for 22 weeks of every year.

In other words, the annual physical is a poorly thought-out strategy for applying modern knowledge of preventive medicine in family practice.

The approach to prevention called "the periodic health examination" (PHE) provides a more rational strategy for family practice. It is based on the following principles:

1. Tests and procedures are repeated at intervals determined by epidemiological evidence, not by arbitrary choice.
2. Where feasible, these are grouped into "packages," so that the number of visits the patient has to make are reduced.
3. Maximum use is made of the opportunity for case-finding provided by visits for all purposes. In 1 year, 70% of the practice population is seen at least once. The average number of visits for each patient is about four per year. In the course of 5 years, virtually the whole population of the practice will pass through the physician's office. A relatively straightforward procedure like detection of hypertension can be performed almost entirely as a case-finding maneuver.
4. Screening tests and procedures are not included unless there is good evidence for their effectiveness. For example, there is no justification for including a chest X-ray.

Since the periodic health examination makes a more efficient use of time and resources than the annual examination, the strategy can be applied to the whole practice population. The whole practice team, including family practice nurse and public health nurse, can participate in the process. Review of studies on scheduled PHEs found that they improve delivery of some recommended services and reduce patient worry (Boulware, Barnes, Wilson, et al., 2007). From the perspective of the family physician, the extra time that is normally provided for the PHE allows for becoming more acquainted with the patient and his or her context, thus building a stronger patient–physician relationship.

The Organizational Tools

To practice preventive medicine in an organized way, the practice needs a well-designed record system. Two types of records are required:

1. For the individual patient. If all visits to the physician are to be used for case-finding, the physician should be able to see at a glance from the patient's record which preventive procedures the patient has had and which procedures are needed in any particular year. This can be done by means of a flow chart. Different types of flow charts can be used for different age and sex groups.

2. For the whole practice population. Unless there is some system for monitoring preventive procedures in the whole population, there will be no way of knowing whether the practices' preventive targets have been achieved or not. There will be no way of knowing which children remain unimmunized, which adults have not had a blood pressure reading, which women have not had a Pap smear or mammography, or which diabetics have not attended for follow-up.

Record-keeping in family practice has progressed rapidly with the increasing use of electronic record systems. It remains true, however, that some practitioners have not completed the transition to these systems and remain with paper-based records. Even with simple paper records, many useful tools have been developed to enable tracking of preventive medicine procedures. One useful system is the practice age/sex register. A simpler method is to attach a colored tag or sticker to the chart when a particular procedure has been done. A red tag on the chart could mean that the blood pressure had been recorded in the years 2011 or 2012. By quickly looking through all the charts at the end of 2013, one could then identify those patients who had not had a blood pressure reading done in the previous 2 years. This method can also be used for identifying patients who are at special risk.

Computerized record systems used in family practice have made possible preventive medicine reminders tailored to the patient to appear on the screen at the time of the visit. So, for example, if a woman has not had a mammogram in the recommended time frame, when she is visiting for a prescription renewal, a prompt appears on her electronic record and the physician is able to use the visit to remind her of the importance of having the test done.

Electronic patient records also make it easy to derive aggregate data from a practice population, fulfilling the second requirement mentioned. Family physicians with such systems are able to quickly obtain a list of all diabetic patients in their practice and even display the average hemoglobin A1C for that cohort of patients. Insurance companies and government health insurance plans are using the achievement of preventive medicine benchmarks, such as this, to provide incentives to practitioners. In addition, a family physician can introduce a program to increase the uptake of, for example, influenza vaccinations and measure the degree of success by comparing practice-based immunization rates before and after.

Preventive Procedures for Specific Conditions

Excellent online resources detailing recommended preventive procedures are available from the Canadian Task Force on Preventive Health Care (www.ctf-phc.org/) and the US Preventive Services Task Force (www.ahrq.gov/clinic/usp-st5x.htm). These databases are updated and are relevant to family physicians.

NOTES

1. For additional reading, see the excellent series of articles in the *Canadian Medical Association Journal* (Marshall KG, 1996: May 15, June 15, July 15, and August 15).
2. These figures assume a cutoff score of 4.0 ng/ml. Attempts to improve this screening method include measuring the velocity of change observed in multiple measurements and fractionating the level of PSA into free and total.

REFERENCES

Acheson LS, Wang C, Zyzanski SJ, et al. 2010. Family history and perceptions about risk and prevention for chronic diseases in primary care: A report from the Family Healthware™ Impact Trial. *Genetics in Medicine* 12:212–218.

AGREE (Appraisal of Guidelines for Research and Evaluation). http://www.agreetrust. org/.

Antonovsky A. 1979. *Health, Stress and Coping.* San Francisco, CA: Jossey-Bass.

Antonovsky A. 1987. *Unravelling the Mystery of Health.* San Francisco, CA: Jossey-Bass.

Armstrong D. 1995. The rise of surveillance medicine. *Sociology of Health and Illness* 17:393–404.

Boulware LE, Barnes GJ, Wilson RF, et al. 2007. Systematic Review: The Value of the Periodic Health Evaluation. *Annals of Int Med* 146(4):289–300.

Burgers JS, Cluzeau FA, et al. 2003. Characteristics of high-quality guidelines: evaluation of 86 guidelines developed in ten European countries and Canada. *International Journal of Technology Assessment in Health Care* 19(1):148–157.

Burke BL, Arkowitz H, Menchola M. 2003. The efficacy of motivational interviewing: A meta-analysis of clinical trials. *Journal of Consulting and Clinical Psychology* 71(5):843–871.

Canadian Medical Association Office for Public Health. 2001. *Health Promotion and Injury Prevention.* http://www.cma.ca/index.cfm/ci_id/3391/la_id/1.htm.

Collins R, Peto R, MacMahon S, et al. 1990. Blood pressure, stroke, and coronary heart disease. II. Short-term reductions in blood pressure: Overview of randomized drug trials in their epidemiologic context. *Lancet* 335:827–838.

Cook RJ, Sackett DL. 1995. The number needed to treat: A clinically useful measure of treatment effect. *British Medical Journal* 310:452–454.

Curry S, Grossman DC, Whitlock EP, Cantu A. 2014. Behavioral counseling research and evidence-based practice recommendations: U.S. Preventive Services Task Force Perspectives. *Annals of Internal Medicine* 160:407–413.

Dales LG, Friedman GD, Collen MF. 1979. Evaluating periodic multiphasic health check-ups: A controlled trial. *Journal of Chronic Disease* 32:385.

Dubos R. 1980. *Man Adapting.* New Haven, CT: Yale University Press.

Feinstein AR. 1988. Scientific standards in epidemiologic studies of the menace of daily life. *Science* 2(242):1257–1263.

Foss L, Rothenberg K. 1987. *The Second Medical Revolution: From Biomedicine to Infomedicine.* Boston, MA: Shambhala.

Fradet Y. 2007. Should Canadians be offered systematic prostate cancer screening?: YES. *Canadian Family Physician* 53(6):989–992.

Freed LA, Benjamin EJ, Levy D, et al. 2002. Mitral valve prolapse in the general population: The benign nature of echocardiographic features in the Framingham Heart Study. *Journal of the American College of Cardiology* 40(7):1298–1304.

Galen RS, Gambino SR. 1975. *Beyond Normality: The Predictive Value and Efficiency of Medical Diagnoses*. New York: John Wiley.

Gordon I. 1958. That damned word health. *Lancet* 2:638–639.

Greaves D. 2004. The creation of partial patients. In: *The Healing Tradition: Reviving the Soul of Western Medicine*. Oxford: Radcliffe Publishing.

Grol R. 2001. Successes and failures in the implementation of evidence-based guidelines for clinical practice. *Medical Care* 38(8 Suppl. 2):1146–1154.

Grol R, Thomas S, Roberts R. 1995. Development and implementation of guidelines for family practice: Lessons from the Netherlands. *Journal of Family Practice* 40(5):435–439.

Grol R, van Weel C. 2009. Getting a grip on guidelines: How to make them more relevant for practice. *British Journal of General Practice* 59(56):e143–e144.

Hayes MV. 1992. On the epistemology of risk: Language, logic and social science. *Social Science & Medicine* 35(4):401–407.

Hepner AD, Ahmadi-Kashani M, Movahed MR. 2007. The prevalence of mitral valve prolapse in patients undergoing echocardiography for clinical reason. *International Journal of Cardiology* 123(1):55–57.

Holland WW, et al. 1977. A controlled trial of multiphasic screening in middle age: Results from the SE London screening study. *International Journal of Epidemiology* 6:357.

Hollnagel H, Malterud K. 1995. Shifting attention from objective risk factors to patients' self-assessed health resources: A clinical model for general practice. *Family Practice* 12(4):423–429.

Idler EL. 1992. Self-assessed health and mortality: A review of studies. In: Maes S, Leventhal H, Johnston M, eds., *International Review of Health Psychology*. New York: John Wiley & Sons.

Keys A, Menotti A, Aravanis C, et al. 1984. The seven countries study: 2,289 deaths in 15 years. *Preventive Medicine* 13(2):141–154.

Labrecque M, Légaré F, Cauchon M. 2007. Should Canadians be offered systematic prostate cancer screening? NO. *Canadian Family Physician* 53(6):989–992.

Laupacis A, Sackett DL, Roberts RS. 1988. An assessment of clinically useful measures of the consequences of treatment. *New England Journal of Medicine* 318:1728–1733.

Leventhal H, Brissette I, Leventhal, EA. 2003. The common-sense model of self-regulation of health and illness. In: Katouzian, HD, Cameron LD, Leventhal H, eds., *The Self- regulation of Health and Illness Behaviour*. London: Routledge.

Lorig K, Mazonson PD, Holman HR. 1993. Evidence suggesting that health education for self-management in patients with chronic arthritis has sustained health benefits while reducing health care costs. *Arthritis and Rheumatism* 36:439–446.

McCormick J. 1994. Health promotion: The ethical dimension. *Lancet* 344:390–391.

Moore WS, Barnet HJM, Beebe HG, et al. 1995. Guidelines for carotid endarterectomy: A multidisciplinary consensus statement from the Ad Hoc Committee, American Heart Association. *Stroke* 26:188–201.

Mossey JM, Shapiro E. 1982. Self-rated health: A predictor of mortality among the elderly. *American Journal of Public Health* 72(8):800–808.

Murphy EA. 1976. *The Logic of Medicine*. Baltimore, MD: Johns Hopkins University Press.

Norris SL, Holmer HK, Ogden LA, Borda BU. 2011 Conflict of interest in clinical practice guideline development: A systematic review. *PLoS ONE* 6(10):e25153.

O'Connor A, Tugwell P. 1995. *Making choices: Hormones after the menopause* (cassette and booklet). University of Ottawa.

Prochaska JO. 1979. *Systems of psychotherapy: A transtheoretical analysis.* Homewood, IL: Dorsey Press.

Rich-Edwards JW, Manson JAE, Hennekens CH, Buring JE. 1995. The primary prevention of coronary heart disease in women. *New England Journal of Medicine* 332:1758–1766.

Rosser WW, Palmer WH, Fowler G, Lamberts H, et al. 1993. An international perspective on the cholesterol debate. *Family Practice* 10(4):431–437.

Ryle J. 1948. The meaning of normal and the measurement of health. In: *Changing Disciplines.* New York: Oxford University Press.

Schroeder S. 2007. We can do better: Improving the health of the American people. *New England Journal of Medicine* 357(12):1221–1228.

Siegrist J. 1993. Sense of coherence and sociology of emotions. Comment on Antonovsky. *Social Science & Medicine* 37:974–979.

Sinatra ST, Teter BB, Dowden J, Houston MC, Martinez-Gonzalez MA. 2014. The saturated fat, cholesterol and statin controversy: A commentary. *Journal of the American College of Nutrition* 33(1):79–88.

Skolbekken JA. 1995. The risk epidemic in medical journals. *Social Science & Medicine* 40(3):291–305.

Skrabanek P, McCormick J. 1990. *Follies and Fallacies in Medicine.* Glasgow: The Tarragon Press.

Sobel DS. 1995. Rethinking medicine: Improving health outcomes with cost-effective psychosocial interventions. *Psychosomatic Medicine* 57:234–244.

Soderlund LL, Madson MB, Rubak S, Nilsen P. 2011. Systematic review of motivational interviewing training for general health care practitioners. *Patient Education and Counseling* 84(1):16–26.

US Preventive Services Task Force. 1996. *Guide to Clinical Preventive Services,* 2nd ed. Baltimore, MD: Williams and Wilkins.

Walter F, Emery J. 2005. Coming down the line-patient's understanding of their family history of chronic disease. *Annals of Family Medicine* 3(50):405–414.

Walter FM, Emery J. 2006. Perceptions of family history across common diseases: A qualitative study in primary care. *Family Practice* 3(5):405–414.

WHO Ottawa Charter for Health Promotion. 1986. An International Conference on Health Promotion, the move towards a new public health; 17–21 November, Ottawa, Geneva, Canada: World Health Organization.

Woolf SH, Harris R. 2012. The harms of screening: New attention to an old concern. *Journal of the American Medical Association* 307(6):565–566.

Yudkin J. 1964. Patterns and trends in carbohydrate consumption and their relation to disease. *Proceedings of the Nutrition Society* 23:149–162.

PART II

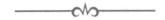

Clinical Problems

The six chapters in Part II are intended to demonstrate an approach to organizing information about common illnesses in a way that is useful to family practitioners and to demonstrate the application of the principles in the first section of the book. Emphasizing the importance of social factors, family influences, and the subjective aspects of illness does not diminish the importance of our biological understanding of disease. The scientific foundation of the family physician's clinical approach is one of the central pillars of the discipline. This biomedical pillar is well delineated in the literature and guidelines and requires our constant attention. The remaining pillars recognize the importance of context, relationships, and personal meaning in both the generation of ill health and its alleviation. These are less often found in standard textbooks and guidelines, though they are prominent in the approach taken in family practice. Properly understanding and applying knowledge in these areas is fundamental to a patient-centered clinical approach.

CHAPTER 11

᭜ᐓᖡ

Respiratory Illness

Respiratory illnesses affect both children and adults and are among the most common reasons for attendance in family practice. Respiratory disease can be roughly categorized into acute and chronic. Acute disease may be principally present in the upper respiratory tract (URTI) or the lower respiratory tract (LRTI), and the latter may be further divided into pneumonia or bronchitis (non-pneumonia LRTI). Chronic respiratory diseases consist of asthma and chronic obstructive pulmonary disease (COPD) or emphysema. There still remains the less common causes of respiratory symptoms such as malignancies and autoimmune diseases, which will not be addressed here.

PREVALENCE IN FAMILY PRACTICE

All told, diseases of the respiratory system account for 10% of visits to physician's offices in the United States in a 1-week period (NAMCS, 2010). The symptom of cough, alone, accounts for 3.1% of such visits. Many of these visits are due to acute illness, but patients attending physicians also have a number of chronic diseases, and among these are asthma (6.8% of all visits) and COPD (3.9% of all visits). In a family practice with a patient enrollment or panel size of 2500 and an age distribution reflecting the US population (including children), Ostbye (2005) and colleagues estimated that there would by 183 patients with asthma and 131 with COPD.

SOCIAL CONTEXT

In most acute infectious diseases there is a well-established negative relationship with socioeconomic status. Poverty and deprivation go hand in hand with disease. In developing countries, acute respiratory infections are the leading cause of death in all age groups (WHO, 2011). The risk of pneumonia is higher where low birth weight, poor nutrition, low income, and indoor air pollution are prevalent (Fried and Gaydos, 2012). Prevalence of asthma, on the other hand, is higher in high-income countries and in urban compared to rural environments. The complex relationship between asthma and economic conditions is not well understood. In the United States, stress and violence are emerging as risk factors (Williams et al., 2009). "Poverty is a complex condition and it is not easy to unravel the effects of the various environmental and lifestyle factors involved in asthma causation, nor indeed the impact of this chronic disease upon the perpetuation of poverty" (Cruz et al., 2010, p. 239). Tobacco consumption, linked to respiratory illness as well as cardiac disease and other conditions, is declining in developed countries but rising in developing ones and is negatively associated with socioeconomic status (Fried and Gaydos, 2012).

FAMILY INFLUENCES

The family is a semi-closed system, with each member having varied exposures outside the home. Depending upon the age of each family member, host resistance will vary, with the very young and very old having relatively less immunity. Further, levels of stress will vary and will affect susceptibility to infection. So, although family members share genetic makeup, the presentation of infective illness will demonstrate characteristics unique to each individual.

A common scenario in families with young children is for a respiratory infection to be introduced into the family system by a young child in school or day care and proceeding to affect other members. Symptomatology may vary from one person in the household to another (Medalie, 1978). Looking at the family as a unit, such undifferentiated respiratory infections may continue over a long period of time.

In a summary of findings, Medalie (1978) points out that consulting rates for URTI in firstborn children is higher than siblings, even though the latter tend to have more such illnesses. This likely reflects increasing parental confidence in recognizing and coping with these events.

Family dynamics, especially stress, have long been observed to influence children's susceptibility to infection (Boyce et al., 1977) and may be a factor in understanding why some children are prone to frequent URTI and other illnesses. These earlier observational studies become easier to explain with the increased understanding of how the immune system is affected by environmental influences including stress (see Chapter 6).

SUBJECTIVE EXPERIENCE

Illness blogs devoted to chronic diseases such as asthma and COPD are common and are a good source of information about the day-to-day lives of patients trying to cope with the limitations imposed by these diseases. In a book that combines the subjective experience of deteriorating lung function with reflection on the importance of a more phenomenological approach in medicine, Havi Carel (2008) describes the way in which her world became more restricted with the onset of chronic illness. Though she was afflicted at a young age (35 years) with a rare disorder (lymphangioleiomyomatosis), her experiences are typical of those with more common chronic lung disorders. "I imagine that this is what it must be like to grow old: to gradually realize that as your body loses capacities your world shrinks too" (Carel, 2008, p. 6). This loss of control necessitated a rethinking of her life and acceptance of asking for help from friends and, sometimes, strangers.

In a qualitative study of COPD patients from an outpatient clinic, all of whom had been identified by their treatment team as experiencing some emotional distress, several themes emerged that are common to many chronic diseases (Ellison et al., 2012). The challenge to the sense of personal identity and the work entailed in constructing a new one is, naturally, accompanied by a sense of loss and grief. As abilities and independence become restricted, confidence in one's self becomes adversely affected. There is a real danger of social isolation and reluctance to ask others for help when, in the case of COPD, there is a strong sense that the problem was brought on by one's own behavior (smoking). There is guilt and a desire to avoid becoming a burden to others, especially the family. For some, there occurs an acceptance that is difficult to distinguish from simply resignation. A reluctance to undertake counseling or antidepressants was observed, though programs in pulmonary rehabilitation were more favorably viewed.

Over time, elderly people with COPD learn various coping strategies (Fraser et al., 2006), but when an exacerbation occurs, a sense of panic ensues. This is often when they seek assistance from the family physician, who must recognize and effectively address the acute anxiety that accompanies increasing dyspnea.

CLINICAL APPROACH
URTI

Upper respiratory tract infections (URTI) are confined to the nasopharynx and perhaps the middle ear cavity. The vast majority of these infections are due to viruses and, in otherwise healthy individuals, will typically resolve in

5–7 days. Many will assume that cough due to acute illness will subside in a week, but in fact the duration may be as long as 18 days. This mismatch between expectations and reality may result in unnecessary use of antibiotics (Ebell, Lundgren, and Youngpairoj, 2013). Symptomatic treatment is all that is necessary, including judicious use of antihistamines, increased fluid intake, and rest. In children with evidence of otitis media, watchful waiting is appropriate, as many of these will resolve on their own with no harmful sequelae. In those children in whom pain and/or fever persists past 48 hours, antibiotics such as amoxicillin are indicated. In a family practice where the parents of children with significant symptoms and anxiety are present, the practitioner may reasonably provide a prescription for an antibiotic with instructions that if the symptoms don't clear spontaneously, they should fill it and begin treatment. This type of delayed prescribing strategy has been found to reduce the use of antibiotics (Little, 2005).

Many patients will seek medical attention for acute respiratory illnesses for relief of symptoms, but also due to an underlying, unstated, fear that something more serious, such as pneumonia, is present. Careful attention by the physician to the patient's symptoms and the onset of his or her illness, as well as sensitive inquiry about the patient's own ideas and fears and a careful physical examination, will ensure that the physician and patient arrive at common ground about how to proceed. When treating children, it is particularly important to understand the parent's fears and assist in developing a plan that gives the parent a sense of control over the situation.

LRTI

Lower respiratory tract infections (LRTI) are less common than URTI, but fear of them often lies behind patients seeking treatment. As in most infectious diseases, physicians will be aware of the seasonal variations they typically demonstrate, and it is common for clusters of cases to occur in a practice. Those patients who have underlying chronic respiratory conditions such as asthma and COPD are vulnerable to complications such as LRTI at these times.

A patient presenting with a new onset or a worsening cough with either dyspnea, wheezing, chest pain, or an auscultation abnormality as well as reported fever (> 38° C), or perspiring, or headache or myalgia, will raise suspicion of an LRTI. The clinician's clinical judgment is important here, as past experience with the patient must not be ignored. Clinical prediction rules, such as summarized in Table 11.1, may be useful as well. Bronchitis (infection in the bronchial passages) is understood to differ from pneumonia (infection in the lung parenchyma) at the level of tissue pathology, but clinically may be difficult to distinguish, and an X-ray may be necessary to clarify the diagnosis. Bronchitis is most often due to viral infection and will resolve without

Table 11.1 CLINICAL PREDICTION RULE
FOR PNEUMONIA

Finding	Points
Rhinorrhea	-2
Sore throat	-1
Night sweats	1
Myalgia	1
Sputum all day	1
Respiratory rate > 25	2
Temperature > or = 100°F	2

Score	No. with Score	With pneumonia
-3	140	0%
-2	556	0.7%
-1	512	1.6%
0	323	2.2%
1	136	8.8%
2	58	10.3%
3	16	25.0%
> or = 4	11	29.4%

Based on Diehr P, Wood RW. Bushyhead J, et al. 1984. Prediction of pneumonia in outpatients with acute cough: a statistical approach. *Journal of Chronic Disease* 37:215–225.

antibiotics, though bronchodilators may be helpful in alleviating symptoms. Patients with pneumonia require antibiotics for resolution. For this reason, making an accurate diagnosis is important. Nevertheless, family physicians tend to see illnesses early in their course and the diagnosis may be more challenging since changes visible on X-ray may not be present at that point. Once again, the physician's clinical judgment based on general experience as well as prior history with the patient is crucial.

Pneumonia of sudden onset with a cough productive of sputum (typical pneumonia) is usually due to Streptococcus pneumonia or sometimes Hemophilus pneumonia. The chest X-ray most often shows lobar consolidation. If there are no comorbidities and the patient does not require hospitalization, a macrolide (e.g., azithromycin, clarithromycin) is usually recommended, but in those areas of the world where macrolide resistance is increasing, doxycycline is a better choice. When comorbidities (e.g., COPD, diabetes, renal failure, alcoholism, congestive heart failure, asplenia, or immunosuppression) are present, either a combination of a beta lactam (e.g., high-dose amoxicillin) and a macrolide (e.g., azithromycin) or a fluoroquinolone (e.g., levofloxacin, moxifloxacin) alone is recommended. Treatment is for a minimum of 5 days or until the patient is afebrile and clinically stable for 48–72 hours. Atypical pneumonia (due to Mycoplasma, viruses, or Chlamydia) is generally of a more gradual onset, the cough is dry and paroxysmal, and the X-ray shows diffuse consolidation. Treatment consists of a macrolide. The practitioner will need to keep abreast of the recommendations in his or her area, as these may differ depending on antibiotic resistance (Mandell, Wunderink, Anzueto, et al., 2007; Lim, Baudouin, and George, 2009).

In an attempt to identify clinical features relevant to prognosis in LRTI, a longitudinal study of 247 adults with pneumonia was carried out in the Netherlands (Hopstaken, Coenen, Butler, et al., 2006). Physicians felt that 89% of patients were clinically cured by 28 days, but 43% of those patients continued to have symptoms and only 51% considered themselves to be cured. Nineteen percent of them were still experiencing functional limitations. Those with a prior history of asthma tended to have prolonged courses of recovery. Having knowledge of the natural history of diseases is important to avoid overtreatment and to provide patients with accurate information regarding expectations.

When illness is severe, the family practitioner will need to make a decision about whether a patient can no longer be treated in the community and needs hospital admission. Tools such as the Pneumonia Severity Index (Fine, Auble, and Yealy, 1997) and the CURB-65 (Boersma, van der Eerden, Karalus, et al., 2003) can help with this decision. The CURB-65 takes account of confusion, urea (BUN > 7mmol/L or 20 mg/dL), respiratory rate (> 30 breaths/ minute), blood pressure (systolic < 90 mmHg or diastolic < 60 mmHg), and age > 65. A CURB-65 score of 2 should be considered for hospital admission.

Biomarkers for pneumonia, such as procalcitonin, may hold promise in the future for determining which patients may benefit from antibiotics, but at present are probably not practical for community-based practitioners (Schuetz, Albrich, and Mueller, 2011).

CHRONIC RESPIRATORY DISEASE
Asthma

Asthma is understood to be due to an inflammatory disorder of the airways, usually presenting with sudden cough, shortness of breath, sputum production, wheezes, and airflow limitation that is variable in character. Exogenous and endogenous stimuli cause a variable degree of hyper-responsiveness to the airways. In children over the age of 6 and in adults, diagnosis relies on a careful history and spirometry. It is essential, then, that family physicians have access to or can provide spirometry by qualified individuals. In children under the age of 6 in which spirometry is not possible or reliable, diagnosis depends upon a careful history that includes family history and risk factors for asthma, as well as physical examination (Lougheed et al., 2012). In cases of frequent exacerbations or difficult courses of illness, referral to a pediatrician or a colleague with added training is prudent. Noninvasive testing, such as sputum cell counts and exhaled fractional concentration of nitrous oxide, in adults may play a role in diagnosis in special cases, but are generally outside the realm of family practice.

Unusual presentations of asthma must be kept in mind. These include cough variant asthma when nighttime cough may be the only symptom, and cough and shortness of breath with activity, as in exercise-induced asthma. The latter may be the first presentation in children.

As in any chronic disease, patient education is an important first step in the therapeutic approach to asthma. Careful instruction in the proper use of inhaled medications is essential. Self-management by an educated patient is the ultimate goal. Central to this is a strong patient–physician relationship. Written action plans are a key element of self-management and when combined with self-monitoring and regular medical review are effective in aiding patients coping with asthma. Sample action plans are available from the Global Initiative for Asthma (GINA, 2013). Such action plans are developed with the patient and outline how to respond to episodes of loss of control and when to seek medical assistance.

Medical therapies in asthma may be loosely divided into controller medications (e.g., inhaled corticosteroids), which are taken daily to prevent attacks and improve lung function, and reliever medications (e.g., salbutamol), which are taken to cope with an acute episode. Asthma can be classified as controlled, partly controlled, and uncontrolled by whether symptoms are present in the daytime or nighttime, and by any limitation of activities, frequency of use of rescue inhaler, and/or measured peak flow or forced expiratory volume (Global Initiative for Asthma [GINA], 2015).

Due to the underlying inflammatory nature of asthma, inhaled corticosteroids (ICS) are the mainstay of chronic management. Asthma in most children and adults can be controlled with low doses of inhaled corticosteriods (ICS) inhalation. Patients must also be instructed in the proper use of short-acting beta agonists (SABA) for acute exacerbations. Regular use (> 3 times/week) of a SABA indicates inadequate control. If control is not achieved with low-dose ICS, it is acceptable to either increase to a medium dose or add a long-acting beta agonist (LABA) or leukotriene receptor antagonist (LTRA). Examples of LABA are formoterol or salmeterol, and LTRAs include montelukast and pranlukast. In children with poor control on low-dose ICS, it is recommended to increase to a medium-dose ICS.

Acute exacerbations can be classified by symptoms and signs (Figure 8 in GINA, 2015) and the treatment adjusted accordingly. Once an acute exacerbation is over, it is important to review the situation with the patient and optimize therapy. In addition to the environmental triggers that may have led to an exacerbation, the family physician must become aware of the emotional and family factors.

COPD

Chronic obstructive pulmonary disease (COPD) is common, preventable, and treatable. Airflow limitation is progressive and exacerbated by airway irritants, which also cause a chronic inflammation of the airways. The presence of other comorbidities and acute exacerbations contribute to overall severity in any given individual. Dyspnea and cough with sputum characterize the symptoms of COPD, but spirometry is necessary to confirm the diagnosis. An FEV_1/FVC ratio of less than 0.70 confirms the diagnosis. Tobacco smoking is the most common etiological agent, but indoor and outdoor air pollution or exposure to occupational irritants also play a role. Heredity plays a role in those with alpha-1 antitrypsin deficiency. Based on history and physical findings as well as comorbidities, COPD must be distinguished from asthma, congestive heart failure, bronchiectasis, tuberculosis, and obliterative bronchiolitis.

Once the diagnosis is made, the patient's airflow restriction can be classified as mild, moderate, severe, or very severe (Global Initiative for Chronic Obstructive Pulmonary Disease [GICOPD], 2013, Table 3). Evaluating the number of exacerbations per year can also help in developing the therapeutic approach to the patient.

Clearly, cessation of airway irritants is important not only for prevention, but also for reducing exacerbations and slowing the progression of the disease. In this regard, those patients who smoke may need assistance in quitting, and this may involve both counseling (see Chapter 9 regarding motivational interviewing) and nicotine replacement therapy. A review of occupational exposure is warranted in some cases. Maintaining physical activity must be encouraged in all COPD patients. This can be challenging when there are comorbidities such as osteoarthritis or symptomatic ischemic heart disease.

Bronchodilators, including beta$_2$ agonists, anticholinergics, and, in some cases, theophylline all may play a role in reducing symptoms, depending on the patient and the availability of these agents. Long-acting bronchodilators reduce the number of exacerbations and improve pulmonary function. Inhaled corticosteroids alone are not indicated, but when combined with a long acting beta$_2$-agonist (LABA) reduce exacerbations more than either component alone in patients with moderate or severe COPD, but carry a slightly higher risk of pneumonia. Methyxanthines such as theophylline have fallen out of favor due to the narrow therapeutic window and side effects, but may still play a role in individual cases.

All patients with COPD should receive annual influenza vaccination. Pneumococcal vaccine is also indicated. Formal pulmonary rehabilitation programs, if available, can improve exercise tolerance and reduce symptoms. As the disease progresses, when arterial oxygen falls below 7.3 kPa (55 mmHg), long term oxygen is indicated as it has been shown to increase survival.

COPD frequently occurs with other morbidities such as cardiovascular disease (chronic ischemia, heart failure, atrial fibrillation, and hypertension), osteoporosis, diabetes, and lung cancer (Case 11.1). The presence of these diseases adds to the overall allostatic load and reduces quality of life. Generally, the existence of comorbidities does not alter the pharmacological approach to COPD. Depression and anxiety are common and often missed comorbidities

---

CASE 11.1

Jane L was an 82-year-old widowed woman, living alone when she presented late in the summer with increasing cough and shortness of breath. When she was 21 she had had tuberculosis and underwent a right lobectomy. She was also being treated for asthma, osteoporosis, hypertension, and lipid disorder. There was recent construction around her home and it was a season of high pollen count, so an exacerbation of asthma was not entirely unexpected. Her prescription for salbutamol puffer was renewed and she was asked to return if she failed to improve or worsened. Ten days later she once again presented, this time with increasing shortness of breath and cough productive of brownish-yellow sputum. Her chest examination revealed scattered wheezes and her capillary oxygen saturation was 92%. A chest X-ray showed only the previous right lobectomy, but no sign of infection. Ipratropium puffer was added to her treatments and she continued with Symbicort (budenoside-formeterol) spray as well. However, 2 days later she became very fatigued and short of breath. There were, once again, diffuse scattered wheezes on auscultation of her chest, but no crackles. The capillary oxygen saturation was 96%. Because of how ill she looked and the persistence of her symptoms, she was started on clarithromycin 500 mg twice daily. Four days later, when next seen, she felt much better, but when she awoke that morning became very anxious at her level of fatigue and felt palpitations. She was worried that she would have difficulty looking after herself. This time on examination, there were audible crackles in the right lower chest and her capillary oxygen level was only 88%, but improved to 92% after administration of her puffers. She was started on a short course of prednisone and another chest X-ray was ordered. This showed pneumonia in the right lower lobe. Two weeks later her symptoms had largely resolved, but she had developed oral thrush that was treated with nystatin oral rinses.

in those with COPD. Their presence adds greatly to the individual's ability to adapt to his or her changing physiological status. In a systematic review, anxiety was present in 13%–46% of outpatients with COPD and was more common in women (Willgross and Yohannes, 2013). Depression is estimated to be present in up to 42% of patients with COPD (Maurer, Rebbapragada, Borson, et al., 2008). It is critical that family physicians be aware of and develop a therapeutic approach to depression and anxiety in COPD patients. This may include psychotherapy, cognitive behavioral therapy, pulmonary rehabilitation, and psychopharmacology.

Healthy nutrition is important for all patients with chronic diseases. Patients with COPD are prone to weight loss as the disease progresses. The ability of nutritional supplements that are rich in anti-inflammatories, such as omega-3 polyunsaturated fatty acids, to reduce inflammation and improve function is unclear at present.

In end-stage COPD, provision of appropriate palliative care by a physician known to the patient is invaluable and can help allay the attendant anxiety and suffering.

REFERENCES

Boersma WG, van der Eerden MM, Karalus N, Laing R, Lewis SA, Lim WS. 2003. Defining community acquired pneumonia severity on presentation to hospital: An international derivation and validation study. *Thorax* 58(5):377–382.

Boyce WT, Jensen EW, Cassel JC, Collier AM, Smith AH, Ramey CT. 1977. Influences of life events and family routines on childhood respiratory tract illness. *Pediatrics* 60(4):609–615.

Carel, Havi. 2008. *Illness*. Stocksfield Hall, UK: Acumen.

Cruz AA, Bateman ED, Bousquet J. 2010. The social determinants of asthma. *European Respiratory Journal* 35:239–245.

Diehr P, Wood RW. Bushyhead J, et al. 1984. Prediction of pneumonia in outpatients with acute cough: a statistical approach *J Chronic Disease* 37:215–225.

Ebell MH, Lundgren J, Youngpairoj S. 2013. How long does a cough last? Comparing patients' expectations with data from a systematic review of the literature. *Annals of Family Medicine* 11(1):5–13.

Ellison L, Gask L, Bakerly ND, Roberts J. 2012. Meeting the mental health needs of people with chronic obstructive pulmonary disease: a qualitative study. *Chronic Illness* 8(4):308–320.

Fine MJ, Auble TE, Yealy DM Hanusa BH, Weissfeld LA, Singer DE, Coley CM, Marrie TJ, Kapoor WN. 1997. A prediction rule to identify low-risk patients with community-acquired pneumonia. *New England Journal of Medicine* 336:243–250.

Fraser DD, Kee CC, Minick P. 2006. Living with chronic obstructive pulmonary disease: Insiders' perspectives. *Journal of Advanced Nursing* 55(5):550–558.

Fried BJ, Gaydos LM, eds. 2012. *World Health Systems: Challenges and Perspectives*. Chicago: Health Administration Press.

Global Initiative for Asthma (GINA). 2015. *Pocket Guide for Asthma Management and Prevention (for Adults and Children Older Than 5 Years).* http://www.ginasthma. org/local/uploads/files/GINA_Pocket_2015.pdf.

Global Initiative for Chronic Obstructive Pulmonary Disease (GICOPD). 2013. http:// www.goldcopd.org/uploads/users/files/GOLD_Pocket_2013_Mar27.pdf.

Hopstaken RM, Coenen S, Butler CC, Nelemans P, Muris JWM, Rinkens PELM. 2006. Prognostic factors and clinical outcomes in acute lower respiratory infections: A prospective study in general practice. *Family Practice* 23(5):512–519.

Lim WS, Baudouin SV, George RC, Hill AT, Jamieson C, LeJeune I, Macfarlane JT, Read RC, Roberts HJ, Levy ML, Wani M, Woodhead MA, Pneumonia Guidelines Committee of the BTS Standards of Care Committee. 2009. BTS guidelines for the management of community acquired pneumonia in adults: Update 2009. *Thorax* 64(Suppl 3):iii1.

Little P. 2005. Delayed prescribing of antibiotics for upper respiratory tract infection: With clear guidance to patients and parents it seems to be safe. *BMJ* 331(7512):301–302.

Lougheed MD, Lemiere C, Ducharme FM, Licskai C, Dell SD, Rowe BH, FitzGerald M, Leigh R, Watson W, Boulet L-P, Canadian Thoracic Society Asthma Clinical Assembly. 2012. Canadian Thoracic Society 2012 guideline update: Diagnosis and management of asthma in preschoolers, children and adults. *Canadian Respiratory Journal* 19 (2):127–164. http://www.respiratoryguidelines.ca/sites/all/files/2012_CTS_Guideline_Asthma.pdf.

Mandell LA, Wunderink RG, Anzueto A, Bartlett JG, Campbell GD, Dean NC, Dowell SF, File TM Jr, Musher DM, Niederman MS, Torres A, Whitney CG, Infectious Diseases Society of America, American Thoracic Society. 2007. Infectious Diseases Society of America/American Thoracic Society consensus guidelines on the management of community-acquired pneumonia. *Clinical Infectious Diseases* 44(Suppl 2):S27.

Maurer J, Rebbapragada V, Borson S, et al. 2008. Anxiety and depression in COPD: Current understanding, unanswered questions and research needs. *Chest* 134:43–56.

Medalie JH, ed. 1978. *Family Medicine: Principles and Applications.* Baltimore, MD: Williams and Wilkins.

National Ambulatory Medical Survey (NAMCS). 2010. *Summary Table.* http://www. cdc.gov.

Ostbye T, Yarnell KSH, Krause KM, Pollak KI, Gradison M, Michener JL. 2005. Is there time for management of patients with chronic diseases in primary care? *Annals of Family Medicine* 3(3):209–214.

Schuetz P, Albrich W, Mueller B. 2011. Procalcitonin for diagnosis of infection and guide to antibiotic decisions: Past, present, future. *BMC Medicine* 9:107.

Willgross TJ, Yohannes AM. 2013. Anxiety disorders in patients with COPD: A systematic review. *Respiratory Care* 58(50):858–866.

Williams DR, Sternthal M, Wright RJ. 2009. Social determinants: Taking the social context of asthma seriously. *Pediatrics* 123(Suppl 3): s174–184.

World Health Organization (WHO). 2011. *The Top Ten Causes of Death.* http://www. who.int/mediacentre/factsheets/fs310/en/index1.html.

CHAPTER 12

༄

Musculoskeletal Pain

Musculoskeletal pain covers a very wide variety of ailments. Bruusgaard and Brage (2002) offer this simple classification:

- Strain-related musculoskeletal complaints, including soft-tissue rheumatism, both localized as tendonitis and myalgia, and widespread as chronic myofascial pain (CMP) and fibromyalgia.
- Inflammatory musculoskeletal complaints, including rheumatoid arthritis and ankylosing spondylitis (AS). We would add polymyalgia rheumatic (PMR) to this group.
- Degenerative musculoskeletal complaints, including osteoporosis and osteoarthritis.
- Other musculoskeletal complaints, including injuries, deformities, infections, and tumors.

This leaves out low back pain (LBP), which may be strain related or may occur as a result of degenerative changes.

This chapter will not deal with acute pain that usually resolves with analgesics, rest, and time. Also, although musculoskeletal pain, sometimes of a chronic nature, occurs in children, it will not be discussed here. Inflammatory and degenerative musculoskeletal disorders have well-developed, widely disseminated therapeutic approaches. Similar to the reasoning presented by Bruusgaard and Brage, therefore, this chapter will focus on the first category, soft tissue pain.

PREVALENCE IN FAMILY PRACTICE

Varying terminology and definitions are challenging when examining prevalence figures for musculoskeletal pain. Many studies focus primarily on localized pain, such as low back or neck pain. Chronic widespread pain (CWP) or chronic myofascial pain (CMP) is any long-lasting, widespread pain thought to be muscular or soft tissue in origin. Fibromyalgia syndrome (FMS) is defined by the American College of Rheumatology as consisting of three dimensions: a duration of at least 3 months; widespread pain (that is, axial pain, pain on both the right and left side, and pain above and below the waist); positive tender points (TP) in at least 11 of 18 specified anatomical areas (), though this strict definition was originally developed for research purposes and has less relevance in the clinical domain (Fitzcharles, Ste-Pierre, and Pereira, 2011). Chronic myofascial pain (CMP) is distinguishable from FMS in that it is characterized by a taut band in the affected muscle, a trigger point (TrP), and a local twitch response in the taut band when the trigger point is stimulated. Fibromyalgia syndrome (FMS), as mentioned, has tender points, but stimulation of them does not radiate as is the case with trigger point (TrP). Because radiating pain is a delayed reaction, it is necessary to maintain pressure on the point for 5–10 seconds to distinguish the two. Gerwin (2001) distinguishes between primary myofascial pain syndrome (MPS) (myogenic headache, neck pain, shoulder pain, low back pain, piriformis syndrome, knee pain, and ankle pain) and those secondary to other conditions (he includes fibromyalgia in the secondary category, along with other chronic conditions such as rheumatoid arthritis, acute trauma, hypothyroidism, vitamin B_{12} deficiency, and others). In terms of developing a therapeutic approach, it may be more useful to distinguish acute pain from chronic pain, as the available modalities are quite different. It is understood that acute pain converts to chronic pain due to a phenomenon known as central sensitization, or remodeling of central processes in response to peripheral stimulation. It follows that a rapid and adequate response to acute pain is necessary to prevent progression to chronic pain. Nevertheless, how rapidly the conversion from acute pain to chronic pain occurs will depend on a host of factors, such as the underlying injury, personal and occupational demands, personal past history including prior experiences with pain, family history, and comorbidities (i.e., allogenic load).

A population-based prevalence study in the Netherlands (Picavet and Schouten, 2003) reported rates as follows: low back pain 26.9%; shoulder pain 20.9%; neck pain 20.6%. In most cases these pains were mild and intermittent in nature, but in 30% of cases they interfered with activities of daily living and, in as many as 42% of cases, resulted in visits to their physician.

Generally, population-based prevalence studies find CWP to be more likely reported by women (15%–20%) than men (9%–10%) and to increase with age. Fibromyalgia, with a narrower definition and requirement for physical examination to establish the diagnosis, has lower prevalence figures, 1%–5% in a Canadian study, but increasing with age and six times more common in women than in men, as high as 9%–13% among women (McNally, Matheson, and Bakowsky, 2006). For those over the age of 65, 32% reported pain for 3 or more consecutive years, and 32% had intermittent pain (Thielke, Whitson, Diehr, et al., 2012).

In a family practice with a patient enrollment or panel size of 2500 individuals with an age distribution reflecting the US population (including children) and the known chronic disease prevalence, Ostbye and colleagues estimated that there would be 381 patients with arthritis alone. They did not include the strain-related pains or other musculoskeletal complaints in the classification system of Bruusgaard and Brage (2002). One Swedish study (Andersson et al., 1999) reported that the number of patients presenting to family physicians with pain-related diagnoses rose from 156/1000 per year in 1987 to 193/1000 per year in 1996. Healthcare utilization in general is higher for those with chronic pain.

The National Ambulatory Care Survey of 2010 in the United States reported that diseases of the musculoskeletal and connective tissues accounted for 8.5% of visits to physicians.

Fibromyalgia is often accompanied by disturbances in sleep, fatigue, cognitive dysfunction (poor working memory, free recall and verbal fluency, spatial memory alterations), and mood disorders (depression, anxiety, or both). Also migraine headaches, irritable bowel syndrome, and bladder dysfunctions (interstitial cystitis) are more often seen in those with fibromyalgia than in the general population. The symptoms persist over years, but fluctuate in intensity, with flare-ups often in association with changes in stress. It is understood to be a polysymptomatic distress syndrome and one best managed in the family practice setting (Fitzcharles, Ste-Marie, and Pereira, 2013). The high prevalence of mood disorders in those with a chronic pain syndrome may be an artifact of studies done in tertiary care centers and are not necessarily reflective of those in the general population and family practice (Clauw and Crofford, 2003).

The natural history of fibromyalgia is one of exacerbations and remissions over time, but rarely is there complete resolution. There is some suggestion that the prevalence begins to decline in those in the 55–64-year age group (White and Harth, 2001), but this remains uncertain. Myofascial pain, if inadequately or inappropriately treated, can convert from acute to chronic and can prove to be much more difficult to resolve (Gerwin, 2001).

If severe daily pain occurs in one site, it is more likely to occur in other sites, and the greater the number of painful areas, the greater the likelihood of other comorbidities such as depression. Hence, a strictly biomechanical or injury/overload approach is insufficient alone to explain or direct treatment (Hartvigsen, Natvig, and Ferreira, 2013).

FAMILY FACTORS

Genetic influences on musculoskeletal (MSK) pain has been most extensively studied in low back pain in twins (Ferreira, Beckenkamp, Maher, et al., 2013). It is becoming recognized that heritability is an important component of low back pain and its consequences. There appears to be a genetic component to degenerative disc disease and a move away from seeing this as simply a wear-and-tear phenomenon (Hartvigsen, Neilsen, Kyvik, et al., 2009). A review of all twin studies and low back pain estimates that heritability may account for 40%–44% of the variance in liability to this condition and may be stronger for severe cases. Due to the association of low back pain with other chronic conditions (asthma, diabetes, osteoporosis, osteoarthritis, hypertension, obesity, and patients' own estimates of their health), it has been suggested that it is a response to a general decline in health (Ferriera, Beckenkamp, Meyer, et al., 2013). This has significant implications for therapeutics (see discussion later in this chapter).

Early life events appear to play a significant role in the predisposition to pain syndromes as well as other illnesses later in life. The Adverse Childhood Events (ACE) study serves to illuminate the relationship between events early in life and adult morbidities. Increased knowledge of how external events help to mold the central nervous system, which in turn is related to how one perceives and interacts with and interprets one's world, has led to greater understanding of the complexity of human health and well-being.

It has long been observed that early life events, especially exposure to physical and psychological abuse, is associated with multiple symptoms and disorders throughout life. Intimate partner violence can be both a triggering and a perpetuating factor in chronic MSK pain. There is an association between victimization and fibromyalgia (van Houdenhove et al., 2001), and this frequently has its roots in childhood.

It has been suggested that interactions between genetic and environmental factors have a final common pathway or central nervous system dysfunction (Clauw and Chrousos, 1997). Epigenetic factors are those environmental pressures that serve to turn on or suppress gene function. Both genetic and epigenetic factors are active in childhood and set the stage for further neurological and psychological development.

Due to the generalist nature of family practice and the tendency to attend to all members of a family, family physicians are likely to see these associations in their day-to-day practice. However, patients will not often volunteer this information, and it is imperative that the physician make sensitive inquiry and earn an atmosphere of trust that will enable them to bring it forward. Awareness of how commonly family and social factors are associated with symptoms that cross the boundaries between mind and body reinforces the need to think beyond this arbitrary cultural dichotomy (see Chapter 6, "Philosophical and Scientific Foundations of Family Medicine").

SOCIAL CONTEXT

Other factors that predict the development or persistence of either widespread or regional pain include greater age, a family history of chronic pain, low social support, being an immigrant, being in a lower socioeconomic class, and performing manual labor (Clauw and Crofford, 2003).

The 1958 British Cohort Study followed participants from the time of birth in 1958 into adulthood. At age 45, the prevalence of forearm, low back, knee, and chronic widespread pain generally increased with a threefold increased risk in those in the lowest social class. Social class in childhood was also related to pain in adulthood, but was less strongly associated than adult social class. The latter was partly explained by poor adult mental health, psychological distress, adverse life events, and lifestyle factors (MacFarlane, Norrie, Atherton, et al., 2009).

Chronic widespread pain (CWP) is more common in women, increases with age and lower social status, manual labor, and physical and psychological stress, both in the workplace and in personal life. Work-related MSK pain is more common with physically demanding work, but also occurs, though to a lesser extent, with sedentary work that is monotonous or involves tight time schedules.

As already noted, population-based studies have demonstrated that distress can lead to pain, and pain to distress. In this latter instance, a typical pattern is that, as a result of pain and other symptoms of FMS, individuals begin to function less well in their various roles. They may have difficulties with spouses, children, and work inside or outside the home, which exacerbate symptoms and lead to maladaptive illness behaviors. These include isolation, cessation of pleasurable activities, reductions in activity, and exercise, and so on. In the worst cases, patients become involved with disability and compensation systems that may ensure that they will not improve (Clauw and Crofford (2003). Even in osteoarthritis and rheumatoid arthritis, factors such as formal education, coping strategies, and socioeconomic variables are more important in predicting pain and disability than seemingly objective measures such as erythrocyte sedimentation rate (ESR) and radiographic evidence of joint space narrowing (Hadler, 1996).

SUBJECTIVE EXPERIENCE

In a qualitative study of patients diagnosed with FMS, Raymond and Brown (2000) described a continuum in the illness experience of participants, beginning with the onset of widespread pain and associated symptoms, often associated with a precipitating event. There followed a period, sometimes prolonged, during which there was a search for answers. This often involved extensive medical consultations and investigations that failed to identify a cause for the symptoms in the standard biomedical framework. This phase lasted until the patient received a diagnostic label, which, while initially leading to a sense of relief, also made plain the chronic nature of the illness. Once a diagnosis was made, patients' energies turned from seeking answers to learning how to cope with the limitations imposed by it. There followed a fluctuating course as different strategies were attempted and physical limits were tested out, but gradually these patients were able to settle into a routine that recognized their limits. Support systems were essential in this phase, including organizations such as the Arthritis Society. The role of the patient's family is important in coming to agreement about how to support her in her changing roles and identities. They provided further information and understanding about the condition. A trusted relationship with a family physician providing continuous, comprehensive care during these various phases of the continuum of the illness was essential for aiding the patient. Family physicians benefit their patients by recognizing what phase their patients are in and providing appropriate support. This approach has been found to be relevant to other chronic illnesses (Snadden and Brown, 1992; Hudon, Fortin, Haggerty, et al., 2012).

In a synthesis of literature pertaining to chronic MSK pain (including fibromyalgia), Toye et al. (2013) developed a conceptual framework that helps clinicians understand the experiences of their patients. It emphasizes the pervasive adversarial nature of the world of those in chronic pain as they attempt to find answers for their symptoms and then deal with larger system issues. The main conceptual categories include struggling to define a new "self," reconstructing time to take into account physical limitations, seeking an explanation for suffering, negotiating the healthcare system, proving legitimacy, and, finally, moving forward "alongside" one's pain.

In coming to an understanding of the person's illness experience, it is important to listen carefully to the patient's own description of the pain, as the language of pain, such as the similes and metaphors, frequently provide insight into the emotional content and hidden attribution of the illness. As pointed out by Stensland (2002) citing Vygotsky (1988), "Worries, fears or ideas of mastering a problem come to mind of the patient as voices of different quality." (Stensland, 2002, p. 54). Such language is often contextual and may vary by gender. For example, in describing the limitations imposed by chronic pain, women are more likely to cite inability to use a vacuum cleaner, whereas men are more likely to describe difficulty with using a lawnmower or snow shovel (Johansson and Hamberg, 2002).

For individuals with chronic pain, time can take on a different quality. Dr. Michael Lockshin, a rheumatologist who is considered an expert in the long-term care of those with chronic illness, draws upon categories of time as perceived by the Mayans. In their system, a day was called a *kin* (pronounced *k-e-e-n*),

20 days was a *uinal* (pronounced *we-e-n-al*), one year was a *tun* (*t-oo-n*) and a *katun* (*ka-t-oon*) a much longer and variable period of time. The *katun* is the measure of time most appropriate for consideration in those with chronic illnesses. "On the scale of a *katun* people marry, achieve, see children grow, watch parents die, do or do not become disabled" (Brill and Lockshin, 2009, p. 7). The current era emphasizes speed and immediacy, but chronic illness and healing must be conceived on a longer time scale. Oscar Wilde makes a similar point: "Suffering is one very long moment. We cannot divide it by seasons. We can only record its moods and chronicle their return. With us, time itself does not progress. It revolves. It seems to circle around one centre of pain" (Wilde, 1905, p. 82).

Thinking of the phases of illness and the longer time frame described here will help both the physician and the patient more realistically plan a useful approach.

CLINICAL APPROACH

The approach to the patient with chronic widespread pain must begin with an understanding of the full dimensions of their suffering. From his memoirs, McWhinney (2012) writes:

> Dr. Fred Arthur, a general practitioner in London, Ontario, is an example of a physician who considers the whole person when treating chronic pain. His approach to chronic pain challenges the current (often ineffective) paradigm of treating only tissue injury. He found that after acute low back pain, pain and disability at six months are best predicted not by tissue injury but by psychological and social factors. Even the measured degree of disc displacement can predict no more than 12 per cent of the variance of persistent pain at six months. . . . There is . . . a logical gap between our present understanding of painful injury and the reality of this experience. Arthur's observations over five years led him to generate a new category to replace the focus on tissue injury: *suffering patient*. The focus was therefore on the holistic illness experience. His criteria for suffering included the following: a pain score greater than six, sleep disturbance, the expression of feelings and fears not congruent with clinical findings, and signs pointing to fear or anxiety.
>
> Arthur's clinical method is patient-centred, with a focus on the illness experience, the patient's motivation for the consultation beyond the injury, and gaining common ground with the patient. His key insight is that suffering related to the injury fuses with a problem of living or suffering experienced and repressed in the past, and then is expressed as chronic pain. Arthur postulates that a high pain report reflects extensive brain activations in the limbic and brain stem regions. This concept of "pain" where severe pain reflects significant brain

activations, rather than significant tissue injury, constitutes a paradigm shift for primary care. (McWhinney, 2012, p. 126)

The interaction between MSK pain and other comorbidities, mentioned earlier, means that therapeutic approaches that focus on one entity or morbidity are of limited use (see Chapter 16). For example, recommending physical activity to someone with low back pain, obesity, osteoarthritis, and depression is generally met with resistance and lack of adherence. Patients in such situations, understandably, wonder if the physician truly understands their total life experience.

Newer approaches to diagnosis of FMS reflect a significant change in thinking, similar to Arthur's (Fitzcharles, Ste-Marie, and Pereira, 2013). Patients will generally present with the pain component as the most prominent symptom, and the physician must inquire about related symptoms such as sleep disorders, mood disorders, and cognitive functioning. An appropriate physical examination is necessary, but may be completely normal. Tender points are no longer required to confirm the diagnosis. It is, in fact, not a diagnosis of exclusion but one reached by careful attention to the patient's symptoms and context, including psychological and social stresses. If other diagnoses are being considered, based on the history and physical findings, investigations should be limited to complete blood count, erythrocyte sedimentation rate (ESR), C-reactive protein level, creatine kinase, and thyroid function. Any further testing is determined by the clinical presentation, but excessive and repeated testing is to be avoided as it reduces the patient's confidence and leads to unnecessary expense.

The therapeutic approach to any widespread pain syndrome, including fibromyalgia, incorporates all of the elements of the patient-centered clinical method (Chapter 9). Careful attention must be paid to the patient's illness experience and his or her own interpretation of events. This will generally mean eliciting the patient's narrative and aid in shaping a newer, more positive one. This must take place over a period of time and multiple visits, during which the physician carefully builds a trusting relationship with the patient. This can be challenging, and there are many opportunities to lose focus, especially when there are so many comorbidities that also require the attention of a comprehensive family physician. When the clinician has satisfactorily made the diagnosis, taking time to educate the patient is essential to ensuring confidence and finding common ground, thus helping to maintain adherence to a therapeutic regimen. This regimen must include both nonpharmacologic and pharmacologic elements. Focusing on the patient's functioning and aspirations for health is key. Given the often widespread nature of pain in those with CWP, and frequent comorbidities, even the term *diagnosis* must yield to a multifactorial assessment aimed at identifying those with a high impact of pain and higher likelihood of poor outcome (Hartvigsen, Natvig, and Ferreira, 2013).

In addition to developing a strong therapeutic relationship with the physician, an interdisciplinary approach involving physiotherapy, occupational therapy, social work, and psychology will enhance outcomes and reduce burnout in the physician. Cognitive behavioral therapy (CBT), relaxation, and exercises that emphasize gentle stretching (tai chi, swimming) may be indicated. Recent evidence suggests some commonalities in the approach to the most common musculoskeletal painful conditions, such as low back pain, neck pain, osteoarthritis, fibromyalgia, and widespread pain. Generally, regardless of the location of pain, diagnosis relies more on history and physical findings than on imaging; remaining active and at work improves long-term outcomes; self-management and maintaining levels of exercise and physical activity, along with appropriate pain relief, are of paramount importance (Hartvigsen, Natvig, and Ferriera, 2013).

Generally, pharmacologic approaches are aimed at either reducing pain transmission from the periphery to the brain or increasing downward modulation of incoming pain signals. The former includes anti-inflammatories and opioids as well as physical modalities (i.e., application of heat or cold). The latter may utilize anticonvulsants, opioids, and cannabinoids, as well as massage, transcutaneous nerve stimulation (TNS), and acupuncture.

The class of drugs known as gabapentinoids (gabalin, pregabalin) have been found to be useful for neuropathic pain in general and may be effective in a minority of patients with fibromyalgia (Siler, Gardner, Yanit, et al., 2011).

Antidepressant medications may play a role for more than one reason. By increasing neurotransmitters such as serotonin and norepinephrine, they increase downward pain modulation. In addition, since depression is frequently present with chronic pain, these drugs may aid in improving emotional health and, therefore, resilience. Tricyclic antidepressants (TCA; principally amitriptyline), selective serotonin reuptake inhibitors (SSRIs, including paroxitene, fluoxitene, and sertraline, but apparently not citalopram) have been found to reduce pain, and to improve sleep, depressed mood, and fatigue in those with fibromyalgia (Uceyler, Hauser, and Sommer, 2008). Serotonin reuptake inhibitors (SNRIs, such as duloxitene, milnacipran) appear to have a more modest effect (Hauser, Bernardy, and Uceyler, 2009).

Because CWP and FMS are diagnoses principally based on subjective symptoms, it is not uncommon for issues to arise with respect to claims for disability. Family physicians may have the distinct advantage of knowing the patient prior to the onset of symptoms and thereby are better able to distinguish the patient who becomes enmeshed in secondary gain complications.

The use of opioids for chronic non-cancer pain (CNCP) must be undertaken with extreme caution due to the addictive potential and long-term side effects associated with them. It has been estimated that as much as 30% of people in North America with fibromyalgia take opioids for chronic pain (Fitzcharles,

Ste-Pierre, Gamsa, et al., 2011). Before initiating therapy with opioids, it is important to identify, with the patient, that the goal of therapy is to reduce pain in order to increase function. Keeping an ongoing activity log is central to this. A useful tool for monitoring opioid use is the Pain Assessment and Documentation Tool (PADT) (http://www.caresalliance.org/ResourceList. aspx?userType=6&itemType=11). There are a number of tools available to aid in identifying those patients who are at heightened risk of becoming addicted to opioids (see Opioid Screening Tools). Those at high risk should be referred to a pain specialist if available. Regardless of risk of addiction, all patients receiving opioid medication for a prolonged period of time should be asked to sign a narcotic contract that delineates the rules of their use. Complications of long-term opioid therapy include constipation, physical dependence, and opioid-induced hypogonadism. The physician must anticipate and be prepared to address each of these complications.

REFERENCES

Andersson HI, Ejiertsson G, Leden I, Schersten B. 1999. Musculoskeletal chronic pain in general practice: Studies of health care utilization in comparison with pain prevalence. *Scandinavian Journal of Primary Health Care* 17(2):87–92.

Brill A, Lockshin MD. 2009. *Dancing at the River's Edge: A Patient and Her Doctor Negotiate Life with Chronic Illness.* Tucson, AZ: Schaffner Press.

Bruusgaard D, Brage S. 2002. The magnitude of the problem. In: Malterud K, Hunskaar S., eds., *Chronic Myofascial Pain: A Patient-Centered Approach.* Oxon, UK: Radcliffe Medical Press.

Clauw DJ, Chrousos GP. 1997. Chronic pain and fatigue syndromes: Overlapping clinical and neuroendocrine features and potential pathogenic mechanisms. *NeuroImmunoModulation* 4(3):134–153.

Clauw DJ, Crofford LJ. 2003. Chronic widespread pain in fibromyalgia: What we know and what we need to know. *Best Practice and Research Clinical Rheumatology* 17(4):685–701.

Ferreira PH, Beckenkamp P, Maher CG, et al. 2013. Nature or nurture in low back pain? Results of a systematic review of studies based on twin samples. *European Journal of Pain* 17:957–971.

Fitzcharles M-A, Ste-Marie PA, Pereira JX. 2013. Fibromyalgia: evolving concepts over the past 2 decades. *Canadian Medical Association Journal* 185(13):E645–651.

Fitzcharles M-A, Ste-Pierre PA, Gamsa A, et al. 2011. Opioid use, misuse and abuse in patients labeled as fibromyalgia. *American Journal of Medicine* 124:955–960.

Gerwin RD. 2001. Classification, epidemiology and natural history of myofascial pain syndrome. *Current Pain and Headache Reports* 5:412–420.

Hadler NM. 1996. If you have to prove you are ill, you can't get well: The object lesson of fibromyalgia. *Spine* 21(20):2397–2400.

Hartvigsen J, Natvig B, Ferreira M. 2013. Is it all about pain in the back? *Best Practice & Research Clinical Rheumatology* 27:613–623.

Hartvigsen J, Nielsen J, Kyvik KO, et al. 2009. Heritability of spinal pain and consequences of spinal pain: A comprehensive genetic epidemiologic analysis using a population-based sample of 15,328 twins ages 20–71 years. *Arthritis and Rheumatism* 61:1343–1351.

Hauser W, Bernardy K, Uceyler N, et al. 2009. Treatment of fibromyalgia syndrome with antidepressants: a meta-analysis. *Journal of the American Medical Association* 301:198–200.

Huddon C, Fortin M, Haggerty J, et al.2012. Patient-centered care in chronic disease management: A thematic analysis of the literature in family medicine. *Patient Education and Counseling* 88:170–176.

Johansson E, Hamberg K. 2002. Women in pain: The meaning of symptoms and illness. In: Malterud K, Hunskaar S, eds., *Chronic Myofascial Pain: A Patient-Centered Approach*. Oxon: Radcliffe Medical Press.

MacFarlane GJ, Norrie G, Atherton K, et al. 2009. The influence of socioeconomic status on reporting of regional and widespread musculoskeletal paint: Results from the 1958 British Cohort Study. *Annals of the Rheumatic Diseases* 68:1591–1595.

McNally JD, Matheson DA, Bakowsky VS. 2006. The epidemiology of self-reported fibromyalgia in Canada. *Chronic Diseases in Canada* 27:9–16.

McWhinney IR. 2012. *A Call to Heal: Reflections on a Life in Family Medicine*. Saskatoon, SK: Benchmark Press.

Ostbye T, Yarnell KSH, Krause KM, et al. 2005. Is there time for management of patients with chronic diseases in primary care? *Annals of Family Medicine* 3(3):209–214.

Picavet HSJ, Schouten JSAG. 2003. Musculoskeletal pain in the Netherlands: Prevalences, consequences and risk groups, the DMC$_3$-study. *Pain* 102(1):167–178.

Raymond MC, Brown JB. 2000. Experience of fibromyalgia: Qualitative study. *Canadian Family Physcian* 45(5):1100–1106.

Siler AC, Gardner H, Yanit K, et al. 2011. Systematic review of the comparative effectiveness of antiepileptic drugs for fibromyalgia. *Journal of Pain* 12:407–415.

Snadden D, Brown JB. 1992. The experience of asthma. *Social Science & Medicine* 34:1351–1361.

Stensland P. 2002. Communicating illness experience. In: Malterud K, Hunskaar S, eds., *Chronic Myofascial Pain: A Patient-Centered Approach*. Oxon, UK: Radcliffe Medical Press.

Thielke SM, Whitson H, Diehr P, et al. 2012. Persistence and remission of muscloskeletal pain in community-dweliing older adults: Results from the Cardiovascular Health Study. *Journal of the American Geriatric Society* 60(8):1393–1400.

Toye F, Seers K, Allcock N, et al. 2013. Patients' experiences of chronic non-malignant musculoskeletal pain: A qualitative systematic review. *British Journal of General Practice* 63(617):e829–e841.

Uceyler N, Hauser W, Sommer C. 2008. A systematic review on effectiveness of treatment with antidepressants in fibromyalgia syndrome. *Arthritis and Rheumatism* 59:1279–1298.

Van Houdenhove B, Neerinckx E, Lysens R, et al. 2001. Victimization in chronic fatigue syndrome and fibromyalgia in tertiary care: A controlled study on prevalence and characteristics. *Pyschosomatics* 42(1):21–28.

Vygotsky I. 1988. *Thought and Language*. Cambridge, MA: MIT Press.

White KP, Harth M. 2001. Classification, epidemiology and natural history of fibromyalgia. *Current Pain and Headache Reports* 5:320–329.

Wilde O. 1905 *De Profundis*. London: Methuen.

Opioid Addiction Screening Tools

Current Opioid Misuse Measure (COMM). www.hamiltonfht.ca/docs/public/opioid-maintenanc—comm-opioid-misuse-measure.pdf.

Drug Abuse Screening Test (DAST). www.emcddaeuropa.eu/html.cfm/index3618EN.html.

Opioid Risk Tool (ORT). www.partnersagainstpain.com/printouts/Opioid-Risk_Tool.pdf.

Screener and Opioid Assessment for Patients-Revised (SOAPP-R). nationalpaincentre.mcmaster.ca/documents/soap_r_sample_watermark.pdf.

CHAPTER 13

ᴄᴠᴐ

Depression

Careful consideration was taken before including a chapter on the topic of depression because it may convey the notion that it is a single biological entity, which is not supportable. Like other emotional experiences, including anxiety, the symptoms of depression cannot be separated from the person experiencing them or their biological functions. Conceiving of depression as a stand-alone diagnostic entity repeats the mistake of assuming a division between the mind and the body. However, given the fact that as a diagnostic entity (*DSM-5*, 2013) it represents a substantial component of profiles of family and medical practice, and because the symptoms used to describe depression cut across most of clinical medicine (and indeed, human life in general), it was decided to include a chapter on the topic.

Depression and anxiety frequently coexist, and generalized anxiety disorder may precede a major depression (Dowrick, 2004). Most mood disorders are dealt with at the level of primary care. The current understanding and clinical approach to them is dominated by a model derived from psychiatry, where there are significant differences in patient population and priorities from those in family practice. Family medicine has come under criticism for uncritically accepting this model and for failing to develop a model suitable for the family practice setting (Callahan and Berrios, 2005).[1]

"Distinguishing between depression 'the disease,' depression 'the symptom,' and depression 'the experience' is one of the most difficult problems facing physicians and patients, and we often get it wrong" (Callahan and Berrios, 2005, p. 5). This is perhaps more true in family practice, where the dividing line between normal and abnormal is often indistinct and where the practitioner's knowledge of individual patient characteristics over the life course often provides unique insights into their predicaments. As suggested by Callahan and Berrios (2005, p. 102), "descriptions and classifications of depression constructed in general practice and in secondary or tertiary referral venues may be different, but both are correct." In addition, "[a]ttention must be paid to patients' sufferings, to their emotions, beliefs, and relationships, not only for humanitarian reasons but also because they have an important bearing on the origins of illness" (McWhinney, 2014, p. 26).

PREVALENCE

Emotional symptoms and experiences such as depression (and anxiety) are a normal part of the human experience. Individuals deal with them in a variety of ways. They may talk with family and friends; read one of the burgeoning number of books in self-help; meditate; use herbal therapies; or exercise. Some will be reluctant to approach the healthcare system, fearing that they might acquire an unwanted label. In many parts of the world, being labeled as mentally ill is stigmatizing and has negative implications. Less positive ways in which some may deal with difficult emotions include abuse of alcohol and other substances, as well as family violence and risk-taking behavior. Consequently, in a family practice, there will be a number of people who, if they were administered a standardized depression questionnaire (e.g., Hamilton Depression Scale; Patient Health Questionnaire PHQ 9) will fulfill the criteria for depressive disorder, but will not have been diagnosed as such by their physician. They may deal with their symptoms in one of the previously mentioned ways. They may also experience their distress in various bodily, or somatic, ways and present these symptoms, or what Balint (1964) called "offers," to their family physician. Thus, the number of individuals in a family practice who present to their physician with depressive symptoms will vary with the cultural milieu, the severity of any symptoms, barriers (or lack of) to primary care, personal preferences, and the perceived openness of the physician to discussing emotional issues.

The interpretation of prevalence figures for depression is complicated by the differences in definition and methods or tools used to diagnose the condition. For what is defined as major depressive disorder, the prevalence in the United States over 12 months is estimated to be 7%. Among females it is 1.5 to 3 times higher than males starting in early adolescence. In the 18–29-year age group it is three times higher than in those over the age of 60 (*DSM-5*, 2013, p. 165).

The prevalence of depression in a population varies with socioeconomic status. Jani et al. (2012) estimated that in economically deprived areas the prevalence may be as high as 30%, whereas in more affluent areas the prevalence is 18.5%.

In a study in the Netherlands in the 1980s, Verhaak (1995) recorded all physician visits among a population of 335,000 patients in 105 Dutch general practices over a 3-month period. They selected a random sample of 16,000 of them for further in-depth interviews to understand mental disorders in the community and help-seeking behavior. Over 37% of those interviewed had experienced some form of distress that could be construed as psychosocial in nature, with women, older people, the unemployed, and homemakers having higher rates. Using the GHQ (General Health Questionnaire), 9% of males and 16% of females scored above the threshold for diagnosis of depression. More than half of all patients who experienced some mental distress did not seek help through the formal healthcare system, but those with high GHQ scores were most likely to consult their general practitioner and receive a psychiatric diagnosis.

Using national Electronic Medical Record (EMR) data, the Canadian Primary Care Sentinel Surveillance Network (CPCSSN) estimated lifetime prevalence of depression in family practice to be 13.2%, which compares favorably with a 12.1% estimate from community-based epidemiologic survey (Puyat, Marhin, Etches, et al., 2013).

It has been estimated that about half of the patients consulting with depression are not recognized at the index visit, but 10% are recognized at a subsequent visit and 20% remit spontaneously. The remainder, however, may remain unrecognized for long periods (Paykel and Priest, 1992).

Based on prevalence figures in the United States, Ostbye et al. (2005) estimated that a family practice of 2500 patients with an age and sex profile representative of the US population would have 118 patients with depression at any time.

Depressive disorders often exist in the company of many other problems, such as substance abuse, anxiety, obsessive compulsive disorder, anorexia nervosa, and borderline personality disorder, as well as virtually any major chronic disorder, such as obesity, ischemic heart disease, chronic pulmonary disease, or gastrointestinal and rheumatic problems.

It is important to recognize that most people with mental illness do not seek care. The largest component of incongruous consultations (see Chapter 3) are those who identify themselves as having significant problems and do not go to a physician. For those with depressive symptoms, there may be concerns about feeling stigmatized. Because of presumed under-recognition of the problem, there have been calls to screen for depression. The Canadian Task Force on Preventive Health Care (CTFPHC) does not recommend screening for adults at average risk for depression or those who may be at increased risk (CTFPHC, 2013). The US Preventive Services Task Force (USPSTF, 2009), on the other hand, does recommend screening if staff-assisted depression care supports are in place.

FAMILY FACTORS

A genetic component to depression is supported by the observation that it is more common if there is a family history of treated depression and that it is more common in monozygotic than in dizygotic twins (Kendler, Neale, Kessler et al., 1992; Malhi, Moore, and McGuffin, 2000). The first-degree relatives of individuals with major depressive disorder have a two- to fourfold higher risk of depression themselves. The personality trait of neuroticism (negative affectivity) may contribute to this susceptibility (DSM-5, p. 166).

Environment and coping capacity are at least as important as genetics and neurochemistry in explaining the causes of depression. Adverse events in childhood (ACE) have been associated with a higher risk of depression later in life. In the Canadian Community Health Survey (Afifi, MacMillan, Boyle, et al., 2014) it was found that the prevalence of child abuse was 32% and that all types of abuse (physical abuse, sexual abuse, and exposure to intimate partner violence) were associated with increased risk of mental conditions later in life. In addition, there was an apparent dose–response effect depending on the number of each of the three types of abuse to which an individual was exposed in childhood. For example, the risk of depression was increased 2.6 times with any one of the three types of abuse, but 5.3 times if all three were present in childhood.

About half of all patients with major depression have excessive levels of blood cortisol, suggesting a response to stress that disrupts serotonin and norepinephrine transmission. Most antidepressant drugs are thought to act on either serotonergic or noradrenergic neurotransmitter systems, or both. By blocking reuptake, they increase the availability of these neurotransmitters. These imbalances of endocrine and neurotransmitter systems may in turn reflect changes at the more basic level of gene transmission and brain structure. In affective disorders, 50% of the first episodes are associated with significant stressors, but only 36% of the second or third episodes. Animal studies indicate that an acute stressor can turn on genes for substances that initiate long-term changes in the structure of brain cells (Post, 1992). In the theory of kindling, Post postulates that the trauma of events like childhood bereavement could change the structure of the developing brain, making the person vulnerable to depression when under stress in later life. If each episode increased the vulnerability, later depressive episodes could occur with little or no environmental stimulus. This would also explain the greater severity of depression in women who had had previous episodes (see Brown and Harris, 1978). If this is so, then adequate treatment of early episodes of depression may reduce vulnerability to later attacks.

SOCIAL FACTORS

As stated earlier, the prevalence of depression is higher in economically deprived areas. Interestingly, when international comparisons are made, this effect may be mitigated in those countries where economic disparities are less. The GINI coefficient of income disparity is a number that represents the degree of income disparity between the lowest and highest earners in a country. Countries with a high GINI coefficient (i.e., greater income disparity) have higher rates of depressive illness (Cifuentes, Sembajwe, Tak, et al., 2008).

In an important study of depression in women, Brown and Harris (1978) have shown that social factors are important in all types of depression. Brown and Harris identify three types of factors: those that make a woman more vulnerable to depression, those that precipitate a depression, and those that influence the way the depression will be clinically expressed. Women developing a depression were much more likely than those without depression to have had a traumatic life event in the 9 months before the onset. These events involved loss and disappointment, separation or threat of separation from a key figure, an unpleasant revelation about somebody close, a life-threatening illness in a close relative, and loss of employment.

The key factor is not change in itself, but the meaning that the event has for the person. Also important as precipitating events were major difficulties in life, such as a poor marriage, bad housing, financial problems, or difficulties with children. A traumatic life event or a major difficulty were precipitating factors in 83% of depressions. Minor events could also precipitate depression if they served to bring home to a person the implications of a long-term loss or disappointment.

The factors that made a woman vulnerable to depression were those that tended to isolate her, reduce her supports, and lower her self-esteem. The lack of a confidant, especially the inability to confide in a spouse, was important. Having three or more children at home and not being employed outside the home were factors increasing isolation. Regarding the past, the death of the woman's mother during childhood was the most significant factor.

Whether or not a depression had severe features, such as retardation of thought, was related to three factors. Severe depression was more likely to be associated with past bereavements, such as the death of a parent or sibling during childhood or the death of a spouse several years previously. Less severe depression was more likely to be associated with loss by separation rather than death. Women were more likely to have a severe depression if they were older, if they had had a previous depression, and if a traumatic event occurred after the onset.

The fact that social factors are important in depression does not necessarily mean that all depressed patients have "problems." If they have current problems, these should be identified, but it is counterproductive to be incredulous when a patient and spouse insist that they are happily married and have no major stresses in their lives. After the initial stimulus of a life stressor, recurrent depressions can eventually become autonomous (see the earlier discussion of the theory of kindling).

ILLNESS EXPERIENCE

The concept that neurotransmitter systems are disturbed makes it unnecessary to invoke such mechanisms as somatization to explain the physical symptoms that many depressed patients present. Neurotransmitters circulate widely in the body, and one might expect such a widespread bodily disturbance to be accompanied by pain and other symptoms. Because it is so difficult to describe the anguish of depression, it is not surprising that patients complain first of bodily sensations, which they can express in words. Even a person as articulate as William Styron (1990) found his experience of depression to be indescribable:

> I was feeling in my mind *a sensation close to, but indescribably different from, actual*
> *pain*. . . . That the word "indescribable" should present itself is not fortuitous,
> since it has to be emphasized that if the pain were readily describable most
> of the countless sufferers from this ancient affliction would have been able to
> confidently depict for their friends and loved ones (even their physicians) some
> of the actual dimensions of their torment, and perhaps elicit a comprehension
> that has been generally lacking; such incomprehension has usually been due not
> to a failure of sympathy but to the basic inability of healthy people to imagine
> a form of torment so alien to everyday experience. *For myself, the pain is most*
> *closely connected to drowning or suffocation*—but even these images are off the
> mark. William James, who battled depression for many years, gave up the search
> for an adequate portrayal, implying its near-impossibility when he wrote in *The*
> *Varieties of Religious Experience*: *"It is a positive and active anguish, a sort of psychi-*
> *cal neuralgia wholly unknown to normal life."* (Styron, 1990, pp. 4–5).

John Bentley Mays (1995), noted visual arts critic, described his depressive episodes as the circling of "the black dogs" (a literary metaphor for depression, attributed to Winston Churchill). Raised in a "house of anger," the death of Mays's father when he was 7 and of his mother when he was 12 led to ". . . a curious strategy that would harden into a frigid pattern . . . extinguish every desire to depend, need, want" (p. 9). Struggling with depression as a graduate student and after visiting apartheid-era South Africa, he drew a parallel between totalitarian political regimes and the mind of someone afflicted with depressive illness:

> It was not until much later that I realized that depression is the culture of such
> a society writ small: the self as a tiny modern state, mimicking the totalitarian
> state's boredom and frantic distraction, oppressive and parasitic bureaucracies,
> police forces, its terror that leaves no visible scars. Our intimacies are conducted
> like foreign policy. The depressive issues contradictory demands to himself,

practices seductions meant to subdue and degrade and control others, and unruly forces inside the self. At the heart of our policy is, of course, the modern state's greatest arrogation, its ultimate power over us: the right to judicial murder. Suicide is capital punishment under another name. (p. 51)

Both of these individuals are accomplished authors, able to convey difficult experiences in words. Most of our patients will not be able to express themselves this way, but the value of becoming familiar with such first-person accounts lies in approaching a better understanding of their anguish.

CLINICAL APPROACH
Diagnosis

It is important to distinguish between simple sadness and depressive disorder. Periods of sadness are a common human experience and differ from depression in severity and duration and the extent to which normal functions are affected. At one end of the spectrum, depression is a devastating and potentially fatal disease; at the other, it merges with the inescapable sadness of life. Family physicians are witnesses to a great deal of sadness: the sadness of disappointment, the sadness of loss, the sadness and despair of overwhelming misfortune, and the sadness of old age and mortality. Sadness is not a "disease" to be cured by medication or cognitive therapy. In some ways, sadness in these circumstances may be a personal growth experience, because it invites reflection and self-examination, perhaps also self-forgiveness and healing. Perhaps some of the "depressions" missed by general practitioners are feelings of this kind. The need may not be for cure, but for presence, support, and a listening ear. Kay Toombs, severely disabled by multiple sclerosis, tells of a visit she paid to her physician. She said, "I don't know why I've come to see you." "Yes, you do," he replied, "you came because you wanted to know that somebody gives a damn."

One of the reasons that depression, as defined in *DSM-5*, is missed in general practice is that patients may not be overtly depressed. They are often smiling when they first enter. Those with more severe forms of depression, however, will usually strike the physician as being unhappy, and the first cue may be the physician feeling "this patient makes me feel depressed."

Another reason for missed diagnosis is the occurrence of depression in a member of the family other than the patient being treated at the time: the spouse of a chronically ill or dying patient, or the mother of a disturbed child. This may need a question like "And how are you doing?" to allow the family member to express his or her pain.

The most common diagnostic error we have noted in residents in training is the failure to ask the most sensitive and specific question of all: "Do you feel depressed, low in spirits, down in the dumps?" (It is often necessary to express the question in several ways, because some patients do not identify their feeling as depression.) Instead of asking this question, residents will often ask much less sensitive and specific questions about appetite, constipation, and weight loss, which leave them uncertain about whether or not the patient is depressed.

Once the key question has been asked, other defining attributes of depression can be sought. The following are in approximate order of sensitivity, based on our experience:

1. Sleep disturbance. Nearly all patients have some trouble with sleeping, either difficulty in getting to sleep, frequent waking, or early waking. A patient presenting with difficulty sleeping should prompt the physician to probe for depression.
2. Loss of interest in life. Tasks and hobbies lose their interest; life loses its joy.
3. Loss of concentration. Work takes longer to complete; tasks are postponed.
4. A tendency to worry about small matters, the anxiety often going around and around in the mind like an obsession.
5. Feelings of worthlessness and failure; self-reproach about past failures and supposed defects of character.
6. Bouts of crying or wanting to cry. Patients will often cry during the interview—a strong cue to depression, especially in those not normally prone to crying.
7. Irritability. Patients are often aware of being irritable and feel guilty about the effect on spouse or children.
8. Loss of appetite, constipation. These symptoms are of less diagnostic value because they are shared with many other conditions.

If the patient admits to feeling depressed and other evidence is supportive, the diagnosis can be made on positive grounds. The diagnosis of depression is not made by exclusion. Sometimes the patient insists that he or she is not depressed, even though strong evidence points to this. If the patient is convinced that the symptoms point to some organic disease, he or she may angrily reject the suggestion that the problem is psychogenic. Understanding the patient's fear of a disease is an important component of patient-centered medicine; taking time to come to this understanding and acknowledging its existence contribute to trust in the patient–doctor relationship.

Whatever the nature of the depression, social factors should be assessed in all cases. Prominent among these will be family factors, especially the marital relationship, the quality of family life, and the presence of any problems with children, parents, in-laws, or other relatives. It is important to listen to the patient's life story, both the early experiences and relationships with parents and the more recent life events, especially losses of various kinds such as bereavement, separation, loss of home, or loss of job. The purpose of the inquiry is also to assess the strength and quality of social supports, since these play an important part in recovery.

One of the pitfalls of diagnosis is the co-occurrence of depression with the early stages of organic disease. Carcinoma of the pancreas, hypothyroidism, obstructive sleep apnea (OSA), and pernicious anemia are well known for this. To avoid this pitfall, it is advisable to screen for organic disease, especially in older patients. Physical examination will exclude gross evidence of physical disease. The erythrocyte sedimentation rate (ESR) is a valuable screening test for occult cancer or chronic infection, and complete blood count, serum B_{12}, and tests of thyroid function will be helpful in some patients (Case 13.1).

Another pitfall is the confusion of depression in the elderly with dementia caused by brain failure. Depression in the elderly may present with memory loss and confusion that are entirely reversible by treatment. A trial of antidepressive treatment is advisable before concluding that a patient's symptoms are caused by dementia. Of course dementia and depression may occur together, complicating the diagnosis and therapeutic approach. A family physician's longitudinal experience with a patient can assist in delineating the sequence of onset of cognitive impairment or depressive symptoms.

When depression presents with physical symptoms such as pain, it may be necessary to carry out investigations to identify or exclude organic disease. The need to do these should not delay treatment of the depression. Suicide during investigation is a risk in depressed patients. One of my (IRMcW) own patients committed suicide while awaiting a barium enema for diarrhea and weight loss. When investigations are required, it is advisable to have them done as quickly as possible, so that the patient is spared unnecessary anxiety.

Depressed patients with physical symptoms are especially at risk for spurious diagnosis. The investigation may reveal some "abnormality," which becomes the explanation of their symptoms, while their depression is overlooked—for example, osteoarthritis of the spine to explain backache, hiatus hernia to explain dyspepsia, a colonic diverticulum to explain abdominal pain.

CASE 13.1

An elderly woman asked for a home visit because of extreme fatigue. There was strong evidence of depression, no localizing symptoms, and examination was negative. A tentative diagnosis of major depressive illness was made, and blood was taken for an ESR. The ESR was 80 mm in 1 hour, and further investigation revealed a malignant carcinoma of the stomach.

Physicians who are more likely to recognize depression make more eye contact with patients, are good listeners, and are less likely to interrupt patients. They are also more likely to explore psychological and social issues (Paykel and Priest, 1992). All of these are features of the patient-centered clinical method. Recognition of depression occurs more frequently in consultations that are longer, where the doctor tolerates silence, notices nonverbal behavior, and uses patients' responses in further discussion, and where patients present psychological symptoms early (Paykel and Priest, 1992). The deficiencies probably reflect a lack of awareness of the many faces of depression and inadequate training in interviewing methods. The recognition of depressive illness in patients is influenced by physician factors such as familiarity with the patient, time available, personal beliefs about or experience with depression, and clinical experience. The latter, in turn, consists of familiarity with common clinical patterns and clinical skills, learning what "works" in the real clinical world, understanding the physician's role, and thinking of the whole person (Seong-Yi Baik, Bowers, Oakley, et al., 2008).

The diagnosis of major depressive episode requires the presence of five or more of nine symptoms, present every day for 2 weeks. At least one of the symptoms must be either depressed mood or loss of interest or pleasure (*DSM-5*).

Validated questionnaires, such as Patient Health Questionnaire (PHQ-9), Hamilton Depression Rating Scale (HAM-D), and Beck Depression Inventory (BDI-II), were originally designed as screening tools, but may be an aid to diagnosis or follow-up of treated patients. They are not a substitute for an appropriate patient-centered interview. As physicians gain more experience, these tools may be less necessary, allowing more time to focus on interacting with the patient (Baik, Bowers, Oakley, and Susman, 2008).

Impairment due to depression can be mild to very severe, but in general practice commonly takes the form of physical illnesses, pain, and reduced social and role functioning (*DSM-5*, p. 167).

Evaluation of depressive symptoms can be particularly difficult in the face of comorbidities such as cancer, recent myocardial infarction, diabetes, or the postpartum period when symptoms such as weight loss, fatigue, and sleep disturbance may occur for other reasons. In these circumstances, discerning depression depends more on the non-vegetative symptoms such as dysphoria, lack of pleasure from things or activities that usually are pleasurable, feelings of guilt, difficulty concentrating, and suicidal thoughts (*DSM-5*, 2013, p. 164). Depressive symptoms are more common in those with chronic disorders such as diabetes, cardiovascular disease, and morbid obesity, and are more likely to become chronic. Long-term improvement of depressive symptoms may depend on helping the patient come to terms with the entire spectrum of his or her illnesses and the impact they are having on their lives.

The risk of suicide must always be kept in mind, and sensitive, appropriately timed inquiry into such thoughts explored. Although suicidal ideation and attempts are more common in women, completion is more common in men. Besides gender, higher risk of suicide occurs in the elderly, and those who live alone and in circumstances of profound hopelessness (*DSM-5*, p. 167). Substance abuse adds significantly to suicidal risk. It is important for family physicians to evaluate which patients are at risk of attempting suicide. This evaluation must begin by thinking about this risk in the case of patients who are seriously distressed, as reported by themselves or a family member or friend, and in patients with impaired reality testing, who have expressed complete hopelessness, who have previously attempted suicide, or who have a severe psychiatric disorder (major depression, schizophrenia, borderline or antisocial personality disorder), or a family history of suicide. The question must be asked sensitively, after there has been sufficient time for the patient to develop trust in the physician, and one must evaluate the severity of the intent to commit suicide. Questions may include "What kind of thoughts have you been having?" or "How often are they happening?" Ask about whether there is a plan and access to the means to carry out the plan. Is there a history of impulsive behavior? (Craven, Links, and Novak, 2011).

Treatment

Whatever specific treatment is given, depressed patients have a deeply felt need for reassurance and support. A person experiencing depression for the first time finds it a very disturbing experience. According to Watts (1984, p. 70), after a lifetime of observing depression in general practice, "only someone who has suffered from the illness can fully appreciate the utter devastation it inflicts. . . . In my view, a severe depression is the most painful malady known to man."

The patient may feel that he or she is going insane. It is often an immense relief to be told that he or she is not going mad, that he or she has a very common problem, and that for many, depressions clear completely in a few weeks or months. It is reassuring to be told that the guilt feelings, anxieties, and joylessness are symptoms of depression and will clear when the depression lifts. It is helpful to know that one cannot be expected to alter one's mood by an act of will. The patient will often have been told by unsympathetic family members to "snap out of it" or to "cheer up." The family doctor can also help by explaining to members of the family how they can help the patient.

Besides individual psychotherapy and support, everything possible should þe done to mobilize social supports for the patient. This may include the involvement of the spouse and other relatives, help with children, and the development of contacts outside the home. Cognitive therapy, aimed at altering depressive thought patterns, has been found to benefit depressed patients referred by general practitioners (Teasdale, Fennell, Hibbert, and Amies, 1984). Because this involves 12–16 weekly sessions with someone trained in the method, not all general practitioners will undertake this themselves. It is possible that a modified form could be adapted for general practice. Some family physicians with the necessary extra training may offer this approach to patients referred by colleagues. Other psychotherapeutic approaches for which there is evidence of effectiveness are problem-solving therapy (PST), interpersonal therapy (IPT), and behavioral activation (Akers, Richards, and McMillan, 2011). It is likely that the support given to depressed patients by family physicians already has a cognitive element. The benefits of exercise in depression are well known, and encouraging at least one brisk walk a day should be part of the regimen.

Besides the support provided to all depressed patients, general practitioners have three main management decisions to make: the prescription of antidepressants and other drugs; referral to a psychiatrist, psychologist, or social worker; and admission to the hospital. The main criterion used by family physicians in prescribing antidepressants is the severity of symptoms. The effectiveness of antidepressants in psychiatric outpatients has been well established, but there have been very few trials in general practice. In view of the differences between the two patient populations, this is a serious gap in our knowledge. Because some patients respond very well to explanation and reassurance, it may be wise to wait until the second visit before starting an antidepressant, especially in those with mild depression. In more seriously depressed patients, the follow-up visit must be within days or weeks to ensure that the physician detects any rapid decompensation.

For moderate to severe depression, the selective serotonin reuptake inhibitors (SSRIs) and selective norepinephrine reuptake inhibitors (SNRIs) have largely replaced tricyclic antidepressants (TCAs), monoamine oxidase inhibitors (MAOIs), and reversible monoamine oxidase inhibitors (RIMAs) in family practice. The choice of drug depends on the particular symptoms being experienced by the patient, as well as physician's familiarity with the common side effects and response rate. When anxiety is a prominent symptom, escitalopram, paroxetine, sertraline, and venlafaxine have been shown to be helpful. Bupropion, mirtazapine, and moclobemide are thought to have fewer sexual side effects. They should be cautiously started at low doses, since those individuals with prominent anxiety tend to be very sensitive to side effects such as agitation, and an increase in symptoms from the medication may be misattributed to the underlying disorder. The prudent physician will become familiar with one or two medications in each category.

Once a therapeutic response is obtained, treatment with an antidepressant should continue at least 9–12 months. In the presence of other risk factors such as chronic or recurrent depression, medication should continue for at least 2 years and sometimes longer. When discontinuing antidepressants it is necessary to taper the dose, with at least 1 week between each dose reduction, and to counsel the patient on symptoms of discontinuation. This may include flu-like symptoms, insomnia, nausea, imbalance or dizziness, sensory disturbances, and hyper-arousal or agitation (identified by the acronym FINISH).

When patients do not seem to respond to treatment, it is important to evaluate the level of adherence to the regimen. There may be a low rate of adherence to the use of medication as well as to psychotherapy. This is more likely when depression is complicated by serious medical or psychiatric disorders. Patients may be reluctant to take medication for the long term, fearing addiction, and it is important to find common ground, to provide psycho-education, and to schedule regular follow-up visits. The approach of motivational interviewing may help (see Chapter 10, "The Enhancement of Health and the Prevention of Disease"). If adherence has been assured, nonresponse should prompt a review of the diagnosis. Switching to another medication is a reasonable option, as is combining with another antidepressant in another class. Augmenting agents such as antipsychotic agents (risperidone, olanzapine, or quetiapine) are a further option, but carry the risk of increased side effects (Goldbloom and Davine, 2011) and potentially severe metabolic effects.

Family physicians need to be aware that many of their patients experiencing depression will have tried some form of complementary and alternative medicines (CAM; see Chapter 23). Most common among these is St. John's wort (Hypericum perforatum) and ginkgo. A review of the evidence (Linde, Berner, and Kriston, 2008, updated in 2009) found that St. John's wort was better than placebo and equal to SSRIs in the treatment of major depression with fewer side effects. There were noticeable differences between trials, likely reflecting variation in the components of this herbal product, and this represents the greatest challenge to its use in family practice in countries where botanicals are not well regulated. There may be potentially severe interactions with other medications and inconsistency in the amount of the herb contained in the capsules. If used, the daily recommended dose is 900 mg in three equal doses in a product with a minimum of 2%–5% hyperforin or 0.3% hypericin. It should not be used concurrently with SSRIs or in pregnancy or lactation, and high doses may predispose to photodermatitis. Side effects include stomach upset, allergic reaction, fatigue, dry mouth, restlessness, and constipation (Rakel, 2007). Ginkgo biloba is widely used and recommended by some for resistant depression for those over the age of 50 (Rakel, 2007), but a review of the evidence finds little to support it for this indication (Birks and Grimley Evans, 2009).

The emerging picture of depression is one of an illness in which short- and long-term changes in the central nervous system are coupled in a nonlinear relationship with life experiences and social relationships. The nonlinearity is seen in the capability of any part of the circular chain to produce change. Life events can elicit changes in brain structure, which in turn alter the response to future events. Social isolation increases depression, which in turn increases social isolation (see Case 9.5). Intervention at any point in the circle can be therapeutic: drug therapy, social support, cognitive therapy. Relief from depression can transform the perception of life events from negative to positive.

NOTE

1. Psychiatry has undergone significant changes in the latter half of the twentieth century with the emergence of a paradigm that is described as having four pillars: (1) criteria-based diagnosis (as found in the *DSM*); (2) distinction of severity of illness (as measured by tools such as the Hamilton Depression Inventory); (3) a biomedical model (the catecholamine hypothesis); and (4) the epidemiology of depression in primary care. The applicability of this model to primary care has been questioned, and certainly its transferability has proven problematic. Callahan and Berrios suggest five reasons for difficulty in applying the psychiatric model in family practice: (1) the existence of competing disease priorities in primary care; (2) the uncertainty of the transferability of lessons learned in psychiatric populations; (3) the presence of difficult socioeconomic problems; (4) a discordance in mental healthcare reimbursement; and (5) the role of the patient (Callahan and Berrios, 2005).

REFERENCES

Afifi TO, MacMillan HL, Boyle M, Taillieu T, Cheung K, Sareen J. 2014. Child abuse and mental disorders in Canada. *Canadian Medical Association Journal* 186(9):675.

Akers D, Richards D, McMillan D, Bland JM, Gilbody S. 2011. Behavioural activation delivered by the non-specialist: Phase II randomised controlled trial. *British Journal of Psychiatry* 198:66–72.

Baik S-Y, Bowers BJ, Oakley LD, Susman JL. 2008. What comprises clinical experience in recogniziing depression? The primary care clinician's perspective. *Journal of the American Board of Family Practice* 21(3):200–210.

Balint M. 1964. *The Doctor, His Patient & the Illness*, 2nd ed. London: Pitman Medical.

Berrios GE. 1994. Historiography of mental symptoms and disease. *History of Psychiatry* 5:175–190.

Birks J, Grimley Evans J. 2009. Ginkgo biloba for cognitive impairment and dementia. *Cochrane Database of Systematic Reviews* 2009, Issue 1. Art. No.: CD003120. doi: 10.1002/14651858.CD003120.pub3.

Brown GW, Harris TO. 1978. *Social Origin of Depression: A Study of Psychiatric Disorder in Women*. New York: Free Press.

Callahan CM, Berrios GE. 2005. *Reinventing Depression: A History of the Treatment of Depression in Primary Care, 1940–2004*. New York: Oxford University Press.

Canadian Task Force on Preventive Health Care, Screening for Depression. 2013. http://canadiantaskforce.ca/ctfphc-guidelines/2013-depression/

Cifuentes M, Sembajew G, Tak S, Gore R, Kriegel D, Punnett L. 2008. The association of major depressive episodes with income inequality and the human development index. *Social Science & Medicine* 67(4):520–539.

Dowrick C. 2004. *Beyond Depression: A New Approach to Understanding and Management*. New York: Oxford University Press.

DSM-5: Diagnostic and Statistical Manual of Mental Disorders. 2013. Arlington, VA: American Psychiatric Association.

Craven MA, Links PS, Novak G. 2011. Assessment and management of suicide risk. In: Goldbloom DS, Davine J, eds., *Psychiatry in Primary Care: A Concise Canadian Pocket Guide*. Toronto: Centre for Addiction and Mental Health.

Goldbloom DS, Davine J, eds. 2011. *Psychiatry in Primary Care: A Concise Canadian Pocket Guide*. Toronto: Centre for Addiction and Mental Health.

Kendler K, Neale M, Kessler R, Heath A, Eaves L. 1992. Familial influences on the clinical characteristics of major depression: A twin study. *Acta Psychiatrica Scandinavica* 86:371–378.

Linde K, Berner MM, Kriston L. 2008. St John's wort for major depression. *Cochrane Database of Systematic Reviews* 2008, Issue 4. Art. No.: CD000448. doi: 10.1002/14651858.CD000448.pub3.

Malhi G, Moore J, McGuffin P. 2000. The genetics of depressive disorder. *Current Psychiatric Reports* 2:165–169.

Mays, JB 1995. *In the Jaws of the Black Dogs*. Toronto: Viking, Published by the Penguin Group.

McWhinney IR. 2014. The evolution of clinical method. In: Stewart M, Brown JB, Weston WW, et al., eds., *Patient-Centered Medicine: Transforming the Clinical Method*, 3rd ed. London: Radcliffe Publishing.

Ostbye T, Yarnell KSH, Krause KM, et al. 2005. Is there time for management of patients with chronic diseases in primary care? *Annals of Family Medicine* 3(3):209–214.

Paykel ES, Priest RG. 1992. Recognition and management of depression in general practice: Consesnus statement. *British Medical Journal* 305:1198.

Puyat JH, Marhin WW, Etches D, Wilson R, Elwood Martin R, Sajjan KK, Wong S. 2013. Estimating the prevalence of depression from EMRs. *Canadian Family Physician* 59(4):445.

Rakel D. 2007. *Integrative Medicine*, 2nd ed. Philadelphia: Elsevier.

Seong-Yi Baik, Bowers BJ, Oakley LD, Susman JL. 2008. What comprises clinical experience in recognizing depression? The primary care clinician's perspective. *Journal of American Board of Family Practice* 21(3):200–210.

Teasdale JD, Fennell MJV, Hibbert CA, et al. 1984. Cognitive therapy for major depressive disorder in primary care. *British Journal of Psychiatry* 14(4):400.

US Preventive Services Task Force. 2009. *Depression in Adults: Screening*. http://www.uspreventiveservicestaskforce.org/Page/Topic/recommendation-summary/depression-in-adults-screening?ds=1&s=depression.

Verhaak PFM. 1995. *Mental Disorder in the Community and in General Practice*. Aldershot, UK: Avebury.

CHAPTER 14

cᴧᴐ

Diabetes

The prevalence of type 2 diabetes mellitus (T2DM) is continuing to grow globally and represents an increasingly large disease burden, both as a public health concern and in the general practitioner's office. Complications of poorly controlled diabetes can cause a number of negative medical outcomes for patients. Family physicians must manage and monitor clinical targets, support their patients in self-care, and also be cognizant of the varied ways in which T2DM affects patients' daily lives. This chapter provides a framework for family physicians to approach the screening, diagnosis, and long-term care of patients with T2DM. We will not address type 1 diabetes mellitus (T1DM) here.

PREVALENCE IN FAMILY PRACTICE

Worldwide, there are over 347 million people living with diabetes (types 1 and 2) (WHO, 2013). While most studies do not distinguish between T1 and T2DM, according to the World Health Organization over 90% of diabetics have T2DM. Since the 1980s there has been a twofold increase in the number of adults with diabetes (Danaei et al., 2011). Often, the fastest growing rates are from low- and middle-income countries where healthcare systems are not as robust as in higher income nations. However, North American rates have also shown large increases. In Canada, the prevalence of diagnosed diabetes has increased by 70% over the past decade (PHAC, 2011a). Across Europe, the average prevalence of diabetes in adults is 8.4%, and the number is expected to increase from 55 million to 64 million adults by 2030 (IDF, 2012). In the United States, where diabetes is the seventh leading cause of death, the estimated prevalence is varies between 7.6% and 15.9% depending on race/ethnicity (CDC, 2014). Based on data from the Canadian Primary Care Sentinel

Surveillance Network, the point prevalence of diabetes between 2011 and 2012 in a typical Canadian primary care practice was 7.6%. Over the same 2-year period, the median number of visits by diabetic patients to the family practitioner was 10, compared to 5 visits for a nondiabetic patient (Greiver et al., 2014). The DIASCAN study found that of routine visits to the family physician, just over 16% were for diabetic patients (Leiter et al., 2001). Ostbye and colleagues (2005) estimated that in a family practice of 2500 patients with an average age and sex distribution typical of the United States, there would be 145 individuals with recognized diabetes. Based on Lipscombe and Hux's (2007) study, a family physician may expect to have 10–12 new cases of diabetes each year in his or her practice among patients over the age of 20.

Undiagnosed Diabetes

Importantly, there is a significant proportion of undiagnosed diabetics in primary care practices. In the United States, approximately 7 million people (or 2.5% of the population) have undiagnosed diabetes (CDC, 2011). The Canadian rate of undiagnosed diabetes is estimated to be 2.2% (Leiter et al., 2001). These observations emphasize the importance of comprehensive, effective screening programs.

Aboriginal Populations

Aboriginal communities in North America and Australia are highly vulnerable populations with drastically elevated rates of T1 and T2DM as compared to the non-Aboriginal population. Age-adjusted prevalence rates in these communities are three to five times higher than the general population, and in some communities the prevalence is as high as 26% (Stewart, Bhattacharyya, Dyck, et al., 2013). An Australian study of 15 remote Aboriginal communities determined the age- and gender-adjusted prevalence of diabetes to be just under 15% (Daniel et al., 2002), but ranging as high as 33.1% in some segments of the population (Minges, Zimmet, Magliano, et al., 2011).

Geographic Disparities

It is also relevant to note that in many regions there remain significant geographic disparities in prevalence and acute complications of T2DM. In Canada, there is a measurable east-to-west gradient in the prevalence of diabetes. The eastern Maritime provinces typically have higher rates compared to the western provinces and Quebec. Some of this variation may be linked to other significant variables, such as socioeconomic status (SES), education, and rural location (Ardern and Katzmarzyk, 2007). In Europe, the prevalence of diabetes ranges from less than 4% in countries such as France, Italy, and England, to over 7.5% in Russia, Poland, and Turkey (International Diabetes Federation, 2012).

FAMILY FACTORS

Understanding the various aspects of family influence on the risk, development, and disease progression of T2DM is fundamental for a successful clinical approach by patient and physician. As with patients' personal care habits, socioeconomic circumstances, and lifestyle choices, the influence of family is one area where the family physician should be well versed so that he or she may create, with the patient, a personalized plan of care.

Genetics

The genetics of T2DM is an exceedingly complex area of scientific study, and while research continues to reveal new loci and gene variants that contribute to its polygenic etiology, this research has not led to any clinically relevant treatment targets or therapies as yet. However, this may be the case in the future, and it is prudent to have a basic grasp of the genetics and epigenetics influencing the risk, onset, and progression of T2DM. As an example, a particular variant of the gene TCF7L2 has a verified, reproducible effect on the risk of developing T2DM. Variation at a single nucleotide base of TCF7L2 causes impaired insulin secretion, and patients with this variant have up to twice the risk of developing T2DM compared to individuals without (Zeggini and McCarthy, 2007). Abnormal insulin secretion due to impaired β-cell function is the most common mechanism, but each candidate gene identified to date acts in its own way on the pathways of insulin metabolism (Lyssenko et al., 2008). Mutations in the gene TCF2 alter hepatic transcription factors; a variant of P12A changes the PPAR-γ receptor (target for thiazolidinediones) (Frayling, 2007). As such, each gene identified, along with its corresponding metabolic pathway and protein products, represents a potential target for pharmaceutical therapies (Scott, Mohike, and Bonnycastle, 2007). Although a number of genes have already been identified and population-based studies continue to reveal more, the relative risk for developing T2DM if a sibling has the disease is approximately three or four times, much lower than other familial conditions (e.g., rheumatoid arthritis or Crohn's disease) and the estimate of heritability in a population is less than 15% (Frayling, 2007; Pinney and Simmons, 2012).

This observation speaks to the role of epigenetics—the interactions between genes and the environment (Groop and Pociot, 2013). Epigenetic changes such as DNA methylation and histone modification alter genetic activity and begin *in utero*, and once the DNA's structure is altered, these changes can theoretically extend onward through multiple generations.

Prenatal Environment

Observational studies in humans reveal a strong relationship between the intra-uterine environment and disease later in life. High maternal glucose concentrations are linked to obesity in offspring, independent of the mother's pre-pregnancy body mass index (BMI) (Pinney and Simmons, 2012). An observational study in Pune, India, found that maternal fasting plasma glucose and triglycerides were strong, positive predictors of fetal birth weight. Comparing this population to a British cohort revealed links between maternal nutrition, birth weight, insulin resistance, and adult-onset T2DM in the offspring (Yajnik, 2002). The fundamental relationships between these variables was first highlighted in the early 1990s as the "thrifty phenotype" (today referred to as the Barker Hypothesis). In the specific case of T2DM, it was postulated that poor maternal/fetal nutrition, as well as poor nutrition and growth in infancy, lead to irreversible changes in pancreatic tissues. This abnormal development initiated in the fetus predisposes adults to metabolic abnormalities and T2DM (Hales and Barker, 1992). Interestingly, studies have shown that this risk is most elevated in those adults who were malnourished but experienced subsequent catch-up growth. For example, at 8 years of age, Indian study subjects with the worst cardiovascular risk profiles (including insulin resistance, cholesterol, and blood pressure) were the infants born smallest with a subsequent catch-up in weight, height, and body fat (Yajnik, 2002). One possibility is that a pro-inflammatory and hyperglycemic maternal environment changes the levels of transcription factors, leading to long-term dysfunction of metabolic pathways, and may change hypothalamic neural circuitry in the fetus (Pinney and Simmons, 2012).

Breastfeeding

The maternal–offspring interaction continues after birth, influencing infant health, growth, and development. Breastfeeding is the center of this interaction. Breastfeeding may contribute to as much as a 15% reduction in the incidence of DM (Owen et al., 2006). Even two months of breastfeeding after birth may lower the subsequent risk of T2DM in the infant (Taylor et al., 2014). Further, it was postulated that lower circulating levels of estrogen in women who breastfeed may have a protective effect against the later development of diabetes in the mother. Overall, current evidence suggests that breastfeeding is beneficial for all new mothers, regardless of their current diabetes status (Owen et al., 2006; Taylor et al., 2014).

There are some recognized barriers to breastfeeding. Several social determinants and other demographic variables impact the rates of breastfeeding in the population, including maternal SES (CDC, 2013; Petry, 2013), maternal weight and low infant birth weight (Owen et al., 2006), geography (CDC, 2013), and race. Data from the 2004 American National Immunization Survey indicates that while 71% of Caucasian mothers breastfeed, only 50% of black mothers do (CDC, 2013).

Family Eating Environment

Often caring for multiple members of a single household, family physicians may have unique insights into family habits (see Chapter 4, "The Family in Health and Disease"). The eating environment is only one of these habits, but a growing body of research suggests that it plays an important role in the early development of childhood obesity, insulin resistance, and diabetes. Parental modeling of healthy food behaviors (through regular, shared meals) positively correlates with children's vegetable intake, but sweet snacks and high-calorie drinks correlate with increased television time (Campbell, Crawford, and Ball, 2006). Another cross-sectional survey found that children who have more sit-down dinners with their family are more likely to have a healthy diet, including more fruits and vegetables, less soda, and less saturated/trans fats. Overall, more family dinners translated to a lower average glycemic load at mealtime. Although these studies are all cross-sectional, and thus cannot extrapolate data to make links between family eating habits in youth and adulthood risk of metabolic abnormalities, foods with higher glycemic loads are linked with more rapid rises and falls in blood glucose levels, thus over the long term stressing beta cells and predisposing to insulin resistance and T2DM (Ludwig, 2002). Among Latino children in San Diego, those who had at least four meals a week with their family—whether breakfast, lunch, or dinner—were more likely to consume fruits and vegetables (Andaya et al., 2009). However, in a US sample of 16,000 children, only half of 9-year-olds, and less than one-third of 14-year-olds, ate dinner with their families every night (Gillman, 2002).

As with breastfeeding, the family eating environment is related to other social determinants of health: SES, which influences the ability to afford fresh, healthful foods; parents at work or children attending activity programs during family mealtimes; eating food in front of TV/computer screens; the physical environment, which significantly impacts access to supermarkets selling fresh fruits and vegetables; and social networks and education, which influence our understanding of healthy versus unhealthy foods, how to prepare meals, and so on. It is critical that the family physician understands these variables so that counseling can be provided in the context of the patient's everyday life.

SOCIAL FACTORS

Two mechanisms have been suggested by which social determinants influence health status and outcomes in diabetes. First, these factors impact the incidence and prevalence of T2DM, and are relevant for public health policies and programs. Second, social determinants have a critical influence on the successful medical approach to T2DM (Raphael et al., 2003).

Socioeconomic Status

Socioeconomic status (SES) is a particularly complex factor that encompasses several health determinants, including income, education, the physical environment, and behaviors. An observational study in Manchester, the United Kingdom's third poorest city, found rates of T2DM ranging from 20% to 30% among individuals living in areas with a high prevalence of low income in the inner city (Riste, Khan, and Cruickshank, 2001). The most immediate effect of income on health is a deprivation of material resources, including an inability to purchase healthy foods (Reading and Wein, 2009). Financial barriers are compounded by a lack of reasonable access to nutritional, whole foods. The literature on "food deserts" in urban and suburban centers is robust and reveals several common, global trends. In New York City, the lowest income neighborhoods, made up of predominantly black residents, have the poorest access to supermarkets and convenience stores with fresh fruits and vegetables. The wealthiest neighborhoods have significantly better access, geographically and financially, to supermarkets and convenience stores with healthy food options (Gordon et al., 2011). London, Canada, has relatively poor access to supermarkets regardless of SES, with geographic accessibility becoming worse in the study period of 1961–2005 (Larsen and Gilliland, 2008). Lower SES also makes it less likely that an individual will be identified as having T2DM. In the Manchester study, over half of the participants were previously undiagnosed diabetics (Riste, Khan, and Cruickshank, 2001). Of note, this relationship is true for wealthier nations only. In low- and middle-income countries, T2DM is more prevalent among wealthier individuals (Whiting, Unwin, and Rogic, 2010).

Education is an important variable related to SES. Analysis of mortality within American Cancer Society cohorts between 1959 and 1996 found that there is a strong inverse relationship between educational level and mortality from diabetes, independent of conventional risk factors (Steenland, Henley, and Thun, 2002). Data from the NHANES I found that women with greater than 16 years of education were significantly less likely to develop T2DM than those with less than 9 years of education. However, much of this relationship was accounted for by body size, diet, physical activity, and alcohol/tobacco use (Robbins et al., 2004). Others have found that poor glycemic control was related to age (worse among young adults), minority status, and lack of health coverage, but not education (Ali, Bullard, Imperatore, et al., 2012). Patient care in primary practice must always take into account the demographic context of the patient, including culture, geography, gender, and so on.

Social Support Networks

Support networks can be incredibly useful to patients, and an important factor for the family practitioner to appreciate. Social support can be of two types: support from spouses, family, and friends; as well as support from peers and fellow patients. Group visits to the physician have been found to have a positive effect on lowering HbA1C and lipids, and patients' understanding of their diabetes. Social support groups were the best therapy for improving patients' psychosocial health and overall quality of life (van Dam et al., 2005). Others have found weak evidence for a positive effect on HbA1C; however, it is difficult to draw conclusions from social support studies, as there is little standardization for how to assess a given therapy (Stopford, Winkley, and Ismail, 2013).

At-Risk Populations: Immigrants

Urban centers across the developed world continue to see a high influx of immigrants from developing countries, and they are often at an increased risk of having or developing T2DM. In Ontario, Canada, new immigrants to the province have significantly higher rates of T2DM than local residents. Among the new immigrants, South Asians are at particularly high risk: South Asian men were four times as likely to have T2DM as European or American immigrants (Creatore et al., 2010). Among Arab immigrants to the United States, dysglycemia—including impaired fasting glucose, impaired glucose tolerance, and frank diabetes—was more common if the participants were older at the age of immigration, unemployed, frequently consumed Arabic food, and were less active in Arabic organizations. These factors were all risks independent of BMI and age. For female immigrants, additional risk factors included a lack of employment outside the home, less than a high school education, and illiteracy. Overall, individuals with less acculturation were at greater risk for T2DM, but these results are not consistent with other studies on the topic (Jaber et al., 2010). A comparative study in Sweden between ethnic Swedes and new Turkish immigrants identified Turkish women as a particularly high risk subgroup, and researchers attributed this to a lack of physical activity and low rates of employment outside the home, preventing acculturation (Wändell, Steiner, and Johansson, 2003).

At-Risk Populations: Aboriginals

When discussing the determinants of health in Aboriginal populations, it is important to keep in mind that Aboriginal communities and populations within and between countries are heterogenous, each with their own health concerns and community structures. Common to all populations is a history of strife, dispossession, and cultural upheaval. Compared to non-Aboriginal populations, living conditions, community infrastructure, and public services are typically underdeveloped and inadequate. Specific problems include overcrowding, homelessness, a poor water supply, and, especially relevant for T2DM, poor availability of and access to healthy foods. These intermediate and distal determinants create unique and often challenging healthcare environments (Reading and Wien, 2009). As with new immigrants to urban centers, Aboriginal women are at especially elevated risk. Among Aboriginal children in Saskatchewan, incidence of youth-onset T2DM was 46 per 100,000 in females, versus 30 per 100,000 in males (Dyck et al., 2012).

SUBJECTIVE EXPERIENCE
How Patients View Their Illness

A 2002 study in Guadalajara, Mexico, interviewed 20 patients, with the goal of understanding the layperson's perspectives on the etiology of T2DM. All study participants had had prior interaction with healthcare professionals, but all disregarded the biomedical, physiologic explanations for the origin of diabetes. The subjects did not appreciate any role for exercise, diet, or genetic predisposition. Most commonly, they implicated a strong emotional reaction in response to a stressful, frightening, or adversarial event in their life as the origin of their diabetes: "I had a fright [in my house]. I was frightened because someone told me my brother was seriously ill... and I got frightened, and I came home, and I drank water because my mouth was dry, and there's where it started. . . ." (p. 801). The female participants were more likely to attribute these stressors to events in the home, while the males cited work-related triggers (Mercado-Martinez and Ramos-Herrera, 2002).

Culture and our social milieu are critical in informing our understanding of our personal health and the medical sciences. The perceptions of adults in Guadalajara may differ from those of middle-aged diabetics living in Victoria, British Columbia, or San Diego, California, or elderly patients in Egypt. As an example, a qualitative series of interviews of first-generation Korean-American immigrants living in Maryland can be contrasted to the views of the Mexican subjects. On average, the Korean-American subjects viewed their diabetes as an inherited disease, and thus shared many fears about passing it on to their children. They also felt that changes from a traditional Korean diet negatively impacted their health. For the Korean immigrants, health meant having energy, mental acuity, and control over their illnesses. Public appearance and their image within the local Korean community were paramount, such that many participants kept their diagnosis of diabetes secret from friends and acquaintances in the community (Pistulka et al., 2012). In a review article on women with gestational diabetes including studies from the United States, Canada, Australia, and Tonga, there were common feelings and ideas about their illness across cultures. These were categorized as the emotional response, the loss of a normal pregnancy, privileging the baby, information and healthcare support, and personal control. Many women experienced shock and fear. Understanding of the disease process varied: some women cited physiologic changes in the pancreas, while others explained the diabetes as a result of behaviors—lack of exercise or a poor diet. This review also highlighted that patients from Western countries are more likely to reach for a physiologic explanation, while women living in Africa or parts of the Middle East place blame on spiritual factors (Parsons et al., 2014).

Aboriginal populations in North America tend to blend these sorts of explanations, with a holistic perspective on health and disease. Inviting participants to a traditional talking circle was used as a means to explore an Aboriginal community's perceptions of diabetes and its impact within the community (Struthers et al., 2003). Community members were trained to lead the circles, and participants revealed several important trends. Diabetes is seen as an illness for the individual, the family, and the community. It was described as a "silent killer," and a disease that affected not just the person but also the entire people. Diabetes is understood as a medical disease with a physiologic basis, but there is also an expressed a desire to align this understanding with traditional culture and healing methods. There was a desire to treat diabetes, but often participants felt a conflicting sense of hopelessness about their current and future health. As a result, while they understood the need for diet and exercise changes, they felt that attempting change would be futile (Struthers et al., 2003). In this and other studies, patients want local, group-based therapy within their community as a means of social and emotional support. The Aboriginal participants in the talking circles felt that the group sessions provided a sense of community, and that they were able to understand, often for the first time, the medical information provided (Struthers et al., 2003). In the review on gestational diabetes, a common thread across the included studies was a desire for support groups and exercise "buddies" (Parsons et al., 2014).

To explore the patient perspective, online blogs can be a valuable resource. In all aspects of personal health, people commonly turn to the Internet for information, peer support, and evaluation of medical therapies. As physicians, it is important to remember that our patients will access these resources, and that these resources may not always be accurate or helpful. However, many personal and organizational blogs can be positive sources of advice and emotional support for patients living with chronic conditions like diabetes. There are a myriad of personal blogs available online, written by individuals who themselves have diabetes, parents of children with diabetes, and physicians who care for diabetic patients. Patients share how they were diagnosed, experiences with dietary changes, and use of medications, with the goal of offering emotional support and advice on living with diabetes. For example, one blogger writes about switching to a new blood testing machine: "Yesterday was the end of an era. My blood testing machine and I broke up. Neither of us wanted to end it. My machine had been steadfastly and happily testing my glucose levels for almost five years" (http://asweetlife.org/author/alex/). Another writes about her recent blood sugar low: "I love a good 'diabetes hack' when I hear one—anything that makes this ridiculous disease a teeny tiny bit easier I'm game for. I found myself low on Monday night before bed, standing in front of an open fridge, and I was tempted to shovel 2 to 3 times the appropriate amount of chocolate frosting into my mouth to get out of said low and into my bed quicker" (http://www.irunoninsulin.com/?p=8297).

Expectations for Treatment

There is a paucity of research on the subject of patient expectations from their healthcare providers in terms of their diabetes care. The few studies on this topic provide interesting feedback to healthcare providers, and this may be a relevant area for future research. A focus group in Andalusia, Spain, including patients with both T1 and T2DM, highlighted that desires of patients are relatively simple, and tend toward the non-medical expert skill set of the clinician. For example, participants wanted a physician to show understanding and kindness, and to share information in a collaborative versus an authoritative way. In T2DM specifically, patients expressed a desire to avoid the negative outcomes that they had observed in others living with T2DM (Escudero-Carretero et al., 2007).

Fears

A common theme in qualitative studies on T2DM is patient fears. Fears encompass medical, emotional, and social concerns, including lifestyle modifications, personal health outcomes, and the effect on family. One topic well studied in the literature is fear of hypoglycemia (FoH). Hypoglycemic episodes are a very common fear for patients taking insulin, who worry about accidents, injury, and often have anxiety over the possibility of future episodes. Overall, it is associated with poorer quality of life scores, reduced work productivity, and greater healthcare costs (Fidler, Christensen, and Gillard, 2011). One review emphasizes the negative impact that FoH and hypoglycemic events can have on all aspects of daily life, including relationships, employment, recreation, and driving (Frier, 2008). In a study including 2000 patients from China, Korea, Malaysia, Thailand, and Taiwan, 36% of patients reported a hypoglycemic event in the preceding 6 months, and objective assessment of quality of life using various scales demonstrated a significant, negative impact on daily living (Sheu et al., 2012).

A study of 300 patients in Sweden estimated the direct and indirect costs of hypoglycemic events to be about US$14 per month, per patient. In this study, 37% of the patients reported a hypoglycemic event in the preceding month, although only 2% were severe (Lundkvist et al., 2005). As might be expected, FoH is more common among patients who have a history of hypoglycemic episodes or loss of consciousness, have been on insulin longer, or who have poor control over their blood glucose levels (Wild et al., 2007). Patients may overeat or deliberately take less insulin in order to alleviate their fears of having an episode (Marrero et al., 1997). Blood glucose awareness training and cognitive behavior therapy are both effective options to alleviate FoH (Wild et al., 2007).

Medically, assessing a patient's hypoglycemic risk profile is an important aspect of diabetes care. For example, higher glucose values are often acceptable in elderly patients, as the risks from slightly higher blood glucose are preferable to the risks of falls, arrhythmias, impaired cognitive function, and other injuries associated with hypoglycemic events. This will be addressed in more detail in the following section.

CLINICAL APPROACH

Diabetes care involves all aspects of a patient's life. To continue this care in the long term, every interaction with the patient must be built on an appreciation for the person, rather than a scientific, reductive focus on the pathophysiology of hyperglycemia and beta cells. Guidelines are just that, and the work of the family physician is tailoring those guidelines to the patient before him or her. Several factors must be considered when applying generalized treatment algorithms to the individual patient: the patient's feelings surrounding illness, such as fear of death, worry about drug costs, or despair over an uncertain future; his or her understanding of the medical and physiologic aspects of diabetes; the impact of diagnosis and chronic diabetes on daily functions; and the parient's implicit and explicit expectations for care by the physician.

Screening and Diagnosis

The diagnostic cutoffs for pre-diabetes and diabetes vary depending on national guidelines; sample guidelines from Canada, the United States, Europe, and Australia have been presented in Table 14.1. Of course, family physicians must also understand the risk factors, signs, and symptoms of T2DM in order to appropriately identify at-risk patients for targeted screening. The textbook presentation of T2DM—polydipsia, polyuria, blurry vision, and recurrent urinary tract infections—is relatively rare, but the deleterious metabolic effects of insulin resistance and hyperglycemia can begin well before clinical signs and symptoms are evident to the patient or healthcare provider, emphasizing the importance of having a standardized screening program in place

Table 14.1 DIAGNOSTIC CUTOFFS FOR TYPE 2 DIABETES MELLITUS

	Canada (CDA Primer, 2013)	United States (ADA, 2014)	Australia (RACGP, 2014)	Europe (ESC, 2013)
Fasting* plasma glucose	DM: ≥ 7.0 mmol/L IFG: 6.1–6.9	DM: ≥ 126 mg/dL (7.0 mmol/L)	DM: ≥ 7.0 mmol/L IFG: 6.1–6.9 mmol/L	DM: ≥ 7.0 mmol/L IFG: 6.1–6.9 mmol/L
Random plasma glucose	DM: ≥ 11.1 mmol/L	DM: ≥ 200 mg/dL (11.1 mmol/L)	–	–
HbA1C	DM: ≥ 6.5% Pre-DM: 6%–6.4%	DM: ≥ 6.5% Pre-DM: 5.7%–6.4%	DM: ≥ 6.5% Pre-DM: –	DM: ≥ 6.5% Pre-DM: –
2 h plasma glucose (75-g OGTT)	DM: ≥ 11.1 mmol/L IGT: 7.8–11.0 mmol/L	DM: ≥ 200 mg/dL IGT: 140–199 mg/dL (7.8–11.0 mmol/L)	DM: ≥ 11.0 mmol/L IGT: 7.8–11.0 mmol/L	DM: ≥ 11.1 mmol/L IGT: 7.8–11.0 mmol/L
Comments	Asymptomatic patient with one positive test needs a repeat confirmatory test (FBG, A1C, 2 hr PG in a 75 g OGTT) on another day (preferably the same test repeated) to confirm diagnosis. Symptomatic patient with one positive test.			

*Fasting = no caloric intake for a minimum of 8 hours prior to the test.

(Hu et al., 2002; ADA, 2010). As recommended by the Canadian Diabetes Association (Harris, 2013), all patients should be evaluated each year for risk factors of T2DM (e.g., relatives with T2DM, a history of pre-diabetes, presence of vascular risk factor). Screening using a fasting glucose or HbA1C every 3 years is appropriate for individuals over 40 years, or those at high risk. Screening earlier and more frequently is appropriate for those with additional risk factors or at very high risk using a risk calculator (e.g., Canadian Diabetes Risk Assessment Questionnaire-CANRISK). More frequent screening is appropriate based on individual clinical presentation. A 75 g oral glucose tolerance test should be used for those with borderline fasting glucose or HbA1C, or those at extremely high risk (CDA Primer, 2013) (Table 14.2).

Metabolic syndrome is another fundamental consideration when discussing long-term care for patients with T2DM. Metabolic syndrome is diagnosed if any three of the following five criteria are met: population-specific waist circumference; triglycerides greater than 1.7 mmol/L (or treatment for elevated triglycerides); HDL-C less than 1 mmol/L in males or 1.3 mmol/L in females; systolic blood pressure greater than 130 and/or diastolic pressure greater than 85 (or treatment for blood pressure); and finally, fasting blood glucose greater than 100mg/dL (5.5 mml/L) (Alberti et al., 2009).

Such criteria are fundamental in the practice of family medicine, as the parameters are straightforward and easy to track for patients on a regular basis, and early intervention may have the potential to prevent the development of frank diabetes in motivated patients. Based on the NCEP and WHO definitions of metabolic syndrome, one review calculated that the population-attributable risk of metabolic syndrome to the development of diabetes is anywhere from 30% to 50% (Ford, 2005). Thus, many patients in a given family physician's practice who meet the criteria for metabolic syndrome are likely already diabetic; if they are not, they are certainly at the core of the high-risk group and must be the focus of targeted primary prevention strategies in the clinic. These strategies should include both pharmacologic treatment for lipid and glucose abnormalities, as well as nonpharmacologic-based counseling on nutrition and lifestyle modifications, with referral to allied health professionals as indicated.

Nonpharmacologic Therapies

Education of the patient and the family is of fundamental importance. The patient and key family members should have basic knowledge of the pathophysiology of diabetes, the principles of dietary control and foot care, the actions of insulin and oral drugs, monitoring blood glucose, symptoms of hypoglycemia and ketoacidosis, control of infections, and maintenance of health. Other members of the primary care team, such as nurse practitioners,

Table 14.2 OVERVIEW OF AVAILABLE MEDICATIONS AND STARTING DOSES

Medication	Starting Dose
Insulin	10 units, at bedtime*.
	*This is an appropriate insulin start for an obese patient who is only taking oral agents. From there, the patient can titrate up by 1 unit nightly until desired pre-breakfast glucose is achieved (Gerstein, Yale, et al., 2006).
Metformin (first-line)	500 mg OD or BID, or 850 mg OD Extended release: 1000 mg OD
Alpha-glucosidase inhibitors	
Acarbose	25 mg, OD
DPP-4 inhibitors	
Linagliptin	5 mg, OD
Saxagliptin	5 mg, OD* *Adjust for patients with renal compromise
Sitagliptin	100 mg, OD* *Adjust for patients with renal compromise
GLP-1 inhibitors	
Exenatide	5 µg, BID
Liraglutide	0.6 mg, OD
Secretagogues 1 (sulfonylureas)	
Gliclazide	MR formulation: 30–60 mg, OD a.m. 80 mg, BID
Glimepiride	1 mg, OD
Glyburide	2.5–5 mg, OD
Secretagogues 2 (meglitinides)	
Repaglinide	0.5 mg AC
*Thiazolidinediones**	
*No longer commonly prescribed	
Pioglitazone	15–30 mg OD
Rosiglitazone	4 mg OD
SGLTs	Canagliflozin 100 mg OD

Adapted from the Canadian Diabetes Association Clinical Primer, 2013.

dieticians, and pharmacists, can help ensure optimal care. In many areas, local diabetes education centers and diabetic associations are of great assistance to individuals coping with the disease, and physicians should ensure that their patients are aware of these community- and web-based resources.

As with other chronic conditions, there are several domains of therapy relevant to patients with T2DM, including nonpharmacologic approaches. As family physicians, it is important to remember that, as with other chronic diseases, many patients will make use of complementary and alternative medicines to treat their diabetes. One useful classification describes four categories of therapeutic options (Rakel, 2007).

1. Nutrition. Overall, there is a fair amount of flexibility in designing an appropriate diet for a diabetic patient, and counseling from a dietician is certainly recommended where possible. A weight loss of 5%–10% is a realistic and effective goal. Various dietary combinations of the three macronutrients have been studied for their effect on glucose control in T2DM. Current recommendations are to average 45%–65% carbohydrates, 10%–35% protein, and 20%–35% fat. Low-carbohydrate, high-protein diets are currently being studied, although the literature is so far inconclusive (CDA Primer, 2013). The Mediterranean diet is one of the more popularly recommended diabetic diets. It includes a high proportion of vegetables, whole grains, nuts and legumes, as well as fish, poultry, and olive oil. Red meats and sweets are to be consumed infrequently. Foods with a low glycemic index must be emphasized to assist with weight loss.

2. Exercise. Physical activity can increase insulin sensitivity, improve glucose tolerance, reduce blood lipids, and aid in reducing weight. In a randomized control trial spanning 3 years, overweight American adults were assigned to a diet and exercise intervention, or no treatment. This intervention included dietary counseling, regular meetings with a nutritionist, 30 minutes of daily exercise, and the availability of private sessions with a trainer. At the end of the trial, the incidence of diabetes in the control group was 78 per 1000 person-years, versus 32 per 1000 person-years in the intervention arm. Overall, the incidence of diabetes was reduced by 58% (Tumoilehto et al., 2001).

3. Mind/body therapy. Physiologically, emotional and psychological stresses increase endogenous levels of the hormone cortisol, which in turn increases gluconeogenesis in the liver (Hers, 1985; Agardh et al., 2003; Rosmond, 2003). Mind/body therapy includes self-care, relaxation techniques such as yoga, and social support groups. Patients often express desire for social support groups for the emotional satisfaction and sense of community (Struthers et al., 2003; Parsons et al., 2014). For patients with comorbid depression or anxiety, psychological counseling can also be useful. Cognitive behavior therapy has been shown to lower HbA1C and to improve mood (Snoek and Skinner, 2002). Family and social support may have some therapeutic impact on glycemic control, most often quantified by HbA1C, although the literature on this topic lacks standardized methodology and many associations are not statistically significant (Stopford, Winkley, and Ismail, 2013). Regardless of the degree of impact on the physiologic measures of T2DM, these aspects of diabetes care should not be neglected in regular follow-up.

4. Supplements and botanicals. Common natural remedies purported to positively influence blood glucose include ginkgo, cinnamon, garlic, and green tea. Unfortunately, several herbs marketed for weight loss, including coffee seeds, actually have hyperglycemic effects and will increase fasting glucose and HbA1C.

Pharmacologic Therapies

Several classes of drugs are available for the management of T2DM: biguanides and thiazolidinediones are insulin sensitizers; sulfonylureas increase secretion of insulin, as do meglitinides; alpha-glucosidase inhibitors inhibit digestion of carbohydrates; incretins directly and indirectly stimulate the release of insulin; sodium glucose-linked transporters (SGLT2) contribute to renal glucose reabsorption; and finally, insulin as replacement. In a Canadian sample, 85% of patients on pharmacologic therapy were taking metformin, and just over half used two or more classes of medication (Greiver et al., 2014).

The treatment algorithm shown in Figure 14.1 is a typical approach, adapted from those of the Canadian Diabetes Association, the American Diabetes Association, and the European Association for the Study of Diabetes. As always, the algorithm must be adapted to the particular needs and wishes of the patient. For example, if a patient has high blood sugar, is overweight, and has previously shown an unwillingness or inability to change diet and physical activity practices, the patient and physician may choose to immediately start a medication trial.

An overview of nonpharmacologic and pharmacologic therapies is not complete without a discussion of treatment adherence by patients. In the literature, the prevalence of nonadherence to treatment in T2DM varies. One review cites diabetic adherence anywhere from 36% to 93%, depending on the study and patient population (Cramer, 2004). On average, adherence to insulin regimens was approximately 60%. In one Scottish cohort, only one in three patients adequately adhered (defined as taking medication over 90% of the time) to their oral medication regimen. Socially deprived individuals had poorer adherence (Donnan, MacDonald, and Morris, 2002). Nonadherence has been categorized into three types: (1) failure to fill the prescription and begin taking medications; (2) stopping medications soon after beginning; or (3) noncompliance (Blackburn et al., 2013). Both primary nonadherence and not persisting with therapy are common in diabetes, and several discrete barriers exist. Like other chronic conditions, barriers to good adherence can be organized into domains such as patient factors, provider factors, and system factors (Blackburn, Swidorvich, and Lemstra,

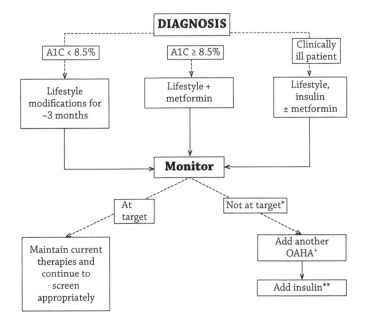

Figure 14.1:
Basic treatment algorithm for glycemic control in T2DM.
*Goal is to attain glycemic target within 3–6 months of diagnosis. Physician should consider changing agents if HbA1C is > 7%. **Insulin can be started at any stage of illness/active treatment. It can be introduced as part of long-term disease control, or it can be used transiently (pregnancy, surgery, illness, or other stressors). + Prior to adding insulin, one may add, adjust, or intensify oral agents. See Table 14.2 for a brief overview of insulin and OAHAs.

2013). As previously discussed, fears of hypoglycemic events may prevent some patients from using their insulin appropriately. Nonadherence in an urban Ugandan population of mixed type 1 and type 2 diabetics was almost 30%, and was closely related to female gender, poor comprehension of the medications, and cost (Kalyango, Owino, and Nambuya, 2008). Seeking concordance or common ground between the patient and the physician with respect to problems, roles, and goals improves adherence (see Chapter 9, "Clinical Method").

Treatment Targets and Adherence

For consistency, the clinical treatment targets have also been provided using Canada, the United States, Australia, and Europe as examples (Table 14.3). Critically, the literature on diabetes consistently reveals that even if patients are prescribed an appropriate treatment regimen and follow it adequately, this does not necessarily translate into glucose control that meets treatment targets. A Lithuanian study including 770 Type 2 diabetics and 95 Type 1

Table 14.3 CLINICAL TREATMENT TARGETS FOR TYPE 2 DIABETES MELLITUS

	Canada (CDA Primer, 2013)	United States (ADA, 2014)	Australia (RACGP, 2014)	Europe (ESC, 2013)
Blood pressure	< 130/80 mmHg	< 140/80 mmHg	< 130/80 mmHg	< 140/85 mmHg
Cholesterol	LDL-C < 2.0 mmol/L	Overt CVD, LDL: < 70 mg/dL (3.9 mmol/L) No CVD, LDL: < 100 mg/dL (5.5 mmol/L)	Total < 4.0 mmol/L LDL-C < 2.0 HDL ≥ 1.0	LDL < 1.8 mmol/L
Plasma glucose	FPG: 4–7 2hPP: 5–10 Frail elderly: 5–12	FPG: 70–130 mg/dL 2hPP: < 180	FPG: 6–8 2hPP: 8–10	FPG: < 7.2 2hPP: < 9–10
HbA1C	Majority: ≤ 7.0% Frail elderly; advanced comorbid: 7.1%–8.5%	< 7%	< 7%	< 7%

diabetics calculated that the average HbA1C was 8.5% for those taking oral anti-diabetic agents, versus 9.2% in patients solely on insulin. This was postulated to reflect a decreasing ability to control diabetes with increasing disease duration (Norkus et al., 2013). A US survey of primary care practices similarly found that the vast majority of diabetic patients are not meeting guidelines set forth by the American Diabetes Association. The mean HbA1C was 7.6%, with 40% of patients achieving an A1C less than 7%. Thirty-five percent of patients were considered to have good blood pressure control (less than 130/85), and 43% had LDL-C less than 100 mg/dL. Overall, less than 7% of patients included in the study achieved all three treatment targets (Spann et al., 2006).

Across 479 Canadian primary care practices, 13% of patients met the three targets. While double the US numbers, this still reflects poor disease control given that the vast majority of patients were prescribed anti-diabetic, anti-hypertensive, and/or lipid-lowering agents (87%, 83%, and 81%, respectively). Addressing lipid and blood pressure targets, in addition to glycemic control, is a critical component of successful long-term diabetes care. Across all cohorts, patients with higher A1Cs were more likely to be treated aggressively, but this did not translate into better glucose control. In the Canadian sample, in patients who achieved an HbA1C less than 7%, 37% were prescribed non-insulin anti-hyperglycemic agents (of whom half were taking only metformin), 20% took insulin alone, and 20% were prescribed insulin and one or more oral agents (Leiter et al., 2013).

As previously stated, these data may reflect increasing difficulty with disease control as the duration of illness progresses. Part of this trend may reflect a decline in the proportion of functioning b-cells in the pancreas (Figure 14.2).

But ascribing all of the blame to pathophysiology may be an oversimplification. Canadian physicians identified poor patient adherence (to diet, medication regimens, etc.) as the greatest barrier to reaching treatment targets. Poor adherence, in turn, may be related to medication costs, lack of communication between patient and physician, patient fears about medications, patient denial of illness, depression, or social concerns. Communication between patient and physician is a key component of ongoing care that may highlight these issues. So-called nonconcordant comorbidities may play a significant role in failing to achieve targets (see Chapter 16, "Multimorbidity"). Constraints on physician's clinic time were also identified as a significant barrier to diabetes management (Leiter, Berard, Bowema, et al., 2013). Inclusion of other health professionals in the basic primary care practice can ameliorate some problems introduced by lack of physician time. The Iranian Diabetes Society ran a 12-week telephone follow-up for 61 patients with T2DM. Those in the intervention group received regular phone calls from a nurse to discuss diet, exercise, medications, blood glucose monitoring, and foot care. At the end of the study, these patients' HbA1C had decreased by almost 2%, compared to a drop of 0.4% in the control group (who had only received an education session at the beginning of the study) (Nesari et al., 2010).

Nurse practitioners may also be an effective way to improve adherence and outcomes in diabetes care. Among primary care clinics in New Jersey

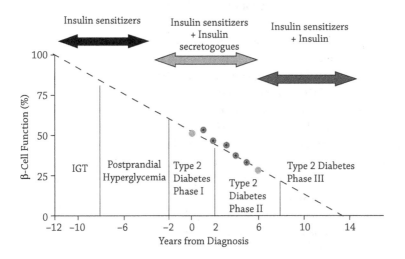

Figure 14.2:
Stages of Type II Diabetes.
Reprinted with permissions from Lebovitz H. 1999. Insulin secretogogues: Old and new. *Diabetes Review* 7:139–153.

and Pennsylvania, those with nurse practitioners were more likely to monitor HbA1C, lipids, and microalbuminuria, and patients of these practices were more likely to be treated for abnormal laboratory values (Ohman-Strickland et al., 2008). The St. Joseph's Primary Care Diabetes Support Program in London, Ontario, employs three physicians, two nurse practitioners with special training in diabetes care, two part-time nurses, two dieticians, and one social worker, who all work together to provide comprehensive health care to their patient population of just under 4000 individuals with diabetes. Approximately half of these patients take both oral anti-hyperglycemic agents and insulin. After 6 months of tracking, HbA1C had decreased by 0.87% in type 2 diabetics, from 8.61% (Reichert, Harris, and Harvey, 2014).

A positive and respectful relationship between patient and physician and other healthcare providers is also an important aspect of successful diabetes care. With such a foundation, it becomes possible to engage and involve the patient directly in his or her own care (Golin, DiMatteo, and Gelberg, 1996).

Even though physicians do set appropriate targets for diabetic disease markers (Leiter et al., 2013), self-care for diabetes involves significant and often drastic behavioral changes to fundamental aspects of daily living—diet, physical activity, and consistent awareness of blood glucose can be difficult for patients (Golin, DiMatteo, and Gelberg, 1996). In addition to glucose monitoring, medication prescription, and regular diabetic physicals, a positive and supportive relationship between patient and physician is a critical component of successful diabetes care.

Diabetes in the Elderly

Caring for frail[1] elderly patients with diabetes presents a unique clinical scenario within diabetes care. In this patient population, relaxed blood glucose targets are the rule, as the primary goal of treatment is to prevent hypoglycemic events (CDA, 2013), as warning symptoms of hypoglycemia may go unnoticed, with serious negative health outcomes, including stroke, falls, or cardiac ischemia (Eld2). Under the Canadian guidelines, HbA1C should be targeted at 8.5% or less, and fasting plasma glucose may range from 5.0 to 12.0 (CDA Primer, 2013). For very ill patients, or those living in nursing facilities, diabetes management may not be adequate. A comparative study of nursing homes in the Greater Toronto area versus those in a community in British Columbia, Canada, found that nursing homes with diabetes-educated staff and hypoglycemia treatment protocols were much better equipped to prevent and treat diabetes in their residents. In the diabetes-educated facilities, over 90% of residents had their HbA1C assessed in the previous 6 months, compared to 68% in the facilities without specific diabetes protocols (Clement and Leung, 2009). Nutritional education and aerobic and/or resistance exercises are all useful adjuncts in this patient population. Metformin is a reasonable first-line choice for oral hyperglycemic medication if renal function is adequate, although no randomized trials in this population have been done (CDA Primer, 2013).

Comorbidities

Long-term patient care in family practice increasingly means being the primary healthcare provider for the treatment and management of comorbid conditions (see Chapter 16, "Multimorbidity"). While diabetic-focused visits are becoming more common, they must still reflect a comprehensive approach to care. When intermediate targets are tied to remuneration, the physician runs the risk of becoming too focused on these targets, at the expense of seeing the whole patient. For example, depression is common in diabetics, and may need to be addressed before the patient can cope with other demands. Appropriate care may involve encouraging the patient, under these circumstances, to set up separate appointments at the clinic for health concerns unrelated to his or her diabetes. In some cases, other health concerns may distract from essential diabetic care issues in a time-limited encounter. Smoking and alcohol consumption (and cessation where appropriate) is also a critical point of discussion with the diabetic patient. This should be discussed in the context of overall health, but also as specific risk factors for progression of diabetes. If the family physician is the only clinician in the circle of care who has a detailed understanding of the patient's social circumstances and other health issues, he or she is uniquely specialized to address behaviors like smoking that straddle both social and health domains. An interdisciplinary high-functioning healthcare team may provide improved health outcomes.

In North American populations, patients with T2DM may have 1.3 times as many comorbid conditions compared to patients without T2DM. The difference in the rate of comorbidities is significant between diabetics and nondiabetics except in patients greater than 80 years old (Greiver et al., 2014). In an average North American practice, the most common comorbidities unrelated to diabetes were hypertension (57%), osteoarthritis (28%), and chronic back pain (23%). Although these comorbidities do not necessarily share a physiologic etiology with T2DM, their presence certainly impacts clinical management. If a patient has severe hip OA and T2DM, it is difficult to implement a physical activity regimen.

The most common comorbidities related to T2DM were coronary artery disease (19%), neuropathy (19%), and nephropathy (16%) (Spann et al., 2006). Table 14.4 outlines the recommended screening guidelines for common diabetic complications. Diabetic flow charts can improve the clinician's ability to track these important variables.

Table 14.4 SCREENING FOR COMPLICATIONS IN TYPE 2 DIABETES MELLITUS

Cardiovascular disease	• Begin screening for any patient with the following characteristics: over 40 years old, end-organ damage, cardiac risk factors, or a patient less than 30 years old with diabetes for greater than 15 years. • These patients require a baseline resting ECG. • All patients require examination of pedal pulses. • Control of blood pressure may be more important than control of glucose in preventing diabetic angiopathy.
Neuropathy	• Begin screening feet at diagnosis for peripheral neuropathy, and repeat annually with 10 gm monofilament or 128-Hz tuning fork. • Once the ankle reflex is absent, it is highly likely that there is microangiopathy in the foot, with its attendant risk of complications. • Symptoms of autonomic neuropathies such as gastroparesis need to be screened regularly.
Chronic kidney disease (CKD)	• An albumin:creatinine ≥ 2 mg/mmol, and/or eGFR <60 mL/min. • Begin screening at diagnosis, and continue annually if no evidence of CKD. • If CKD identified, monitor progression every 6 months.
Foot care	• Foot exams should be performed at least once yearly from the time of diagnosis, based on the patient risk profile. • Proper foot and nail care and orthotics are also an important consideration.
Retinopathy	• If no retinopathy, screen every 1–2 years. • If retinopathy is present, a screening interval is established based on disease severity.

Adapted from Canadian Diabetes Association Clinical Primer, 2013.

Family physicians and associated healthcare teams play an essential role in meeting the worldwide health burden that diabetes represents. The provision of community-based, comprehensive, and continuous care, with a focus on patient and family, represents the optimal way of detecting diabetes and assisting patients in coping with it.

NOTE

1. For an in-depth discussion and classification of the frail elderly, please see the Canadian Diabetes Association's Clinical Practice Guidelines on "Diabetes in the elderly," published in the *Canadian Journal of Diabetes* 2013. 37:S347–S348.

REFERENCES

Agardh EE, Ahlbom A, Andersson T, et al. 2003. Work stress and low sense of coherence is associated with Type 2 diabetes in middle-aged Swedish women. *Diabetes Care* 26(3):719.

Alberti KGMM, Eckel RH, Grundy SM et al. 2009. Harmonizing the metabolic syndrome: A joint interim statement of the International Diabetes Federation Task Force on Epidemiology and Prevention; National Heart, Lung, and Blood Institute; American Heart Association; World Health Federation; International Atherosclerosis Society; and International Association for the Study of Obesity. *Circulation* 120:1640–1645.

Ali MK, Bullard KM, Imperatore G, Barker L, Gregg EW. 2012. Characteristics associated with poor glycemic control among adults with self-reported diagnosed diabetes: National Health and Nutrition Examination Survey, United States, 2007–2010. *MMWR* suppl 61:32–37.

American Diabetes Association. 2010. Diagnosis and classification of diabetes mellitus. *Diabetes Care* 33:S62.

American Diabetes Association. 2014. Standards of medical care in diabetes—2014. *Diabetes Care* 37:S14.

Andaya AA, Arrendondo EM, Alcaraz JE, et al. 2009. The association between family meals, TV viewing during meals, and fruit, vegetables, soda, and chips intake among Latino children. *Journal of Adolescent Health* 44(5):431.

Ardern CI, Katzmarzyk, PT. 2007. Geographic and demographic variation in the prevalence of the metabolic syndrome in Canada. *Canadian Journal of Diabetes* 31(1):34.

Azimi-Nezhad M, Ghayour-Mobarhan M, Parizadeh MR, et al. 2008. Prevalence of type 2 diabetes mellitus in Iran and its relationship with gender, urbanisation, education, marital status and occupation. *Singapore Medical Journal* 49(7):571.

Blackburn DF, Swidorvich J, Lemstra M. 2013. Non-adherence in type 2 diabetes: Practical considerations for interpreting the literature. *Patient Preference and Adherence* 7:183.

Canadian Diabetes Association Clinical Practice Guidelines Expert Committee. 2013. Diabetes in the elderly. *Canadian Journal of Diabetes* 37:S184.

Campbell KJ, Crawford DA, Ball K. 2006. Family food environment and dietary behaviors likely to promote fatness in 5–6 year-old children. *International Journal of Obesity* 30:1272.

Centers for Disease Control and Prevention (CDC). 2006. Racial and socioeconomic disparities in breastfeeding—United States, 2004. *Morbidity and Mortality Weekly Report* 55(12):335.

Centers for Disease Control and Prevention (CDC). 2014. National Diabetes Statistical Report, 2014 http://www.cdc.gov/diabetes/pubs/statsreport14/national-diabetes-report-web.pdf

Clement MC, Leung F. 2009. Diabetes and the frail elderly in long-term care. *Canadian Journal of Diabetes* 33(2):114.

Cramer JA. 2004. A systematic review of adherence with medications for diabetes. *Diabetes Care* 27(5):1218.

Creatore MI, Moineddin R, Booth G, et al. 2010. Age- and sex-related prevalence of diabetes mellitus among immigrants to Ontario, Canada. *Canadian Medical Association Journal* 182(8):781.

Danaei G, Finucane MM, Lu Y, et al. 2011. National, regional, and global trends in fasting plasma glucose and diabetes prevalence since 1980: Systematic analysis of health examination surveys and epidemmiological studies with 370 country-years and 2.7 million participants. *The Lancet* 378:31.

Daniel M, Rowley KG, McDermott R, O'Dea K. 2002. Diabetes and impaired glucose tolerance in Aboriginal Australians: Prevalence and risk. *Diabetes Research and Clinical Practice.* 57(1): 23–33.

Donnan PT, MacDonald TM, Morris AD. 2002. Adherence to prescribed oral hypogly-caemic medication in a population of patients with Type 2 diabetes: A retrospective cohort study. *Diabetic Medicine* 19:279.

Dyck R, Osgood N, Gao A, et al. 2012. The epidemiology of diabetes mellitus among First Nations and non-First Nations children in Saskatchewan. *Canadian Journal of Diabetes* 36:19.

Escudero-Carretero MJ, Prieto-Rodríguez M, Fernández-Fernández I, et al. 2007. Expectations held by Type 1 and 2 diabetes mellitus patients and their relatives: The importance of facilitating the health-care process. *Health Expectations* 10(4):337.

European Commission, Directorate Public Health and Risk Assessment. 2004. *EU Project on Promotion of Breastfeeding in Europe. Protection, Promotion, and Support of Breastfeeding in Europe: A Blueprint for Action.* http://europa.eu.int/comm/health/ph_projects/2002/promotion/promotion_2002_18_en.htm

European Society of Cardiology. 2013. ESC guidelines on diabetes, pre-diabetes, and cardiovascular diseases developed in collaboration with the EASD. *European Heart Journal* 34:3035.

Fidler C, Christensen TE, Gillard S. 2011. Hypoglycemia: An overview of fear of hypoglycemia, quality-of-life, and impact on costs. *Journal of Medical Economics* 14(5):646.

Ford ES. 2005. Risks for all-cause mortality, cardiovascular disease, and diabetes associated with the metabolic syndrome. *Diabetes Care* 28:1769–1778.

Frayling TM. 2007. Genome-wide association studies provide new insights into type 2 diabetes aetiology. *Nature Reviews Genetics* 8:657.

Frier BM. 2008. How hypoglycaemia can affect the life of a person with diabetes. *Diabetes Metabolic Research and Reviews* 24:87.

Gillman MW, Rifas-Shiman SL, Frazier L, et al. 2000. Family dinner and diet quality among older children and adolescents. *Archives of Family Medicine* 9:235.

Golin CE, DiMatteo MR, Gelberg L. 1996. The role of patient participation in the doctor visit. *Diabetes Care* 19(10):1153.

Gordon C, Purciel-Hill M, Ghai NR, et al. 2011. Measuring food deserts in New York City's low-income neighborhoods. *Health & Place* 17:696.

Greiver M, Williamson T, Barber D, et al. 2014. Prevalence and epidemiology of diabetes in Canadian primary care practices: A report from the Canadian Primary Care Sentinel Surveillance Network. *Canadian Journal of Diabetes* 38:179.

Groop L, Pociot F. 2013. Genetics of diabetes: Are we missing the genes or the disease?. *Molecular and Cellular Endocrinology* 382:726.

Hales CN, Barker DJP. 1992. Type 2 (non-insulin-dependent) diabetes mellitus: The thrifty phenotype hypothesis. *Diabetologia* 35:595.

Harris SB (Ed.). 2013. *Prevention and Management of Type 2 Diabetes in Adults: A Clinical Primer.* Toronto: Elsevier.

Harris SB, Bhattacharyya O, Dyck R, Hayward MN, Toth El. 2013. Type 2 diabetes in Aboriginal peoples. *Canandian Journal of Diabetes* 37(suppl.1):s191–s196.

Health Canada. 2014. *Infant Feeding.* http://www.hc-sc.gc.ca/fn-an/nutrition/infant-nourisson/index-eng.php.

Hers HG. 1985. Effects of glucocorticosteroids on carbohydrate metabolism. *Agents and Actions* 17(3):248.

Hu FB, Stampfer MJ, Haffner SM, Solomon CG, Willett WC, Manson JE. 2002. Elevated risk of cardiovascular disease prior to clinical diagnosis of Type 2 diabetes. *Diabetes Care* 25(7):1129.

International Diabetes Federation Europe. 2012. *Diabetes at a Glance, 2012.* https://www.idf.org/sites/default/files/IDF_EUR_5E_Update_FactSheet1_0.pdf

Jaber LA, Brown MB, Hamad A, et al. 2003. Lack of acculturation is a risk factor for diabetes in Arab immigrants in the U.S. *Diabetes Care* 26(7):2010–2014.

Lebovitz H. 1999. Insulin Secretogogues: Old and new. *Diabetes Review* 7:139–153

Kalyango JN, Owino E, Nambuya AP. 2008. Non-adherence to diabetes treatment at Mulago Hospital in Ugana: Prevalence and associated factors. *African Health Sciences* 8(2):67.

Larsen K, Gilliland J. 2008. Mapping the evolution of "food deserts" in a Canadian city: Supermarket accessibility in London, Ontario, 1961–2005. *International Journal of Health Geographics* 7(16).

Leiter LA, Berard L, Bowering CK, et al. 2013. Type 2 diabetes mellitus management in Canada: Is it improving?. *Canadian Journal of Diabetes* 37:82.

Leiter LA, Ross SA, Barr A, et al. 2001. Diabetes screening in Canada (DIASCAN) study. *Diabetes Care* 24(6):1038.

Lipscombe LL, Hux JE. 2007. Trends in diabetes prevalence, incidence and mortality in Ontario, Canada, 1995–2005: A population based study. *Lancet* 369(9563):750.

Ludwig DS. 2002. The glycemic index: Physiological mechanisms relating to obesity, diabetes, and cardiovascular disease. *Journal of the American Medical Association* 287(18):2414.

Lundkvist J, Berne C, Bolinder B, et al. 2005. The economic and quality of life impact of hypoglycemia. *European Journal of Health Economics* 6:197.

Lyssenko V, Jonsson A, Almgren P, et al. 2008. Clinical risk factors, DNA variants, and the development of Type 2 diabetes. *New England Journal of Medicine* 359(21):2220.

Marrero DG, Guare JC, Vandagriff JL, Fineberg NS. 1997. Fear of hypoglycemia in the parents of children and adolescents with diabetes: Maladaptive or healthy response? *The Diabetes Educator* 23(3):281.

Mercado-Martinez FJ, Ramos-Herrera IM. 2002. Diabetes: The layperson's theories of causality. *Qualitative Health Research* 12:792.

Minges KE, Zimmet P, Magliano DJ, Dunstan DW, Brown A, Shaw JE. 2011. Diabetes prevalence and determinants in Indigenous Australian populations: A systematic review. *Diabetes Research and Clinical Practice* 93(2):139–149.

Nesari M, Zakerimoghadam M, Rajab A, et al. 2010. Effect of telephone follow-up on adherence to a diabetes therapeutic regimen. *Japan Journal of Nursing Science* 7:121.

Norkus A, Ostrauskas R, Zalinkevicius R, et al. 2013. Adequate prescribing of medication does not necessarily translate into good control of diabetes mellitus. *Patient Preference and Adherence* 7:643.

OECD. 2014. *OECD Family Database.* www.oecd.org/social/family/database; http://www.oecd.org/els/family/43136964.pdf.

Ohman-Strickland PA, Orzano AJ, Hudson SV, et al. 2008. Quality of diabetes care in family medicine practices: Influences of nurse-practitioners and physician's assistants. *Annals of Family Medicine* 6(1):14.

Ostbye T, Yarnell KSH, Krause KM, Pollak KI, Gradison M, Michener JL. 2005. Is there time for management of patients with chronic diseases in primary care? *Annals of Family Medicine* 3(3):209–214.

Owen CG, Martin RM, Whincup PH, et al. 2006. Does breastfeeding influence risk of type 2 diabetes in later life? A quantitative analysis of published evidence. *American Journal of Clinical Nutrition* 84:1043.

Parsons J, Ismail K, Amiel S, Forbes A. 2014. Perceptions among women with gestational diabetes. *Qualitative Health Research* 24(4):575.

Petry R. 2013. Breastfeeding and socioeconomic status: An analysis of breastfeeding rates among low-SES mothers. *Poverty and Human Capability Studies Capstone.* http://shepherdconsortium.org/wp-content/uploads/2013/04/Petry.2013. POV-423-Capstone.pdf.

Pinney SE, Simmons RA. 2012. Metabolic programming, epigenetics, and gestational diabetes mellitus. *Current Diabetes Reports* 12:67.

Pistulka GM, Winch PJ, Park H, et al. 2012. Maintaining an outward image: A Korean immigrant's life with Type 2 diabetes mellitus and hypertension. *Qualitative Health Research* 22(6):825.

Public Health Agency of Canada. 2011. *Diabetes in Canada: Facts and Figures from a Public Health Perspective.* http://www.phac-aspc.gc.ca/cd-mc/publications/ diabetes-diabete/facts-figures-faits-chiffres-2011/index-eng.php

Rakel D. 2007. *Integrative Medicine,* 2nd ed. Philadelphia: Saunders.

Raphael D, Anstice S, Raine K, et al. 2003. The social determinants of the incidence and management of type 2 diabetes mellitus: Are we prepared to rethink our questions and redirect our research activities? *International Journal of Health Care Quality Assurance Incorporating Leadership in Health Services* 16(3):10–20.

Reading C, Wein F. 2009. *Health inequalities and social determinants of Aboriginal peoples' health.* Prince George: National Collaborating Centre for Aboriginal Health.

Reichert SM, Harris S, Harvey B. 2014. An innovative model of diabetes care and delivery: The St. Joseph's primary care diabetes support program (SJHC PCDSP). *Canadian Journal of Diabetes* 38:212.

Riste L, Khan F, Cruickshank K. 2001. High prevalence of type 2 diabetes in all ethnic groups, including Europeans in a British inner city: Relative poverty, history, inactivity or 21st century Europe? *Diabetes Care* 24(8): 1377–1383.

Robbins JM, Vaccarino V, Zhang H, Kasl SV. 2004. Socioeconomic status and diagnosed diabetes incidence. *Diabetes Research and Clinical Practice* 68(3):230.

Rosmond R. 2003. Stress induced disturbances of the HPA axis: A pathway to Type 2 diabetes?. *Medical Science Monitor* 9(2):RA35.

Royal Australian College of General Practitioners. 2014. *General Practice Management of Type 2 Diabetes—2014–15.* Royal Australian College of General Practitioners, Melbourne, Australia.

Scott LJ, Mohlke KL, Bonnycastle LL. 2007. A genome-wide association study of Type 2 diabetes in Finns detects multiple susceptibility variants. *Science* 316(5829):1341.

Sheu WH, Li-Nong J, Nitiyanant W, et al. 2012. Hypoglycemia is associated with increased worry and lower quality of life among patients with Type 2 diabetes treated with oral antihyperglycemic agents in the Asia-Pacific region. *Diabetes Research and Clinical Practice* 96:141.

Snoek FJ, Skinner TC. 2002. Psychological counseling in problematic diabetes: Does it help? *Diabetic Medicine* 19:265.

Spann SJ, Nutting PA, Galliher JM, et al. 2006. Management of Type 2 diabetes in the primary care setting: A pratice-based research network study. *Annals of Family Medicine* 4(1):23.

Steenland K, Henley J, Thun, M. 2002. All-cause and cause-specific death rates by educational status for two million people in two American cancer society cohorts, 1959–1996. *American Journal of Epidemiology* 156(1):11.

Stopford R, Winkley K, Ismail K. 2013. Social support and glycemic control in type 2 diabetes: A systematic review of observational studies. *Patient Education and Counselling* 93:549.

Struthers R, Hodge FS, Geishirt-Cantrell B, De Cora L. 2003. Participant experience of talking circles on Type 2 diabetes in two northern plains American Indian tribes. *Qualitative Health Research* 13:1094.

Taylor JS, Kacmar JE, Mothnagle M, Lawrence RA. 2014. A systematic review of the literature associating breastfeeding with Type 2 diabetes and gestational diabetes. *Journal of American College of Nutrition* 24(5):320.

van Dam HA, van der Horst FG, Knoops L, et al. 2005. Social support in diabetes: A systematic review of controlled intervention studies. *Patient Education and Counseling* 59:1.

Wändell PE, Steiner KH, Johansson SE. 2003. Diabetes mellitus in Turkish immigrants in Sweden. *Diabetes & Metabolism* 29:435.

Whiting D, Unwin N, Roglic G. 2010. Diabetes: equity and social determinants. In: *Equity, Social Determinants and Public Health Programmes.* Eds. Blas E, Kurup AS. World Health Organization, Geneva.

Wild D, von Maltzahn R, Brohan E, et al. 2007. A critical review of the literature on fear of hypoglycemia in diabetes: Implications for diabetes management and patient education. *Patient Education and Counseling* 68:10.

World Health Organization. 2015. *Diabetes Fact Sheet.* http://www.who.int/mediacentre/factsheets/fs312/en/

Yajnik CS. 2002. The lifecycle effects of nutrition and body size on adult adiposity, diabetes and cardiovascular disease. *Obesity Reviews* 3:217.

Zeggini E, McCarthy MI. 2007. TCF7L2: The biggest story in diabetes genetics since HLA? *Diabetologia* 50:1.

CHAPTER 15

☙

Obesity

Obesity is variously described as a health concern, a risk factor, or a disease. There seems little doubt that increasing weight is characteristic of many countries around the world, whether they are of low, middle, or high income. Some have described the increase in obesity and overweight individuals as an *epidemic*. This term leads to an unfortunate perception that it is the result of some external agent spread among the population, whereas it may more usefully be thought of as arising in the interaction between biology, family, culture, economics, and environment. The use of the term *obesity epidemic* has been criticized as rooted in ideology and politics rather than science (Gard and Wright, 2005).

Obesity is a recognized risk factor for other risk factors that impact on health, including hypertension, dyslipidemia, Type 2 diabetes mellitus (T2DM), metabolic syndrome, ischemic heart disease, cancer, obstructive sleep apnea (OSA), pulmonary disease, and fatty liver disease. Aside from these risk factors, it has also been associated with an increased risk of low self-esteem and depression.

For purposes of classification, an individual is defined as obese if the body mass index (BMI) is greater than or equal to 30 kg/m². Those with a BMI greater than or equal to 25 kg/m² are considered to be in the overweight or pre-obese category. Waist circumference, when adjusted for ethnicity and gender, is sometimes added, as centrally abdominal fat has prognostic value. Such a classification is more useful for population-based studies, but has limited applicability in clinical work. The Edmonton Obesity Staging System (Sharma, 2009) takes into account other health conditions and is a more useful guide in the general practitioner's office (see Table 15.1).

Table 15.1 EDMONTON OBESITY STAGING SYSTEM

Stage	Description	Management
0	No apparent obesity-related factors (e.g., blood pressure, serum lipids, fasting glucose, etc., within normal range), no physical symptoms, no psychopathology, no functional limitations and/or impairment of well-being	Identification of factors contributing to increased body weight. Counseling to prevent further weight gain through lifestyle measures including healthy eating and increased physical activity.
1	Presence of obesity-related subclinical risk factors (e.g., borderline hypertension, impaired fasting glucose, elevated liver enzymes, etc.), mild physical symptoms (e.g., dyspnea on moderate exertion, occasional aches and pains, fatigue, etc.), mild psychopathology, mld functional limitations and/or mild impairment of well-being	Investigation for other (non-weight-related) contributors to risk factors. More intense lifestyle interventions, including diet and exercise to prevent further weight gain. Monitoring of risk factors and health status.
2	Presence of established obesity-related chronic disease (e.g., hypertension, type 2 diabetes, sleep apnea, osteoarthritis), limitations in activities of daily living and/or well-being	Initiation of obesity treatments, including consideration of all behavioral, pharmacological, and surgical treatment options. Close monitoring and management of comorbidities as indicated.
3	Established end-organ damage such as myocardial infarction, heart failure, diabetic complications, incapacitating osteoarthritis, significant psychopathology, significant functional limitations in activities of daily living and/or well-being	More intensive obesity treatment, including consideration of all behavioral, pharamacological, and surgical treatment options. Aggressive management of comorbidities as indicated.
4	Severe (potentially end-stage) disabilities from obesity-related chronic diseases, severe disabling psychopathology, severe functional limitaions and/or severe impairment of well-being	Aggressive obesity management as deemed feasible. Palliative measures including pain management, occupational therapy, and psychosocial support.

Reprinted with permission from Sharma AM, Kushner RF. 2009. A proposed clinical staging system for obesity. *International Journal of Obesity* 33(3):289.

PREVALENCE

In the United States, as of 2011–2012, 39.4% of Americans met the criteria for obesity using the previously noted definition, with African-Americans having the highest age-adjusted rate of 47.8% (Ogden, Carroll, and Kit, 2014). Among children and adolescents the prevalence is estimated to be 17%.

Since the 1970s the proportion of Americans in the overweight category has increased from 46% to 64.5%.

Prevalence of obesity in Canada is significantly lower at 24.1% for adults, though the difference was somewhat lessened if only non-Hispanic white adults were compared in both countries (Statistics Canada, Health Fact Sheets). Using the World Health Organization cutoff criteria for children and adolescents 5–17 years of age, 19.8% were in the overweight category and 11.7% obese (Roberts, Shields, de Groh, et al., 2012).

The figures for Europe are generally lower than in North America. The International Obesity Task Force (IOBTF) keeps current data on the prevalence of obesity around the world (http://www.worldobesity.org/iotf/obesity/). A consistent observation has been that prevalence has been on the rise both in adults and in children and adolescents.

FAMILY FACTORS

Obesity is thought to have a polygenic inheritance pattern and this may account for as much as 30%–40% of adult variability in weight.

Our relationship to food is learned in the womb (Adams, Ferraro, and Brett, 2012) and continues to be developed in our family of origin. Food taste preferences are established in the first year of life and have an effect in later childhood (Grimm, Kim, Yaroch, et al., 2014). It is a complex relationship involving emotions of love and comfort and sometimes power and tension. Much of this lifelong interaction is rooted in the preverbal period of a person's life. This has significant implications for any clinical approach. Families that eat dinner together with no television distraction tend to have lower rates of obesity (Wansin and Van Kleef, 2014). Such family meals may be a proxy for the level of family organization and stability, and where there is dysfunction in a family, there is also stress. Chronic stress in children may contribute to weight problems in a number of ways, including raised cortisol levels, irregular access to nutritious food, learning poor eating habits, and eating as a way of coping.

Being slim as an adult is linked to childhood experiences (Bevelander, Kaipainen, Swain, et al., 2014). Adults with lower BMIs had certain childhood experiences in common, including family meals prepared using fresh ingredients; parents who talked to their children about nutrition; engaging in outdoor physical activities with their families; sleeping a healthy number of hours on weeknights; and having many friends. Adults with higher BMIs, on the other hand, held the following childhood experiences in common: food being used as a reward or punishment; having obese parents or grandparents; drinking juice or soda more than water; and parents who restricted their food intake.

Maternal smoking during pregnancy increases the risk of obesity in children. Other confounders include maternal obesity, excessive weight gain in pregnancy, low birth weight, and not being breastfed (Ino, 2010). The efficacy of breastfeeding as a preventive measure against childhood obesity has recently come under question, but there remain many compelling reasons to encourage it (Harder, Bergmann, and Kallishnigg, 2005; Casazza, Fontaine, Astrup, et al., 2013).

Cultural values are transmitted in the family, and these include attitudes toward "ideal" body image and approach to what foods are desirable and appropriate. Many cultures do not share the predominant Western view that "normal" weight and even thinness is associated with health. In some regions of the world, being thin is a sign of poor nutrition or poor health and is highly undesirable. Among African-Americans living in the United States, a large body size is more acceptable than is commonly the case among whites (Kittler, Sucher, and Nelms, 2012).

SOCIAL FACTORS

Although men are more likely to be overweight or obese than women, the latter tend to be more concerned about their weight. This emphasis on women's weight has led to its development as a feminist issue and to the emergence of "size activists" or "fat activists" (Rothblum and Soloway, 2009).

Socioeconomic status has been negatively correlated with obesity in a number of studies (Jeffery, Forster, and Folsom, 1989; Martikainen and Marmot, 1999). Those in lower income categories may have a higher prevalence of obesity for a number of reasons, including easier access to "fast foods" and less access to parks and recreational facilities (Reidpath, Burns, Garrard, et al., 2002). The chronic stress of living in poverty may also contribute to unhealthy weight gain through the influence of chronically raised glucocorticoids, which may predispose to an increase in "comfort food" (heavy in sugar and fat) and to greater abdominal or central obesity (Dallman, Pecoraro, and Akana, 2003).

Education, like socioeconomic status (to which it is closely linked), is negatively associated with obesity, at least in women. For men the association with education is not evident (Centers for Disease Control and Prevention).

Age is sometimes cited as related to obesity, as weight tends to increase gradually over a person's lifetime until about the seventh decade.

It is commonly assumed that everyone who is obese wants to change and, for the most part, that would be correct. However, it is important for general practitioners to recognize that many people have come to an acceptance of their weight, and social support does exist for them, as demonstrated by what are dubbed "fat acceptance sites" and blogs[1] and even what has been dubbed a "fat subculture," which may help dispel some of the discrimination felt by many (Rothblum and Soloway, 2009).

Some ethnic groups, such as Native Americans, African-Americans, and those of Hispanic background, are at higher risk of obesity. New immigrants are also at higher risk, beginning about 10 years after arrival.

SUBJECTIVE EXPERIENCE

We all construct life narratives that help to make sense of our situation and the decisions we have made or are making. It is important for the physician who is trying to understand his or her patient to be familiar with the patient's predominant narrative. In a study examining the discourse of individuals involved in weight loss surgery (Throsby, 2007) that began with the simple question "Tell me the story of your weight," a number of themes came to the fore. Many gave expression to the notion that they had inherited a "fat gene" or that they possessed an innate difference in metabolism compared to other, thinner people. In essence, their body does not respond to food the way other people's bodies respond. Also prominent was that they were "chunky" or "chubby" as children and, as a result, being obese as an adult was somewhat inevitable. Interestingly, this idea is also central to the notion that one of the appropriate responses to the obesity epidemic is to tackle childhood obesity. At third major narrative line is the imposition of certain life events, making it difficult to follow a "normal diet." These events might consist of illness or injury or major changes such as divorce, bereavement, new parenthood, new relationships, moving to a new house, or leaving school. Among men, employment changes leading to a more sedentary lifestyle or increased mobility leading to more "fast foods" were common. Also the pressures of adopting a "masculine diet" of high carbohydrates and alcohol in large quantities were cited by some. Women's narratives tended to emphasize the use of food as a comfort measure for both positive and negative events.

Individuals coping with weight problems may not feel well supported by their physician or the healthcare system more generally, with physicians rarely raising the issue with them (Wadden et al., 2000).

In a qualitative study (Kirk, Price, Penney, et al., 2014) that involved 22 individuals living with obesity in an eastern Canadian province, several themes emerged. Feelings of shame and guilt were common and, in subtle ways, their experience with healthcare providers sometimes reinforced these feelings. They expressed feelings of frustration and demoralization from repeated failures to lose weight. Frequently expressed was the fact that they knew what they had to do, but were overwhelmed by barriers to taking these measures. As stated by one individual living with obesity, "It's not the diet; it's the mental part of it that [we] need help with, and I don't have any support anywhere for it" (Kirk, Price, Penney, et al., 2014, p. 793).

The individuals surveyed felt that the support they needed was lacking or was not easily accessible. Health professionals interviewed in the same study also expressed frustration and difficulty understanding the complexities of the issue of obesity in their patients.

A second major theme was a feeling of lack of support from the healthcare system as a whole, and this was expressed by both individuals living with obesity and providers of health care. For the providers there was frustration that, though they were expected to act in the role of expert, they did not feel well prepared.

The third theme was difficulty with the prevailing medical management discourse, which sometimes led to conflicting messages. Many practitioners expressed that obesity in itself is not a disease. They found it easier to deal with obese patients if they had another comorbidity. Presumably, it is easier to address weight loss if the focus is on hypertension or diabetes.

Patients' expectations of physicians is that they will support them by providing dietary advice, and help with setting realistic weight-loss goals and an exercise prescription (Potter, Vue, and Croughan-Minihane, 2001).

CLINICAL APPROACH

It is common to conceive of obesity and overweight problems as simply related to calories in and calories out, and this "simple physics" approach is characteristic of most weight-loss programs as well as the biomedical approach. The rather poor long-term results of this approach lie in failing to recognize that our relationship with food is much more complex. The physician and the patient–doctor relationship lie at the nexus of a complex interplay of largely unspoken habits, past and current relationships with family, self-identity, and stress. The continuity and comprehensiveness of care that are possible in family practice lead to circumstances in which it is feasible to effectively initiate and support the changes necessary to a bring about weight loss. Unfortunately, physicians tend to fail to address weight issues, though patients would welcome their opening the discussion (Wadden, 2000; Heintze, Sonntag, Brinck, et al., 2012).

Physicians' tendency to ignore the problem may be due to personal experiences with their own problems with attempting weight loss; previous lack of success with patients and hence a fear of failure; or a belief that obesity is not a medical problem itself, but rather a lifestyle choice or due to a lack of self-discipline, leading to a tendency to blame/shame patients. Physicians may feel a great deal of frustration, having learned an approach based on a medical model that often does not work and, as a result, feeling powerless to help their patients with this problem (Kirk, Price, Penney, et al., 2014). They may feel they lack the time and resources to properly counsel their patients and that raising the issue may threaten the patient–doctor relationship.

Whether physicians perceive themselves to be obese influences their approach to weight problems in patients. Keeping in mind the shortcomings of self-reports, the prevalence of obesity among physicians is lower than in the general population, averaging in the 7%–8% range (Brotons, Bjfrkelaund, Bulc, et al., 2005; Frank and Segura, 2009). Family physicians whose own BMI is in the normal range were found to be more likely to engage their obese patients in a discussion about their weight and felt greater confidence in providing advice about weight loss and exercise than overweight or obese physicians. Further, patients were more confident in such advice if it came from physicians with normal BMIs (Bleich, Bennett, and Gudzune, 2012).

In a study of discourse between physicians and overweight patients about their weight, it was found that when physicians used techniques from motivational interviewing (praise, collaboration, and evoking change statements), patients lost more weight after 3 months than following conversations characterized by interview techniques that were inconsistent with motivational interviewing (judging, confronting, providing advice without first seeking permission). The difference in weight after 3 months, while not great (1.6 kg), emphasizes the importance of physician–patient communication to outcomes (Pollak, Alexander, and Coffman, 2010).

The 5 As approach (Table 15.2), originally developed for smoking cessation counseling, has been adapted for use in weight counseling (Vallis, Piccinini-Vallis, Sharma, and Freedhoff, 2013). It begins with requesting of the patient permission to discuss weight (**A**sk). It is important that this be done in a nonjudgmental way. Next comes **A**ssess, using BMI and waist circumference, and a discussion of how the individual's weight affects his or her psychological, social, and physical functions. Here the Edmonton Obesity Staging System usefully takes into account comorbid conditions as an aid in planning (Sharma and Kushner, 2009). Food diaries carefully reviewed with the patient will provide insight into his or her pattern of eating. Unless a family physician has taken extra training in evaluating dietary intake, he or she may elect to have these reviewed by a dietitian or nurse with extra training. There are mobile applications that some patients may find useful. The physician must also inquire about alcohol intake, as it is an often hidden source of calories. The 4 Ms framework is a mnemonic that helps to assess psychosocial and root-cause factors to help the physician achieve a more holistic understanding. It covers possible mental, mechanical, metabolic, and monetary barriers with which a patient may need to cope. The next step is to **A**dvise again, beginning by seeking the patient's permission to offer advice. It is helpful at this point to emphasize that even a modest 5%–10% weight loss has benefits, and this makes it easier for the patient to envision success than to aim for a weight in the "ideal" BMI range. Treatment options to be discussed include changes in lifestyle, behavioral and

Table 15.2 THE FIVE AS OF OBESITY MANAGEMENT

A	Definition	Rationale
Ask	Ask permission to discuss weight; be nonjudgmental; explore readiness for change	Weight is a sensitive issue; avoid verbal cues that imply judgment; indication of readiness might predict outcomes.
Assess	Assess BMI, WC, obesity stage; explore drivers and complications of excess weight	BMI alone should never serve as an indicator for obesity interventions; obesity is a complex and heterogeneous disorder with multiple causes;drivers and complications of obesity will vary among individuals.
Advise	Advise on health risks of obesity, benefits of modest weight loss, the need for a long-term strategy, and treatment options	Health risks of excess weight can vary; avoidance of weight gain or modest weight loss can have health benefits; considerations of treatment options should account for risks.
Agree	Agree on realistic weight-loss expectations and targets, behavioral changes using the SMART framework, and specific details of the treatment options	Most patients and many physicians have unrealistic expectations; interventions should focus on changing behavior; providers should seek patients' "buy-in" to proposed treatment.
Assist	Assist in identifying and addressing barriers; provide resources and assist in identifying and consulting with appropriate providers; arrange regular follow-up	Most patients have substantial barriers to weight management; patients are confused and cannot distinguish credible and noncredible sources of information; follow-up is an essential principle of chronic disease management.

BMI: body mass index; SMART: specific, measurable, achievable, rewarding, timely; WC: weight circumference
From Vallis M, Piccinini-Vallis H, Sharma AM, Freedhoff Y. 2013. Modified 5 As: Minimal intervention for obesity counseling in primary care. *Canadian Family Physician* 59:27–31.

psychological counseling, medications, and bariatric surgery. Having covered these options, it is important to come to agreement (**A**gree) on the treatment plan. In the patient-centered clinical method (see Chapter 9), this step is designated *finding common ground*, and this has been found to be most important in determining adherence to the plan and ultimately to outcomes (Stewart, Brown, Donner, et al., 2000; Stewart, Brown, Weston, et al., 2014). Focusing on weight management goals rather than weight itself is most useful. Once agreement is reached, the physician must be prepared to **A**ssist the patient in reaching his or her goal. This means helping the patient identify those factors in his or her life that can facilitate reaching the goal, as well as barriers. In family practice it is important to consider who in the household attends to shopping for food and preparing it. It does little good to discuss these issues with one individual if someone else in the family is responsible for these aspects of home life. Counseling may be far more useful if both individuals are involved and supportive of the plan. The physician should be familiar with reliable and credible resources, either in the patient's local community or on the primary care team, and make this information available to the patient.

Five key points for the physician to keep in mind and to convey to the patient are the following:

1. Obesity is a chronic condition. It didn't accumulate overnight, nor will it come off overnight. Hence a long-term plan is needed.
2. Managing obesity is about health and a sense of well-being and not about numbers on a scale. Physicians must assist their patients in avoiding this trap.
3. Early intervention in addressing root causes and removing barriers is needed.
4. The meaning of success will be different for each person.
5. The "best" weight for an individual may not be the "ideal" weight.

Interventions in childhood can be effective and bear great benefits in the long term. They must involve the whole family. Frequently parents do not fully recognize obesity in their children, and this may be particularly true for their sons; they also do not recognize their own weight problems.

The physician's approach to comorbid problems also influences weight. Smoking cessation, one of the most important behavioral changes an individual can make, typically leads to a 4–5 kg weight gain over the following months. Medications that have been linked to weight gain include antidepressant medications (SSRIs, tricyclics, lithium), antipsychotics (olanzapine, clozapine, risperidone), anti-epileptics (valproate, gabapentin, carbamazepine), steroids (hormonal contraceptives, corticosteroids, progestational steroids), adrenergic antagonists, serotonin antagonists, and diabetic medications (sulfonylureas, thiazolidinediones, insulin). When these medications are in use and obesity is an identified problem, it may be desirable to find alternatives. Many times practical alternatives may not be available. For example, insulin may be necessary for controlling diabetes, in which case the goal is not to focus on attaining an ideal BMI, but rather on increased physical activity, sense of wellness, and self-esteem. Meaningful goals are more likely to arise out of a patient–physician relationship that is nonjudgmental and trusting.

Exercise Prescriptions

Attention to diet must be accompanied by appropriate exercise. It is not sufficient to simply encourage to a patient to "get more exercise." It is important to be specific about the intensity and duration of exercise. Improvements in health and fitness require at least 150 minutes of brisk exercise/week, but for weight loss it must be at least 60–90 minutes a day. Petrella and colleagues (2003), in a randomized controlled trial involving elderly, community-dwelling individuals in both urban and rural practices, demonstrated the effectiveness of an exercise prescription in family practice. Fitness, as determined by VO2 max, improved by 11% after 6 months and was maintained at 12 months in the intervention group. Further, there were statistically significant improvements in blood pressure, BMI, and confidence in exercise in the intervention group. Any exercise program must be pragmatic and take into account other comorbidities if it is to be helpful. Some patients prefer to exercise alone and others in groups, and these preferences must be taken into account. Activity guides such as that available from the National Heart, Lung and Blood Institute (Table 15.3) can be useful in illustrating what is meant by moderate physical activity.

Medications

The only available medication for which there is evidence of efficacy in treating obesity is orlistat, which works by reducing the absorption and digestion of fats by inhibiting the gastric and pancreatic lipase. It must be combined with patient adherence to a low-fat diet to lessen the common side effect of loose, greasy stools. There was a 2.9-kg weight loss over 1 year for those who were able to take it compared to a placebo group (Rucker et al., 2007). Research continues in this area, and doubtless more drugs will be brought to the market to reduce weight, but family physicians will need to continue to be skeptical that there is a pharmaceutical "solution" to what is a complex biological, family, cultural, and environmental issue.

Surgery

Bariatric surgery is effective in helping to achieve weight loss in a select population. Those with a BMI greater than 35 kg/m^2 and with severe comorbidities or a BMI greater than or equal to 40 and who have made strong attempts to lose weight through diet, exercise, and behavioral changes may be considered as candidates for a surgical approach. A psychological assessment is needed to determine the ability of the patient to cope with the changes and

Table 15.3 EXAMPLES OF MODERATE AMOUNTS OF PHYSICAL ACTIVITY*

Common Chores	Sporting Activities	
Washing and waxing a car for 45–60 minutes	Playing volleyball for 45–60 minutes	Less Vigorous, More Time#
Washing windows or floors for 45–60 minutes	Playing touch football for 45 minutes	
Gardening for 30–45 minutes	Walking 1¾ miles in 35 minutes (20 min/mile)	
Wheeling self in wheelchair for 30–40 minutes	Basketball (shooting baskets) for 30 minutes	
Pushing a stroller 1½ miles in 30 minutes	Bicycling 5 miles in 30 minutes	
Raking leaves for 30 minutes	Dancing fast (social) for 30 minutes	
Walking 2 miles in 30 minutes (15 min/mile)	Water aerobics for 30 minutes	
Shoveling snow for 15 minutes	Swimming laps for 20 minutes	
Stairwalking for 15 minutes	Basketball (playing a game) for 15–20 minutes	
	Jumping rope for 15 minutes	
	Running 1½ miles in 15 minutes (15 min/mile)	More Vigorous, Less Time

*A moderate amount of physical activity is roughly equivalent to physical activity that uses 3–6 METs (metabolic equivalents) where 1 MET is the energy involved in sitting quietly (1 calorie/2.2 lb. body weight).
Some activities can be performed at various intensities; the suggested durations correspond to expected intensity of effort
Adapted from National Heart, Lung and Blood Institute. *Practical Guide to the Identification, Evaluation and Treatment of Overweight and Obesity in Adults.*

consequences of this surgery. Unless a person is prepared to change his or her fundamental relationship with food, there is a high risk of failure of the procedure over time. A review of three randomized control trials and three prospective cohort studies comparing surgery with nonsurgical management found greater weight loss and reduced comorbidities (diabetes and hypertension) and better health-related quality of life after 2 years following surgery. Effects after 10 years were less clear (Colquitt, Picot, Loveman, and Clegg, 2009). Surgeons and their team attend to the short-term complications and side effects, but family physicians need to be aware of the long-term side effects. These vary depending on what procedure was carried out. The Roux-en-Y gastric bypass may result in dumping syndrome, consisting of cramps, diarrhea, malaise, and sweating if the individual consumes foods such as ice cream or soda that are high in osmolality. In the long term, postsurgical patients must take supplements, including vitamin B_{12}, calcium, vitamin D, and sometimes iron. Ferritin levels must be monitored. Medications used for other medical conditions may have altered concentrations due to reduced absorption. Frequent monitoring of blood levels may be necessary as a result.

Complementary and Alternative Medicine

Many people seek over-the-counter dietary supplements for weight loss. Most of these have no evidence of being efficacious, and some, such as ephedra-containing compounds, should only be used with caution due to possible side effects.

Policy Issues

Family physicians may find themselves personally, or through their colleges, motivated to engage overweight and obesity at a community or even national level, through advocating or supporting policy measures intended to address issues related to food supply and exercise. In this view, obesity in a population is more a failure of policy than of personal will. This has led to draft guidelines from the World Health Organization that daily sugar consumption be no more than 10% of total energy intake per day, but that a reduction to 5% would be more beneficial. Five percent of total recommended intake amounts to 25 gm (5–6 teaspoons) for women and 35 gm (7–8 teaspoons) for men. Because much of the daily intake of sugar is hidden in foods, efforts to improve the labeling of food to make nutritional content more evident are another policy alternative being explored.

NOTE

1. See, for example, Fierce, Freethinking Fatties at http://fiercefatties.com/philosophy/.

REFERENCES

Adams KB, Ferraro ZM, Brett KE. 2012. Can we modify the intrauterine environment to halt the intergenerational cycle of obesity? *International Journal of Environmental Research and Public Health* 9:1263–1307.
Bevelander KE, Kaipainen K, Swain R, Dohle S, Bongard JC, Hines PDH, Wansink B. 2014. Crowdsourcing Novel Childhood Predictors of Adult Obesity. *PLOS one* 9(2):e87756.
Bleich SN, Bennett WL, Gudzune KA, Cooper LA. 2012. Impact of physician BMI on obesity care and beliefs. *Obesity* 20(5):999–1005.

Brotons C, Bjfrkelund C, Bulc M, et al. on behalf of the EUROPREV network. 2005. Prevention and health promotion in clinical practice: The views of general practitioners in Europe. *Preventive Medicine* 40:595–560

Casazza K, Fontaine KR, Astrup A, et al. 2013. Myths, presumptions and facts about obesity. *New England Journal of Medicine* 368:446–454.

Centers for Disease Control and Prevention. 2014. *Fact Sheet Adult Overweight and Obesity.* http://www.cdc.gov/obesity/adult/index.html.

Colquitt JL, Picot J, Loveman E, Clegg AJ. 2009. Surgery for obesity. *The Cochrane Library.* http://onlinelibrary.wiley.com/doi/10.1002/14651858.CD003641.pub3/full.

Dallman MF, Pecoraro N, Akana SF, et al. 2003. Chronic stress and obesity: A new view of "comfort food." *Proceedings of the National Academy of Sciences* 100(20):11696–11701.

Frank E, Segura C. 2009. Health practices of Canadian family physicians. *Canadian Family Physician* 55:810–811.

Gard, M, Wright J. 2005. *The Obesity Epidemic: Science, Morality and Ideology.* London: Routledge.

Grimm KA, Kim SA, Yoroch AL, Scanlon KS. 2014. Fruit and vegetable intake during infancy and early childhood. *Pediatrics* 134(Suppl 1): 563–569.

Harder T, Bergmann R, Kallischnigg G, Plagemann A. 2005. Duration of breastfeeding and risk of overweight: A meta-analysis. *American Journal of Epidemiology* 163:397–403.

Heintze C, Sonntag U, Brinck A, et al. 2012. A qualitative study on patients' and physicians' visions for the future management of overweight or obesity. *Family Practice* 29:103–109.

Ino T. 2010. Maternal smoking during pregnancy and offspring obesity: Meta-analysis. *Pediatrics International* 52(1):94–99.

Jeffery RW, Forster JL, Folsom AR, et al. 1989. The relationship between social status and body mass index in the Minnesota Heart Health Program. *International Journal of Obesity* 13(1):59–67.

Kirk SFL, Price SL, Penney TL, et al. 2014. Blame, shame, and lack of support: A multilevel study on obesity management. *Qualitative Health Research* 24(6):790–800.

Kittler PG, Sucher KP, Nahikian-Nelms M. 2012. *Food and Culture.* Belmont, CA: Wadsworth, Cengage Learning.

Martikainen PT, Marmot MG. 1999. Socioeconomic differences in weight gain and determinants and consequences of coronary risk factors. *American Journal of Clinical Nutrition* 69:719–726.

National Heart, Lung and Blood Institute. 2000. *The Practical Guide: Identification, Evaluation and Treatment of Overweight and Obesity in Adults.* NIH Publication Number 00-4084.

Ogden CL, Carroll MD, Kit BK, Flegal KM. 2014. Prevalence of childhood and adult obesity in the United States, 2011–2012. *JAMA* 311(8):806–814.

Petrella RJ, Koval, JJ, Cunningham DA, Paterson DH. 2003. Can primary care doctors prescribe exercise to improve fitness? The step test exercise prescription (STEP) project. *American Journal of Preventive Medicine* 24(4):316–322.

Pollak, KI, Alexander SC, Coffman CJ, Tulsky JA, Lyna P, Dolor RJ, Ostbye T. 2010. Physician communication techniques and weight loss in adults: Project CHAT. *American Journal of Preventive Medicine* 39(4):321–328.

Potter MB, Vu JD, Croughan-Minihane M. 2001. Weight management: What patients want from their primary care physician. *J. Fam Pract.* 59(6):513–518.

Reidpath DD, Burns C, Garrard J, Mahoney M, Townsend M. 2002. An ecological study of the relationship between social and environmental determinants of obesity. *Health & Place* 8(2):141–145.

Throsby K. 2007. "How could you let yourself get like that?": Stories of the origins of obesity in accounts of weight loss surgery. *Social Science & Medicine* 65(8):1561–1571.

Roberts KC, Shields M, de Groh M, Aziz A, Gilbert J. 2012. Overweight and obesity in children and adolescents: Results from the 2009 to 2011 Canadian Health Measures Survey. *Statistics Canada Health Reports* 23(3): 37–41.

Rothblum E, Soloway S. 2009. *The Fat Studies Reader*. New York; London: New York University Press.

Rucker D, Padwal R, Li SK, et al. 2007. Long term pharmacotherapy for obesity and overweight: Updated meta-analysis. *BMJ* 335:1194–1199.

Sharma AM, Kushner RF. 2009. A proposed clinical staging system for obesity. *International Journal of Obesity* 33(3):289.

Statistics Canada Health Fact Sheets. 2014. *Adult Obesity Prevalence in Canada and the United States*. http://www.statcan.gc.ca/pub/82-625-x/2011001/article/11411-eng.htm.

Stewart MA, Brown JB, Donner A. 2000. The impact of patient-centered care on patient outcomes. *Journal of Family Practice* 49(9):796–804.

Stewart MA, Brown JB, Weston WW, McWhinney IR, McWilliam CL, Freeman TR. 2014. *Patient-Centered Medicine: Transforming the Clinical Method*, 3rd ed. London; New York: Radcliffe Publishing.

Vallis M, Piccinini-Vallis H, Sharma AM, Freedhoff Y. 2013. Modified 5 As: Minimal intervention for obesity counseling in primary care. *Canadian Family Physician* 59:27–31.

Wadden TA, Anderson DA, Foster GD, Bennett A, Steinberg C, Sarwer DB. 2000. Obese women's perceptions of their physicians' weight management attitudes and practices. *Archives of Family Medicine* (9):854–860.

Wansink B, Van Kleef E. 2014. Dinner rituals that correlate with child and adult BMI. *Obesity* 22(5):e91–e95.

CHAPTER 16

✧

Multimorbidity

There has been a worldwide increase in life expectancy in the course of the twentieth century (Gaydos, 2012) that, in part, may be attributable to improvements in public health and the wider determinants of health, as well as improvements in the therapy of diseases. Concomitantly, there has been an increase in people coping with more than one disease: multimorbidity (MM). Family physicians, focused on the individual rather than specific diseases or organ systems, are the principal medical professionals who address patients with MM.

The first challenge in considering MM lies in its definition. Wide differences exist in the definitions of MM used in various research studies. Early studies focused only on chronic diseases, which had some disadvantages. For example, myocardial infarction and ischemic heart disease could be counted twice in the same individual. Also, focusing on diseases made dealing with risk factors, such as hyperlipidemia, problematic. Focusing on health conditions rather than diseases may be more useful. The usual definition of two or more chronic conditions occurring at the same time leads to a number of potential interpretations. For example, the World Health Organization defines chronic conditions as "health problems that require ongoing management over a period of years or decades." This leaves the time frame vague. The European General Practice Research Network recently offered the following definition: "Any combination of a chronic disease with at least one other acute or chronic disease or biopsychosocial factor (associated or not) or somatic risk factor" (LaReste, Nabbe, Manceau, et al., 2013, p. 321). Clearly, this very broad definition is so inclusive as to test the limits of usefulness.

A clinical definition has been offered that defines MM as "a state by which the clinician, along with the patient and/or family faces the multiplicity of long-term conditions experienced by the patient." The same authors point out that any operational definition for research purposes should specify

(a) the number of clinical conditions considered, and (b) which conditions are counted (Mercer, Salisbury, and Fortin, 2014, p. 2). However, for practice it is preferable to not set a limit on the number or type of conditions to be counted, for reasons that will become evident.

It is important to remember that diagnostic categories are professional constructs. No disease occurs separate from other diseases or from the person experiencing them. MM, like any individual disease category, is but one way of representing ill health (see Chapter 6, "Philosophical and Scientific Foundations of Family Medicine"). By its very definition, it tends to be disease-centric. The list of diseases and conditions that are commonly considered may be seen as the biomedical view of human aging. The utility of the concept of MM lies in whether it can improve the care of individuals, including patients' positive experience of their care, improved quality of life and functioning, reduced hospitalizations, and reduced mortality. This concept and the accompanying polypharmacy help us understand the increasing complexity of health care and are especially relevant to the general practitioner, as the commitment to the patient is not restricted to a particular disease or treatment modality.

Despite these difficulties in definition, interest in MM has increased, as it has been associated with more medical consultations, polypharmacy, emergency utilization, hospital length of stay, and mortality (Librero, Peiro, and Ordinana, 1999; Fortin, Bravo, Hudon, et al., 2006; Broemeling, Watson, and Prebtani, 2008; Diederichs, Wellman, Bartels, et al., 2012).

PREVALENCE

Prevalence figures vary widely (3.5%–98.5%) depending on several factors: the definition used, whether the focus is only on the elderly or includes all age groups, and the method of data collection (Fortin, Bravo, Hudon, et al., 2005; Fortin, Stewart, Poitras, et al., 2012). The number of diseases or health conditions that are counted, not surprisingly, has an effect on prevalence estimates. The more diseases that are considered, the higher the prevalence. It stands to reason that since family practice tends to deal with a large number of diseases at low frequency, the most comprehensive studies deal with all chronic diseases rather than a smaller list. Approaches to estimating prevalence include surveys, administrative data sets, consecutive patient visits to general practitioners, or chart review. They may be population-based or practice-based and, at the practice level, may be based on patient visits or record review. Administrative data sets may yield lower figures than surveys and record reviews. It has been suggested that patient record review may be the most accurate method (Fortin, Bravo, Hudon, et al., 2005).

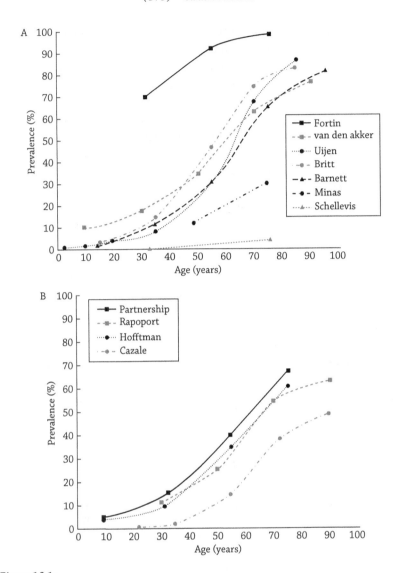

Figure 16.1:
(A) Multimorbidity reported in primary care settings. (B) Multimorbidity reported in the general population.

Reprinted with permission from Mercer SW, Salisbury C, Fortin M. 2014. *ABC of Multimorbidity*. Oxford: John Wiley and Sons.

Surveys of the general population find lower prevalence estimates than those in family practice samples (Fortin, Bravo, Hudon, et al., 2005; Fortin, Hudon, Haggerty, et al., 2010) (Figure 16.1), but may find higher estimates for younger people and for symptom-based diagnoses (Violan, Foguet-Boreu, Hermosilla-Perez, et al., 2013) leading to a call for including the patient perspective in any approach to multimorbidity. Patient self-reports on disease burden tend to incorporate more biopsychosocial constructs in older people, suggesting that counts of health conditions need to be supplemented by assessment of the limitations that accompany them (Bayliss, Ellis, and Steiner, 2009).

All prevalence estimates of MM must include mental disorders, as they are present in 29% of individuals with multiple chronic conditions.

In an Australian study involving 375 general practitioners who recorded the number of chronic diseases in 8707 patients seen in their practices, it was found that 66.5% had at least one chronic condition and 44.5% had two or more. As the number of diseases needed to fulfill the definition increased, the prevalence decreased to 3% if six or more conditions were considered. There was high concordance between patients whether one used Chronic Illness Rating Scale (CIRS) domains, ICPC-2, or ICD-10 chapters to categorize diseases. Prevalence rates increased if the list of chronic conditions increased. With MM defined as two or more from a list of 12 conditions, the prevalence estimate meant that every second patient seen by a family physician fulfilled the definition of MM. Using three or more conditions as the definition meant that every fourth patient meant the criteria. The authors recommend that the label complex MM be used when there is ". . . the co-occurrence of three or more chronic conditions affecting three or more different body systems within one person without defining an index chronic condition." This definition results in lower prevalence estimates and greater differentiation among older patients (Harrison, Britt, Miller, et al., 2014, p. e004694).

A systematic review of 39 studies of MM involving more than 70 million patients in 12 countries found prevalence estimates varying between 12.9% and 95.1%. Consistently, prevalence was higher in women, and increased with age and with lower socioeconomic status (Violan, Foguet,-Boreu, and Flores-Mateo, 2014). In economically deprived areas, MM tends to occur at younger ages and to be more likely to involve mental health problems (Barnett, Mercer, Norbury, et al., 2012). A summary of Australian prevalence studies reported that when eight or more chronic conditions are considered, about 50% of adults aged 45–65 had more than one chronic disease, and this rose to 80% in those over age 75 (Erny-Albrecht and McIntyre, 2013). In 2010, 15.5% of visits to doctors' offices in the United States dealt with three or more medical conditions (National Ambulatory Care Medical Survey, 2010).

Severity

The impact of MM on the family physician's work and on the patient's quality of life and capabilities depends not only on prevalence but also on the types of diagnoses. Some recognized conditions have greater impact than others. Often risk factors such as hypertension and hyperlipidemia are listed as diseases, though they have little direct effect on the individual's quality of life beyond appointments with healthcare providers, the cost of prescribed medications, and lifestyle changes. This is quite distinct from coping with advanced emphysema or osteoarthritis. The Cumulative Illness Rating Scale (CIRS) is used to capture the element of severity. An electronic version of CIRS, adaptable to electronic health records, has been developed and found to be reliable and valid (Fortin, Steenbakkers, Hudon, et al., 2011). The Charlson Index, on the other hand, addresses mortality in those with MM. Disease burden can also be measured as impact on health service utilization, including physician visits at the primary care level, use of secondary care services such as hospitalizations, and the cost of all of these.

Clusters

To help make sense of complex clinical challenges and, perhaps, set the stage for useful clinical guidelines, it may be useful to identify common clusters of health conditions that frequently occur together. Such clusters can be considered as specific disease entities (e.g., diabetes, hypertension, hyperlipidemia) or broader categories (e.g., cardiovascular/metabolic or anxiety/depression/ psychological conditions). Clustering in this way makes sense as treatments may often be complementary within a given cluster. When a patient has diagnoses in different clusters, he or she may be considered as having complex MM, as treatments between clusters may compete for time and attention. As is frequently the case, such clusters are in the eye of the beholder and may represent the "clinical gaze" more than the view of the individual patient. For example, diseases that used to be progressively fatal, such as some types of breast cancer or HIV-AIDS, have become chronic diseases with current treatment, but, for patients, still carry more significant meaning than many other chronic conditions.

Some clusters, such as those with musculoskeletal pain, impaired hearing, or vision, diabetes, or depression, may be associated with work difficulties and thereby affect income as well as physical quality of life (Bayliss, 2014).

A typology (Piette and Kerr, 2006) that is useful for thinking about clusters in MM is *clinically dominant conditions*: those that are so complex or serious that they eclipse other health problems. These may be subdivided into end-stage disease (e.g., late-stage renal failure, advanced dementia, or metastatic lung cancer); severely symptomatic diseases (e.g., class IV heart failure, severe depression); and recently diagnosed serious illnesses (e.g., rheumatoid arthritis, breast cancer). This typology distinguishes between chronic conditions that are *concordant* (those that represent parts of the same overall pathophysiologic risk profile, such as hypertension, coronary artery disease, peripheral vascular disease, and diabetes) and *discordant* (those whose treatments are not directly related to either their pathogenesis or management), such as a combination of asthma, prostate cancer, chronic low back pain, and diabetes. It is also useful to think in terms of those diagnostic clusters that are *symptomatic* (such as depression, arthritis, angina, and gastroesophageal reflux disease) and those that are *asymptomatic* (such as hypertension, hyperlipidemia, and poor glycemic control). Such a typology may be useful for organizing health care and for research, but it leaves out the patient's perspective.

FAMILY FACTORS

There often is a heavy burden assumed by the families of those with complex MM as they become the primary caregivers and, frequently, advocates, for their loved ones. Family members sometimes face great challenges in attempting to provide care as well as continue with employment, and they report great frustrations with long wait times for recommended tests and appointments (Gill et al., 2014). They report the need to serve as the "point person" in helping their family member navigate a fragmented and confusing system and experience distress at watching the effect of these challenges on the patient. Frustration and feelings of helplessness in the face of things that are beyond their control were also expressed (Gill et al., 2014).

SOCIAL FACTORS

As mentioned in the previous clinical chapters, chronic disease tends to be negatively associated with socioeconomic status (SES), so it is not surprising that MM also shows a similar association. The onset of chronic diseases in those in higher SES categories tend to be delayed to later in life when compared to those in lower SES categories (House, Lepkowski, Kinney, et al., 1994; Barnett, Mercer, Norbury, et al., 2012). Advanced age, female gender, and lower education have been independently associated with MM in a Swedish study in which the most common chronic disorders were cardiovascular and mental diseases (Marengoni, Winblad, Karp, et al., 2008).

Age, sex, income, and family structure have been found to be independently associated with MM (Agborsangaya, Lau, Lahtinen, et al., 2012), and economic deprivation in childhood is associated with adult MM, even after controlling for socioeconomic and demographic characteristics (Tucker-Seeley et al., 2011). Further, in geographic areas of low SES, MM occurs at a younger age and exhibits a higher prevalence of depression, drugs misuse, anxiety, dyspepsia, pain, coronary heart disease, and diabetes when compared to areas of higher SES (McLean, Gunn, and Guthrie, 2014).

SUBJECTIVE EXPERIENCE

What is listed as chronic conditions and diseases in medical terminology familiar to physicians may carry a much different meaning to patients. For example, some types of breast cancer and HIV-AIDS are now in the domain of chronic conditions but, to the patient, are freighted with meaning not typical of most other chronic conditions. "Having concurrent clinically defined conditions (MM) does not mean they are experienced as such . . . participants [in the study] do not necessarily see themselves as having discrete diseases nor do they highlight the difference between decline [aging] and disease" (Ong et al., 2014, p. 314). Living with chronic illnesses requires individuals to negotiate practical, everyday functions in the face of significant barriers. They alter biographical or life-narratives and challenge self-identity as a result. The challenge to one's self-identity represents an ongoing existential struggle. There are moral overtones, as well, in that individuals strive to be perceived as "legitimate" and responsible users of the healthcare system and their medications as a way of trying to be "normal" (Townsend et al., 2006; Townsend, 2012).

Physicians' records typically list a patient's diseases and drugs they have been prescribed. If the physician is only using a "clinical eye," this perception may invoke a series of impressions and clinical tasks that fail to take into account the individuality of the person. The individual is more likely to perceive his or her issues as symptoms that affect function, rather than using disease labels (Bayliss, 2014).

Those coping with multiple chronic conditions experience frustration with long waits for investigations and appointments, sometimes with multiple specialists. There may be poor communication between various healthcare providers, which makes it more difficult for them to do necessary self-care. In the words of one patient,

> And I've always thought of a cardiologist as being a person who doesn't worry just about your heart pressures but also about the swelling in my feet. I just found out last fall that he thinks it's the problem of my family physician . . . anyway these silos are almost like people are hard-wired into them. (Gill et al., 2014, p. 79)

Individuals' experiences of coping with MM include the hardship imposed by symptoms such as reduced mobility, physical limitations, pain, fatigue, dizziness, shortness of breath, insomnia, sexual dysfunction, depression, anxiety, anger, irritability, resentment, loneliness, feelings of humiliation, and inadequacy. These may lead to family disruptions, including marital breakup and reduced ability to participate in family activities (Noel et al., 2005; Bayliss, Edwards, Steiner, et al., 2008).

The expectations of patients with MM are

1. Convenient access to healthcare providers, preferably one who knows them well;
2. Continuity of care, meaning someone who knows them and whom they know well (this may even take precedence over convenience);
3. Clear communication of care plans, including supplementary written material;
4. Individualized and coordinated care provided by someone who knows them well; and
5. Being heard and understood. This requires a physician who can listen actively and has a caring attitude (Bayliss, Edwards, and Steiner, 2008).

Polypharmacy

Not surprisingly, drugs occupy a central part of the lives of those coping with chronic illnesses and one of the most common ways they interact with their family physician. For many, drug use entails considerable ambivalence. On the one hand, they are seen as necessary to maintain a "normal life," but are also a constant reminder that one is not "normal" (Townsend et al., 2003). Adhering to medication regimens interferes with people's lifestyle and causes side effects as well as problems coordinating them. Medication renewals are a frequent part of visits to the family physician, and patients perceive that they may be a source of conflict with the clinician (Dowell, Williams, and Snadden, 2007; Noel et al., 2005).

Since MM increases with age, the drug effects in the elderly are particularly relevant. These effects can be divided into pharmacokinetics (absorption, distribution, metabolism, and elimination) and pharmacodynamics (the effect of drugs on the body). As people age, there is an increase in the proportion of body fat and a decrease in the proportion of water, which leads to a longer half-life for lipid soluble drugs and a higher concentration of water-soluble ones. Liver volume decreases with age, reducing the metabolism of many drugs (e.g., benzodiazepines, morphine, lipid-soluble beta-blockers), again prolonging their half-life. Renal clearance of drugs also declines with age, and this results in about a 10% reduction each decade in glomerular filtration rate (GFR). Most measurements of GFR do not take into account the muscle bulk and will overestimate the renal function in the frail elderly. Pharmacodynamically, in addition to altered pharmacokinetics, aging results in changes to individual sensitivity to many drugs. Prominent in this category are benzodiazepines, the effects of which can lead to confusion and falls (Riley, Avery, and Jackson, 2009).

CLINICAL APPROACH
Challenges

As the number of chronic diseases and medications administered rises, family physicians are frequently challenged with sorting out symptoms. Does the onset of new symptoms or the worsening of existing ones represent progression of one or more diseases, a new disease, a drug(s) side effect, the decline of organ functions with aging, or all of these? A useful term to name this challenge is *confluent morbidity* (Upshur and Tracy, 2008). To the clinician, the onset of a new acute condition in an elderly patient with several chronic conditions and a variety of medications presents one of the most difficult diagnostic challenges in medicine.

In a meta-ethnographic study of qualitative research on the perception of general practitioners regarding MM, four areas of difficulty were highlighted: the disorganization and fragmentation of the healthcare system; the inadequacy of guidelines and evidence-based medicine; challenges in trying to deliver patient-centered care; and barriers to shared decision-making (Sinnott, McHugh, Browne, et al., 2013).

Guidelines generally are specific to single diseases and do not address MM or take into account quality of life and patient preferences (Boyd, Darer, Boult, et al., 2005; Fortin, Contant, Savard, et al., 2011; Hughes, McMurdo, and Guthrie, 2013). There are recommendations to try to overcome this problem (Guthrie, Payne, Alderson, et al., 2012), but achieving them will take some time. In any case, the application of guidelines will be of limited use in many situations. With any chronic disease, the context, the particulars of the patient, and the patient's preferences take on greater importance and become paramount when multiple chronic diseases are present.

Solutions

A number of approaches to these challenges have been recommended. The American Geriatrics Society has set five domains to guide the clinical approach to problems faced by patients with multiple problems. These are patient preferences, interpreting the evidence, prognosis, clinical feasibility, and optimizing therapies and care plans (American Geriatrics Society, 2012). For each domain, suggestions are provided on how they inform practice. The sequence will vary depending on the patient's situation.

An approach designed specifically for primary care recognizes three core principles to guide realistic treatment goals shared by the patient and the physician. A visit to the family physician may be triggered by a new symptom or a change in disease or context. The first principle is a thorough interaction assessment, taking into account the possibility of drug–drug, drug–disease, or disease–disease interactions. It is important to keep an updated list of all identified diseases, as well as all other physicians and therapists involved in the patient's care. The interaction assessment involves ongoing monitoring of mental health, psychological and cognitive status, as well as any changes in social status and contextual changes that may have an impact on the need for assistance with activities of daily living. The second principle is to set priorities around planned treatments. This must first begin with discussing patient preferences. In the context of the long-term relationship of family physicians and their patients, it must be recognized that patient preferences may change over time with changing circumstances and new diseases or conditions. These preferences must be revisited at regular intervals. The third principle is establishing a care plan that meets shared, realistic goals and takes into account treatment, monitoring, prevention, and self-management (Muth, van den Akker, Blom, et al., 2014).

The management of polypharmacy in family practice deserves much more attention than it has been generally given. Understanding the patient's priorities is essential to achieving common ground around the use of medication. Family physicians who know the family and social context of their patients' lives are in a good position to help them come to terms with both the pharmaceutical and nonpharmaceutical supports that can enable them to function.

It is common for patients on multiple drugs to ask of their physician if they really need to be on all of them. This presents an opportunity to review the individual's experience with them and to aid their understanding of the purpose of each medication. However, it is essential that the physician step out of the disease-centered approach and consider "How does this drug contribute to this person's self-management and the attainment of his or her goals?" (Britten, 2003). Tools such as the START/STOPP criteria can be very helpful in undertaking a medication review, especially in the elderly (Pharmacist's Letter/Prescriber's Letter, 2011).

The development of interdisciplinary teams in family practice hold promise in providing care to patients with multiple, complex morbidities. Innovative models such as the IMPACT model (Tracy et al., 2013), integrated teams for geriatric home care (Counsell, Callahan, Clark, et al., 2007), and case management by integrated nurses in primary care (Boult, Karm, and Groves, 2008; Chouinard, Hudon, Dubois, et al., 2013) are being developed to improve team-based care in these situations.

In developing a clinical approach to MM, a useful concept is that of *salutogenesis* (see Chapter 10). Medical science can offer approaches that are intended to mitigate the pathophysiology of various chronic diseases, but is unable to cure them. Considering ways to increase a patient's sense of coherence and control, and supporting meaningfulness in the face of the multiple challenges of MM, can increase his or her resilience and makes possible a sense of well-being and purpose. This approach is closely linked to the concept of healing as distinct from curing.

At times, the number of chronic conditions and their impact on an individual patient can invoke a feeling in the physician and the patient of being overwhelmed. When faced with the multiple challenges that this entails, the physician must begin with the patient. The emphasis shifts from addressing diseases to the patient's level of function and aspirations, recognizing that even in the face of multiple health challenges, it is possible, with adequate support, to be in balance with one's physical, psychological and social environment—in short, to be healthy.

The optimal clinical approach to MM is the patient-centered clinical method (see Chapter 9). It is imperative that the family physician come to an understanding of the effects of illness on patients' daily functioning, their fears and feelings, their ideas about what is causing their problems, and their expectations of the physician and healthcare system. A patient's problems and priorities will vary over time, as will his or her illness experience, and this requires that a flexible approach be taken by the physician. Achieving common ground between patient and physician is associated with improved outcomes (Stewart et al., 2014) and may be challenging for the physician who needs to recognize that many of the measures recommended in guidelines for disease entities may only be addressed in a long-term trusting relationship, or, sometimes, not at all. "Compromises may be required to account for the patient's context and sometimes progressive implementation of recommendations might represent a good alternative . . ." (Stewart and Fortin, 2014, p. 24). This requires the judicious exercise of what is known today as practical wisdom. Aristotle named it *phronesis* and described it as the primary virtue. Perhaps the Canadian writer Robertson Davies put it most succinctly calling it ". . . that breadth of spirit which makes the difference between the first rate healer and the capable technician" (Davies, 1996, p. 100).

REFERENCES

Agborsangaya CM, Lau D, Lahtinen M. 2012. Multimorbidity prevalence and patterns across socioeconomic determinants: A cross-sectional survey *BMC Public Health* 12:201.

American Geriatrics Society Expert Panel on the Care of Older Adults with Multimorbidity. 2012. Patient-centered care for older adults with multiple chronic conditions: a stepwise approach from the American Geriatrics Society *Journal of the American Geriatric Society* 60(10):1957–1968.

Barnett K, Mercer SW, Norbury M, Watt G, Wyke S, Guthrie B. 2012. Epidemiology of multimorbidity and implications for health care, research and medical education: A cross-sectional study. *Lancet* 380(9836):37–43.

Bayliss EA, Ellis JL, Steiner JF. 2009. Senior's self-reported multimorbidity captured biopsychosocial factors not incorporated into two other data-based morbidity measures. *Journal of Clinical Epidemiology* 62(5):550–557.

Bayliss EA. 2014. How does multimorbidity affect patients? In: Mercer SW, Salisbury C, Fortin C, eds., *ABC of Multimorbidity*, 1st ed. Chichester, West Sussex, UK: John Wiley and Sons.

Bayliss EA, Edwards AE, Steiner JF, Main DS. 2008. Processes of care desired by elderly patients with multimorbidities. *Family Practice* 25:287–293.

Boult C, Karm L, Groves C. 2008. Improving chronic care: The "Guided Care" model. *The Permanente Journal* 12(1):50–54.

Boyd CM, Darer J, Boult J, Fried LP, Boult L, Wu AW. 2005. Quality of care for older patients with multiple comorbid diseases: Implications for pay for performance. *Journal of the American Medical Association* 294(6):716–724.

Britten N. 2003. Commentary: Does a prescribed treatment match a patient's priorities? *BMJ* 327:841–842.

Broemeling AM, Watson DE, Prebtani F. 2008. Population patterns of chronic health conditions, co-morbidity and healthcare use in Canada: Implications for policy and practice. *Healthcare Quarterly* 11:70–76.

Chouinard M-C, Hudon C, Dubois M-F, Roberge P, Loignon C, Tchouaket E, Fortin M, Couture E-M, Sasseville M. 2013. Case management and self-mangement support for frequent users with chronic disease in primary care: Pragmatic randomized controlled trial. *BMC Health Services Research* 13:49.

Counsell SR, Callahan CM, Clark DO, Tu W, Buttar AB, Stump TE, Ricketts GD. 2007. Geriatric care management for low-income seniors: A randomized controlled trial. *Journal of the American Medical Association* 298(22):2623–2633.

Davies, R. 1996. Can a doctor be a humanist? In: Davies R, *The Merry Heart: Selections 1980–1995*. Toronto, ON: McClelland and Stewart.

Diedrichs CP, Wellmann J, Bartels DB, Ellert U, Hoffmann W, et al. 2012. How to weight chronic diseases in multimorbidity indices? Development of a new method on the basis of individual data from five population-based studies *Journal of Clinical Epidemiology* 65:679–685.

Dowell J, Williams B, Snadden D. 2007. *Patient-centred prescribing: Seeking concordance in practice*. Oxford, New York: Radcliffe Publishing.

Erny-Albrecht K, McIntyre E. 2013. The growing burden of multimorbidity. *PHCRIS RESEARCH ROUNDup* Issue 31, August.

Fortin M, Bravo G, Hudon C, Lapointe L, Dubois MF, Almirall J. 2006. Psychological distress and multimorbidity in primary care. *Annals of Family Medicine* 4(5):417–422.

Fortin M, Bravo G, Hudon C, Vanasse A, Lapointe L. 2005. Prevalence of multimorbidity among adults seen in family practice. *Annals of Family Medicine* 3(3):223–228.

Fortin M, Contant E, Savard C, Hudon C, Poitras M-E, Almirall J. 2011. Canadian guidelines for clinical practice: An analysis of their quality and relevance to the care of adults with comorbidity. *BMC Family Practice* 12:74.

Fortin M, Hudon C, Haggerty J, Akker MV, Almirall J. 2010. Prevalence estimates of multimorbidity: A comparative study of two sources. *BMC Health Services Research* 10:111.

Fortin M, Steenbakkers K, Hudon C, Poitras ME, Almirall J, van den Akker M. 2011. The electronic Cumulative Illness Rating Scale: A reliable and valid tool to assess multi-morbidity in primary care. *Journal of Evaluation in Clinical Practice* 17(6):1089–1093.

Fortin M, Stewart M, Poitras ME, Almirall J, Maddocks H. 2012. A systematic review of prevalence studies on multimorbidity: Toward a more uniform methodology *Annals of Family Medicine* 10(2):142–151.

Gaydos LM. 2012. The nature and etiology of disease. In: Fried BJ, Gaydos, LM, eds., *World Health Systems: Challenges and Perspectives*, 2nd ed. Chicago: Association of University Programs in Health Administration; Health Administration Press.

Gill A, Kuluski K, Jaakimainen L, Naganathan G, Upshur R. 2014. "Where do we go from here?" Health system frustrations expressed by patients with multimorbidity, their caregivers and family physicians. *Healthcare Policy* 9(4):73–89.

Guthrie B, Payne K, Alderson P, McMurdo ME, Mercer SW. 2012. Adapting clinical guidelines to take account of multimorbidity. *BMJ* 345:e6341.

Harrison C, Britt H, Miller G, Henderson J. 2014. Examining different measures of multimorbidity using a large prospective cross-sectional study in Australian general practice. *BMJ Open* 4(7):e004694. doi: 10.1136/bmjopen-2013-004694.

House JS, Lepkowski JM, Kinney AM, Mero RP Kessler RC, Herzog AR. 1994. The social stratification of aging and health. *Journal of Health and Social Behavior* 35(3):213–234.

Hughes LD, McMurdo MET, Guthrie B. 2013. Guidelines for people not for diseases: The challenges of applying UK clinical guidelines to people with multimorbidity. *Age and Ageing* 42(1):62–69.

LaReste JY, Nabbe P, Manceau B, Lygidakis C, Doerr C, Lingner H, Czachowski S, Munoz M, Argyriadou S, Claveria A, Le Floch B, Barais M, Bower P, Van Marwijk H, Van Royen P, Lietard C. 2013. The European General Practice Research Network presents a comprehensive definition of multimorbidity in family medicine and long term care, following a systematic review of relevant literature. *Journal of the American Medical Directors Association* 14(5):319–325.

Librero J, Peiro S, Ordinana R. 1999. Chronic comorbidity and outcomes of hospital care: Length of stay, mortality, and readmission at 30 and 365 days. *Journal of Clinical Epidemiology* 52:171–179.

Marengoni A, Winblad B, Karp A, Fratiglioni L. 2008. Prevalence of chronic diseases and multimorbidity among the elderly population in Sweden. *American Journal of Public Health* 98(7):1198–1200.

McLean G, Gunn J, Wyke S, Guthrie B, Watt GC, Blane DN, Mercer SW. 2014. The influence of socioeconomic deprivation and multimorbidity at different ages: A cross sectional study. *British Journal of General Practice* 64(624):e440–e447.

Mercer SW, Salisbury C, Fortin M. 2014. *ABC of Multimorbidity.* Oxford: John Wiley and Sons.

Muth C, van den Akker M, Blom JW, Mallen CD, Rochon J, Schellevis FG, Becker A, Beyer M, Gensichen J, Kirchner H, Perera R, Prados-Torres A, Scherer M, Thiem U, van den Bussche H, Glasziou PP. 2014. The Ariadne principles: How to handle multimorbidity in primary care consultations. *BMC Medicine* 12:223. doi: 10.1186/s12916-014-0223-1.

National Ambulatory Care Medical Survey. 2010. Table 16. http://www.cdc.gov/nchs/data/ahcd/namcs_summary/2010_namcs_web_tables.pdf.

Noel PH, Frueh C, Larme AC, Pugh JA. 2005. Collaborative care needs and preferences of primary care patients with multimorbidity. *Health Expectations* 8(1):54–63.

Pharmacist's Letter/Prescriber's Letter. September 2011. http://www.ngna.org/_resources/documentation/chapter/carolina_mountain/STARTandSTOPP.pdf.

Piette JD, Kerr EA. 2006. The impact of comorbid chronic conditions on diabetes care. *Diabetes Care* 29(3):725–731.

Ong BN, Richardson JC, Porter T, Grime J. 2014. Exploring the relationship between multi-morbidity, resilience and social connectedness across the lifecourse. *Health (London)* 18(3):302–318.

Riley V, Avery T, Jackson S. 2009. Pharmacokinetics and pharmacodynamics. In: Gosney M, Harris T, eds., *Managing Older People in Primary Care: A Practical Guide*. Oxford: Oxford University Press.

Sinnott C, McHugh S, Browne J, Bradley C. 2013. GPs' perspectives on the management of patients with multimorbidity: Systematic review and synthesis of qualitative research. *BMJ Open* 3:e003610.

Stewart MA, Brown JB, Weston WW, McWhinney IR, McWilliam CL, Freeman TR. 2014. *Patient-Centered Medicine: Transforming the Clinical Method*, 3rd ed. London; New York: Radcliffe Publishing.

Stewart MA, Fortin M. 2014. Multimorbidity and patient-centred care. In: Mercer SW, Salisbury C, Fortin M, eds., *ABC of Multimorbidity*.Chichester, West Sussex, UK: Wiley Blackwell, BMJ Books.

Townsend A. 2012. Applying Bourdieu's theory to accounts of living with multimorbidity. *Chronic Illness* 8(2):89–101.

Townsend A, Hunt K, Wyke S. 2003. Managing multiple morbidity in mid-life: A qualitative study of attitudes to drug use. *BMJ* 327:837.

Townsend A, Wyke S, Hunt K. 2006. Self-managing and managing self: Practical and moral dilemmas in accounts of living with chronic illness. *Chronic Illness* 2:185–194.

Tracy CS, Bell SH, Nickell LA, Charles J, Upshur REG. 2013. The IMPACT clinic: Innovative model of interprofessional primary care for elderly patients with complex health care needs. *Canadian Family Physician* 59(3):e148–e155.

Tucker-Seeley RD, Li Y, Sorensen G, Subramanian SV. 2011. Lifecourse socioeconomic circumstances and multimorbidity among older adults. *BMC Public Health* 11:313.

Upshur REG, Tracy S. 2008. Chronicity and complexity: Is what's good for the diseases always good for the patients? *Canadian Family Physician* 54(12):e1655–e1658.

Violan C, Foguet-Boreu Q, Flores-Mateo G, Salisbury C, Blom J, Freitag M, Glynn L, Muth C, Vladeras JM. 2014. Prevalence, determinants and patterns of multimorbidity in primary care: a systematic review of observational studies. *PLoS One* 9(7):e102149.

Violan C, Foguet-Boreu Q, Hermosilla-Perez E, Valderas JM, Bolibar B, Fabregas-Escurriola M, Brugulat-Guiteras P, Munoz-Perez MA. 2013. Comparison of information provided by electronic health records data and population health survey to estimate prevalence of selected health conditions and multimorbidity. *BMC Public Health* 13:251. doi: 10.1186/1471-2458-13-251.

PART III

The Practice of Family Medicine

CHAPTER 17

☙

Home Visits

If I wanted to discover whether a doctor had a vocation for personal care, I should begin by asking what he thought about housecalls.

Fox (1960, p. 751)

House calls are part of the legacy image of general practitioners, harkening back to the time of the "horse and buggy doctor." However, between Fox's statement and current times, the many changes in diseases, demographics, transportation, and technology have fundamentally altered the place of house calls or home visits in family practice. Despite all of this, a basic truth is still contained in Fox's observation. The family physician's willingness to engage patients in their own environment (rather than just the clinic or hospital) conveys, in a unique way, loyalty to the patient–physician relationship.

In the years following World War II, house calls remained a major part of the family physician's work. Influenza epidemics were dealt with in this way. In my (IRMcW) first practice in the 1950s and 1960s, these epidemics would lead to a change from our usual office practice. Patients knew that they were not to leave their homes. Phone calls would start to pour into the office. The office practice would be contained as far as possible, and the partners would divide up the home visits. Patients with complications such as pneumonia would either be transferred to hospital or, if not severe, would be visited daily. It was not unusual for the practice to make 100 home visits a day.

There has been a marked decline in home visits since that time, more noticeably in North America than in Europe, though evident there as well. In the United States in 1950, about 10% of patient encounters in family practice were in the home, and this fell to 1% by 1980 (Kao, Conant, and Soriano, 2009). In 2008 it was reported that family physicians made, on average, one house call per week (American Academy of Family Physicians, 2013). In Canada, 42.4% of family physicians responding to the National Physician Survey in 2010 stated that they offered house calls to their patients. This is down from 48.3% in the 2007 survey, and these figures do not tell us how many house calls were actually made. A survey done in the province of Quebec found that 58.1% of family physicians made house calls, mainly to elderly patients, with 42% seeing fewer than 5 patients each week, spending no more than 2 hours per week on this activity (Laberge, Aubin, Vezina, et al., 2000). Using billing claims data in the province of Ontario, Chan (2002) found that the provision of house calls by family physicians varied by age of practitioner. Fifty-seven percent of older, established physicians provided this service, but only 37% of younger physicians did so. In 1995 in Britain, 10% of all contacts between general practitioners and patients took place in the home (McCormick, Fleming, and Charlton, 1995). In the Netherlands, the proportion of patient contacts that were house calls fell from 17% in 1985 to 8.5% in 2001 (Jones, Schellevis, and Westert, 2004). In Europe, the average weekly number of home visits varied from 44 in Belgium to 2 in Portugal (Boerma, 2003). There are differences in the way practices are organized for home visits. In Europe it is often still the practice to set aside part of each day for home visits. In North America, some doctors set aside a half day each week for visiting patients with chronic illness. Visits for acute problems, however, are often fitted into a full office schedule.

There has been a great deal of concern about the "shrinking scope of practice" and the decline in comprehensiveness of care provided in family practice. In many studies (Chan, 2002; Wong and Stewart, 2010), providing care in a variety of settings, not just in the office, is essential to comprehensive care. Many reasons for this reduction in home visits have been offered. The general move of people from rural areas to the cities, leading to populations with higher density and more reliable transportation, means that it is easier for patients to come to the physician than was the case in the past. Technology, especially in diagnosis, has greatly advanced, and this is often available only in hospitals and outpatient departments. This has had a centralizing influence on the practice of medicine, but advances in point-of-care testing may help to mitigate this in the future. Reluctance to make house calls is also rooted in increased demands in office practice. As Ostbye and colleagues (2005) have pointed out, simply implementing the guidelines of the most common chronic conditions in the average-sized community practice exceeds the time available to the practitioner, leaving less time for home visits. Fear of litigation if there is a mistake in diagnosis or treatment, as well as relatively poor remuneration, also plays a role in the decline in the number of home visits carried out by family physicians. If this trend is to be changed, average practice sizes may need to be reduced and remuneration and support increased.

PRESSURES FOR MORE HOME VISITS

Changes in the healthcare system are now increasing the demand for home care. Elderly people—the largest group receiving home care—are an increasing proportion of the population. Admission to the hospital can be destabilizing for elderly patients, as well as exposing them to the risk of cross-infection. The cost of inpatient care has risen; patients are discharged home earlier; and new surgical techniques have reduced postoperative length of stay. Economic pressures have forced reductions in acute care beds, so that physicians are now faced with managing patients with complex illness in the home who would formerly have been admitted to the hospital.

Medical technologies since 1950 have been mainly a centralizing influence, requiring the concentration of patients in intensive care units. Many of the newer technologies now favor decentralization of care. Self-monitoring of blood glucose and blood pressure can be done in the home; ECG tracings and X-rays can be transmitted across a distance; equipment for home intravenous and subcutaneous therapy has been greatly simplified; and data can be electronically transmitted between home, hospital, laboratory, and office. Finally, many people strongly prefer home care to hospital admission. There is an increasing trend for dying patients to choose to spend their last days at home. Improvements in the medical management of serious disabilities and injuries have increased the number of disabled people of all ages living at home.

TYPES OF HOME VISITS

There are five types of home visits, defined by the underlying problem(s):

1. An acute problem. For example, a frail elderly person who has suffered a stroke. The physician`s role in this case is to make the diagnosis and coordinate the next level of care. This type of home visit is less likely in urban areas where, generally, transportation to a hospital is easily arranged and often occurs before a physician has assessed the patient. In rural and remote areas, family physicians continue to play an important role by making a home visit to make a provisional diagnosis and to determine, with the patient and family, the next steps.
2. The chronically ill and frail patient. Patients who are disabled and face difficulty in transportation are visited on a regular basis by the family physician to monitor their health and ability to cope. They may require the occasional additional visit if a new symptom arises and requires evaluation. The family physician's role in such cases is critical in ensuring that the necessary supports are in place to maintain the patient in his or her home environment. It is here that family practice intersects with other members of the

community service network. The development of team-based primary care also has the potential to expand this aspect of family practice. Some of these models integrate shared care with geriatric services, family physicians, and an interprofessional healthcare team (Counsell, Callahan, Clark, et al., 2007; Moore, Patterson, White, et al., 2012).

3. Similar to the second type of patient are those patients who are actively dying and require palliative care. We consider them a separate category only because there are many programs specifically devoted to palliative care. The goals of therapy are not fundamentally different from the chronically ill and frail patient who, in many cases, becomes a palliative care patient. Palliative care teams, based in the community, and consisting of palliative care physicians, family physicians, and nurses, were found to reduce ED visits and hospital admissions in the last 2 weeks of life, and patients receiving this service were more likely to die at home than was the case with patients who received usual care. Usual care in this case tended to be fragmented and highly variable (Seow, Brazil, Sussman, et al., 2014).

4. Acute and subacute illnesses, such as community-acquired pneumonia, in those with other chronic problems that might otherwise necessitate hospital admission. Admission avoidance programs have been developed and, to some extent, evaluated with mixed results. Generally, in these programs, the family physician works with a team of care providers such as nurse practitioners, respiratory therapists, physiotherapists, and so on. As stated in the name, the motivation for these programs has been to avoid more costly hospital admissions. The Integrating Physician's Services in the Home (IPSITH) project evaluated such an approach in the Canadian setting (Stewart, Sangster, Ryan, et al., 2010). Its purpose was to compare outcomes of a new home care program integrating general practitioners and nurses, measured against usual care. The patients involved were all acutely ill.

The infrastructure consisted of family physicians and their own patients, working with an experienced nurse practitioner, as well as a network of laboratories, diagnostics, pharmacies, and oxygen suppliers. The IPSITH process goals were prompt medical assessment, effective communication, close monitoring, and prompt response to crises.

The program was evaluated through a nonrandomized case comparison of the 82 IPSITH patients with the 82 usual care patients. The program included the usual care providers and the patient's family physicians, and the CCAC case manager, who had overall supervision for all patients. Forty-four family physicians enrolled in the program, and 29 of these enrolled patients. Thirty-nine specialists agreed to provide urgent consultations on request, and 18 agreed to see the patient in the home on request.

The illnesses enrolled by the physicians were skin infections (25), respiratory illness (14), dehydration (12), congestive heart failure (10), functional decline, dementia (3), urinary tract infection (4), gastrointestinal disorders (6), and others (8).

The key findings were that IPSITH was successful, and that the role of the nurse practitioner was crucial as a link between physician and patient. All the process goals were met. Patients strongly preferred home to hospital, as did caregivers, but less strongly. The physicians were somewhat in favor of home care. Time consumed and remuneration were the main barriers. However, most cases needed less than three home visits, and some none at all. The nurse practitioner minimized the need for doctor visits and was key to the success of the program. The team had better outcomes (fewer emergency room visits, and higher patient satisfaction) than the comparison group.

The New Brunswick Extramural Hospital has the legal status of a hospital and operates under the Public Hospitals Act, but is not outreach of an acute hospital (Ferguson, 1994). Patients may be admitted directly or upon discharge from a hospital admission. When applied to chronic disease management, this system is reported to result in an 85% reduction in hospital admissions and 55% decrease in ED visits (New Brunswick Extra-Mural Program: "Hospital Without Walls").

5. Patients recovering from an illness that required hospital admission. Early discharge programs are meant to safely send the hospitalized patient home earlier than usual practice. Just as in the fourth type, the motivation is to reduce hospital bed days and unnecessary readmissions and costs. Of the almost 40,000 patients served by the New Brunswick Extramural Hospital in 2011–2012, 37.1% were for rehabilitation services (The New Brunswick Extra-Mural Program Strategic Plan, 2013–2016). Optimally, the family physician, along with the community support network, is involved in such programs. Both four and five blur the boundary between conventional ideas of primary and secondary levels of care.

Some programs are designed for all of the above: admission avoidance, early discharge (and re-ablement), in-home chronic disease management, and palliative care (factsheet: ageUK, 2014). In the United Kingdom this was named Intermediate Care. At its inception the plan proposed 5000 extra intermediate care beds, to include community hospitals, nursing homes, and purpose-built facilities. An editorial (Wilson and Parker, 2003) explores general practitioners' attitudes toward intermediate care, their participation in schemes, and workload issues. Support of general practitioners as members of primary care trusts (PCTs) is regarded as crucial in the development of intermediate care. The National Service Framework (NSF) for older people believes that intermediate care services need to be integrated across services, including primary care.

An audit of Intermediate Care (National Audit of Intermediate Care Report, 2014) found wide variation and scale of services provided. Note was made that the capacity for this care was insufficient to meet the demand for services. Also, "[t]he proportion of home-based services relying on the service user's own GP for medical care appears high (72%) when reviewed against the levels of care being provided by these services." (p. 7)

The Royal College of General Practitioners (RCGP) and the General Practitioner Committee of the British Medical Association (BMA), in a joint statement, saw opportunities for the integration of care across primary, secondary, and social care boundaries. Threats included the inability of general practitioners to deliver, and diversion from their core functions as generalists. A significant increase of general practitioners would be needed.

The editorial continues to observe that little is known as to "grassroots" general practitioners' support for intermediate care. One survey found that support varied with the medical condition. Terminal care, chest infections, and stroke were supported by 50%–60%.

At the grassroots level, integration can be enhanced by attachment of home care nurses to group practices. This fosters working relationships between nurses and physicians, a factor that is often lacking in large home care organizations.

In home care, the physician is a key member of the team. If the doctor is prepared to be actively involved and to visit the home frequently, a very good relationship can develop with other team members, as well as with the patient and family. If, on the other hand, the physician remains on the sidelines, going only when called, then he or she can very easily become a marginal member of the team. We have seen this happening frequently with terminally ill cancer patients. In the absence of regular visits by the doctor, the main responsibility for care falls on the nurse. The nurse, patients, and family lose confidence in the physician; thus when a crisis occurs, it is not surprising that they seek help from other sources.

Home care means more than doing home visits. It means being prepared to become a member of a team caring for a seriously ill patient at home. It may, in some cases, mean visiting the patient every day, just as the doctor would if the patient were in the hospital. It means going even when there is "nothing to do." Our experience is that when a patient is seriously ill, there is never nothing to do. The most important outcome of the visit may be the support given to the patient, the family, and other members of the team.

When family physicians decline doing home visits as an outreach part of their office practice, other practitioners will fill the gap. Home-based primary care is one such response and aims to attend to patients only in the home (Stall, Nowaczynski, and Sinha, 2013a, 2013b). At this stage of development, it does not address how this integrates with other sectors of the healthcare system, including the patient's family physician. It has the potential to disrupt a long-term patient–doctor relationship at a time when the patient is in most need of it.

As the care of patients with serious illness is increasingly transferred to the home, it is difficult to see how physicians without a commitment to home care will be able to fulfill their commitments to their patients or maintain their clinical skills. It is often said that most home visits can be delegated to nurses. Although this is technically correct, family physicians should ponder the consequences of doing so. Visiting patients at home is one of the means by which bonds between a doctor and a family are forged and strengthened. A firsthand knowledge of the family home gives physicians an understanding of the patient and the family that they can gain in no other way. Moreover, the great enrichment of the doctor's own working life from caring for patients in their homes must not be underrated. Doctors who cut themselves off from home care risk losing their skills in the management of clinical problems such as congestive heart failure and advanced cancer. From the point of view of the patient, home care can be crucial. Norman Cousins, in his book *Anatomy of an Illness* (1979), has movingly described the peace of mind that comes from being cared for at home, even in serious illness.

REASONS FOR HOME VISITS

Most patients managed at home require conventional medical and nursing care, rather than high-level technology. The four highest-volume diagnoses for community home health beneficiaries in the United States in 2000 were diabetes, hypertension, heart failure, and chronic ulcer of the skin. In 2004, five diagnosis-related groups accounted for the majority of hospital discharges of Medicare patients to home health care: rehabilitation, joint procedure, heart failure and shock, pneumonia, and chronic obstructive pulmonary disease (National Association for Home Care and Hospice, 2010). Cancer patients, another large group, were presumably discharged to home hospice care rather than home health care.

ASSESSMENT OF PATIENTS IN THE HOME

Many aspects of clinical assessment are the same, whether done in the home, the office, or the hospital. In some ways, however, one can learn more from an assessment done in the home:

1. The home expresses the values and the history of the family.
2. Functional assessment (activities of daily living) can be done in patients' actual environment—their own stairs, toilet, and kitchen.
3. Hazards in the home can be identified and corrected—for example, by placing bars and rails in places where an elderly person is likely to fall.

4. Review of medications can include those in the medicine cabinet and other places, sometimes revealing duplicate prescriptions or incompatible drugs.
5. The impact on the family can be experienced directly. Physical and emotional exhaustion can be identified in caregivers before breakdown occurs.
6. The organization of the household and its suitability as a place for a patient with complex illness can be assessed directly.

Home visits can deepen a physician's understanding of a family. This enrichment is difficult to establish by conventional research methods because it is essentially subjective. Gray (1978) tells, for example, of a young woman who showed him a drawer full of baby clothes made for the baby she had lost. We have become aware of long-past bereavements by asking about family photographs in the home. Of course, this kind of information can be obtained from a good family history, but its quality is different. The knowledge is visceral. In an address on the importance of home visiting in child health, Cicely Williams (1973) commented that "practical experience in visiting homes and neighborhoods will provide more understanding in a single glance and five minutes of listening than will volumes of written questionnaires." (p. 778)

Researchers in home care note that some patients prefer providers to behave like guests and wish to preserve "face" in their interactions with providers. Often the visit from the family physician is preceded by preparations that convey perhaps more order and the appearance of wellness than is the usual case. We have found that personal care workers and housekeepers may provide a better sense of how a patient is actually coping. It is important to communicate with all members of the home healthcare team, rather than relying solely on one's own observations.

Appearance, dress, posture, voice, and habits (collectively called *habitus*) all depend on context. Illness and disability change the interface between a person's habitus and his or her interaction with the world. In the case of long-term home care, the logics of health care that emphasize expedience, cleanliness, standardization, and fiscal restraint drastically change a person's most private place in the world. As the home becomes cluttered with the paraphernalia of health care, such as commodes, walkers, oxygen tanks, and so on, the appearance of the home changes from a pleasing aesthetic to a very functional one (Angus, Kontos, Dyck, et al., 2005). For the patient, these necessary devices become a constant reminder of his or her physical deterioration (Case 17.1).

HOME CARE TECHNOLOGY

Advances in technology have made it possible to transfer many therapeutic procedures to the home setting:

CASE 17.1

On a home visit to a 76-year-old woman severely disabled by rheumatoid arthritis, osteoarthritis, spinal stenosis, and chronic anxiety disorder, I (TRF) found that one of her greatest sources of distress was the "clutter" of her small apartment. She wanted someone to take it all away and burn it. Assistive devices consisted of a wheeled walker and commode chair. Everything else, such as medications and TV controls, were kept close at hand to where she sat in a chair from which she rarely moved. Even when assistance was available to "clear the clutter," she lacked the mental energy to make the necessary decisions.

- Home parenteral nutrition
- Home enteral nutrition by nasogastric tube
- Drug delivery systems: pumps for administering drugs for diabetes, or cancer pain
- Intravenous (IV) antibiotic
- Blood transfusion
- Respiratory therapy: oxygen concentrators and cylinders, mechanical ventilation, tracheostomy management
- Renal and peritoneal dialysis.

In the United States, infusion therapy is the fastest growing sector of home care, with costs increasing from $1.5 billion in 1988 to $2.6 billion in 1990. Programs typically involve a team that may include nurse IV specialists, clinical pharmacists, infectious disease specialists, and social workers. Patients are trained in aseptic technique and recognition of drug reactions. Twenty-four-hour emergency care is a requirement for this service. Home care is not always provided by these programs, in which case patients have to attend as outpatients.

Home parenteral nutrition (HPN) has been made possible by developments such as the long-term in-dwelling Silastic catheter and has been shown to be cost-effective. Patients usually infuse solutions during a 10- to 12-hour period at night. HPN is organized through hospitals, and a home assessment is carried out to ensure that strict hygiene is observed. Training of patients in the technique takes place in the hospital. The main indications for HPN are as follows:

- Short bowel syndrome
- Nutrition combined with cancer chemotherapy

- Inflammatory bowel disease
- Chronic fistula of digestive tract
- Scleroderma of digestive tract.

HPN may be a long- or short-term therapy. HPN has been growing rapidly in the United States, where companies marketing nutritional support products have become involved in assessing, educating, and treating patients and monitoring the quality of care. Nutritional support teams are well established and typically consist of nurses, physicians, nutritionists, and pharmacists. In the United States in 2002, it was estimated that 39,000 individuals received HPN through Medicare (ASPEN, 2014). Use varies across nations. Usually the use of HPN is short term, but significant numbers of patients are using it long term as well. Complications can include sepsis, occlusions, liver disease, and metabolic bone disease.

Home enteral nutrition (HEN), which is sometimes called tube feeding, is also common. In France, which has a national registry of this service, the prevalence of HEN was 57.3/100,000 population (Lescot, Daudet, Leroy, et al., 2013).

Oxygen therapy is widely available at home, either by cylinder or oxygen concentrator, and is commonly prescribed for COPD. Mechanical ventilation in the home is used for respiratory failure caused by spinal cord injury or neuromuscular disease. It can be provided through a tracheostomy, by external pressure to the chest wall, or by intermittent positive pressure through a nasal mask. France has a national home respiratory care program. Twenty-eight regional organizations serve over 50,000 people with respiratory problems, 1200 of whom, in 1986, required prolonged ventilation assistance; and 12,000 received respiratory care for 12–24 hours a day. Ventilator-dependent patients and their families are vulnerable people and require well-organized support, with the assurance of a rapid response to crises. There is no margin for error, either in the equipment or in the support system (Goldberg and Faure, 1986; Goldberg, 1989, 1990).

Dialysis for end-stage renal disease (ESRD)—either renal or peritoneal (CAPD)—can be carried out in the home. However, home renal dialysis is only possible for the limited number of patients with the necessary home environment and family support. At present, home dialysis (HD) appears to be underutilized in Canada, with a prevalence rate of 4.0% compared to Australia's rate of 30% (Osterlund, Mendelssohn, Clase, et al., 2014).

THE QUALITY OF HOME CARE

The quality of medical care in the home should be as high as or higher than in the hospital. For patients with serious and complex illness, this places special responsibilities on the physician, including the following:

1. Readiness to respond quickly to crises
2. A deputizing arrangement that can provide the same level of service as the attending doctor
3. Maintenance of clinical records that are available to the home care nurse and to deputizing physicians
4. Communication with home care nurses and other team members, and with hospital and community services
5. Maintenance of skills in clinical management, including facility with new technologies—for example, pain control in advanced cancer.

In a systematic review and meta-analysis of five randomized controlled trials comparing admission avoidance hospital at home (HAH) with hospital inpatient care, it was found that there was a nonsignificant decrease in mortality for the HAH patients that reached significance at 6 months. Patients in the HAH also were more satisfied with their care. Patients in the HAH had a nonsignificant increase in admissions (Shepperd, Doll, Angus, et al., 2008).

Turning to early discharge programs, a systematic review and meta-analysis of 13 randomized control trials reported insufficient evidence of a difference in mortality between those patients with early discharge to an HAH, but a significant increase in readmissions for the elderly with multiple complex conditions (Shepperd, Doll, Broad, et al., 2009).

In assessing palliative care in the home, a review of randomized control trials, controlled clinical trials, controlled before and after studies, and interrupted time series found that patients admitted to such programs were more likely to die at home, and experience a reduced symptom burden when compared to usual care (Gomes, Calanzani, Curiale, et al., 2013).

COST OF HOSPITAL IN THE HOME

Admission avoidance HAH was found to be less expensive than admission to an acute care hospital (Shepperd, Doll, Angus, et al., 2008) in two trials, but early discharge HAH cost analyses were mixed (Shepperd, Doll, Broad, et al., 2009). Analyses of the cost-effectiveness of palliative care in the home also had mixed results (Gomes, Calanzani, Curiale, et al., 2013).

It appears that the HAH initiatives are on the increase and that many general practitioners are willing to care for their patients in their home provided that they are aided by nurse practitioners and are suitably remunerated. The idea of the hospital at home would fit well with primary care groups, which are growing in many parts of the world. HAH can provide many kinds of care, from short-term illnesses to long-term disabilities and housebound aged, to the dying. Issues for general practitioners in these models are the need to maintain competence in the field and arrangement for deputizing or being on call.

WHAT ABOUT THE HOMELESS?

Attention to the marginalized of society has always been a core activity of family medicine. Homeless individuals remain a significant issue in our cities and present unique challenges when attending to their needs. In Canada it is estimated that in any year there are between 150,000 and 300,000 homeless individuals (The Homeless Hub). In the United States, in 2013, the point prevalence of homeless individuals was estimated to be 610,042. Two-thirds were in shelters, and the remaining one-third were in unsheltered locations such as under bridges, in cars, or in abandoned buildings (Henry, Cortes, and Morris, 2013). Most do not have a family doctor and face difficulty in accessing basic health care (Khandor, Mason, Chambers, et al., 2011). Programs such as Palliative Education and Care for the Homeless (PEACH) in the city of Toronto seeks to extend palliative care to the homeless (The Homeless Hub). Street medicine is becoming an area of focused practice, and websites exist to share lessons from around the world (Doctors for Homeless).

During the 14 years of my first practice, I have carried out thousands of home visits (IRMcW). There were few patients whose homes I had not visited. As I drove or walked through the town or the surrounding countryside, I received pleasure from thinking of the stories I had heard or the scenes I had witnessed in the houses I passed. Sometimes there would be sadness, and sometimes guilt at one of my failures. We were able to see our housebound patients because our practice only covered 6 miles in each direction. In the times when home visits were the norm, it was natural for practices to have geographic boundaries. In North America now there are many practices scattered far and wide. If we are to rebuild home visits as integral to our practices for our housebound patients, we will need to draw geographic boundaries again. Eventually, these geographic practices could form networks, enabling health services to deal effectively with global pandemics.

REFERENCES

American Academy of Family Physicians. 2013. *Table 6: Average Number of Family Physician Patient Encounters per Week by Setting (as of December 2013).* http:// www.aafp.org/about/the-aafp/family-medicine-facts/table-6.html.   A.S.P.E.N. 2014. *Sustain Home Parenteral Nutrition.* American Society for Parenteral and Enteral Nutrition. http://www.nutritioncare.org/aspen_sustain/about_sustain.

Angus J, Kontos P, Dyck I, McKeever P, and Poland B. 2005. The personal significance of home: Habitus and the experience of receiving long-term home care. *Sociology of Health & Illness* 27(2):161–187.

Boerma WGW. 2003. *Profiles of General Practice in Europe: An International Study of Variation in the Tasks of General Practitioners.* Utrecht, The Netherlands: Nivel.

Chan BTB. 2002. The decline of comprehensiveness of primary care. *Canadian Medical Association Journal* 166(4):429–434.

Counsell SR, Callahan CM, Clark DO, et al. 2007. Geriatric care management for low-income seniors: A randomized controlled trial. *Journal of the American Medical Association* 298(22):2623–2633.

Cousins N. 1979. *Anatomy of an Illness as Perceived by the Patient.* New York: W. W. Norton.

Doctors for Homeless. Sharing street medicine lessons at http://www.doctorsforhomeless.org/.

Factsheet: ageUK. 2014. Factsheet 76. September 2014. http://www.ageuk.org.uk/Documents/EN-GB/Factsheets/FS76_Intermediate_care_and_re-ablement_fcs.pdf?dtrk=true.

Ferguson G. 1994. *The New Brunswick Extra Mural Hospital (EMH), From Dream to Reality.* Fredericton: New Brunswick Department of Health and Wellness.

Fox TF. 1960. The personal doctor and his relation to the hospital: Observations and reflections on some American experiments in general practice by groups. *The Lancet* (April 2) 277(7180):743–760.

Goldberg AI. 1989. Home care for life-supported persons: The French system of quality control, technology assessment and cost containment. *Public Health Reports* 104(4): 329.

Goldberg AI. 1990. Mechanical ventilation and respiratory care in the home in the 1990's: Some personal observations. *Respiratory Care* 35(3):247.

Goldberg AI, Faure EAM. 1986. Home care for life-supported persons in France: The regional association. *Rehabilitation Literature* 47: 3–4, 60–64.

Gomes B, Calanzani N, Curiale V, McCrone P, Higginson IJ. 2013. Effectiveness and cost-effectiveness of home palliative care services for adults with advanced illness and their caregivers. *Cochrane Database of Systematic Reviews* 2013, Issue 6. Art. No.: CD007760. doi: 10.1002/14651858.CD007760.pub2.

Gray DJ. 1978. Feeling at home. *Journal of the Royal College of General Practitioners* 28:6.

Henry M, Cortes A, Morris S. *The 2013 Annual Homeless Assessment Report (AHAR) to Congress.* US Department of Housing and Urban Development. https://www.hudexchange.info/resources/documents/ahar-2013-part1.pdf.

The Homeless Hub. www.homelesshub.ca.

Jones R, Schellevis F, Westert G. 2004. The changing face of primary care: The second Dutch national survey. *Family Practice* 21(6):597–598.

Kao H, Conant R, Soriano T, McCormick W. 2009. The past, present, and future of house calls. *Clinics in Geriatric Medicine* 25(1):19–34.

Khandor E, Mason K, Chambers, C, Rossiter K, Cowan L, Hwang S. 2011. Access to primary health care among homeless adults in Toronto, Canada: Results from the Street Health survey. *Open Medicine* 5(2):94–103.

Laberge A, Aubin M, Vezina L, Bergeron R. 2000. Delivery of home health care: Survey of the Quebec region. *Canadian Family Physician* 46:2022–2029.

Lescot P, Daudet L, Leroy M, Daniel N, Alix E, Bertin E, et al. 2013. Incidence and prevalence of home enteral nutrition in France. *Nutrition Clinique et Metabolisme* 27(4):171–177.

McCormick A, Fleming D, Charlton J. 1995. *Morbidity Statistics from General Practice: Fourth National Study 1991–1992.* London: Her Majesty's Stationery Office.

Moore A, Patterson C, White J, et al. 2012. Interprofessional and integrated care of the elderly in a family health team. *Canadian Family Physician* 58(8): 436–441.

National Association for Home Care and Hospice. 2010. *Basic Statistics about Home Care*. http://www.nahc.org/assets/1/7/10HC_Stats.pdf.

National Audit of Intermediate Care Report. 2014. http://www.nhsbenchmarking.nhs. uk/CubeCore/.uploads/icsurvey/NAIC%202013/NAICNationalReport2013.pdf.

New Brunswick Extra-Mural Program. *Hospital Without Walls*. http://files.canadianhealthcarenetwork.ca/pdf/CHM/ehealthsummit/2012/eHS%202012_09_ Bustard.pdf.

New Brunswick Extra-Mural Program Strategic Plan. 2013–2016. https://www.gnb. ca/0051/0384/pdf/strategic_plan-e.pdf.

Ostbye T, Yarnall KS, Krause KM, Pollak KI, Gradison M, Michener JL. 2005. Is there time for management of patients with chronic diseases in primary care? *Annals of Family Medicine* 3(3): 209–214.

Seow H, Brazil K, Sussman J, Pereira J, Marshall D, Austin PC, Husain A, Rangrej J, Barbera L. 2014. Impact of community based, specialist palliative care teams on hospitalisations and emergency department visits late in life and hospital deaths: a pooled analysis. *BMJ* 348:g3496.

Shepperd S, Doll H, Angus RM, Clarke MJ, Iliffe S, Kalra L, Ricauda NA, Wilson AD. 2008. Hospital at home admission avoidance. *Cochrane Database of Systematic Reviews* 2008, Issue 4. Art. No.: CD007491. doi: 10.1002/14651858.CD007491.

Shepperd S, Doll H, Broad J, Gladman J, Iliffe S, Langhorne P, Richards S, Martin F, Harris R. 2009. Hospital at home early discharge. *Cochrane Database of Systematic Reviews* 2009, Issue 1. Art. No.: CD000356. doi: 10.1002/14651858.CD000356. pub3.

Stall N, Nowaczynski, Sinha SK. 2013a. Back to the future: Home-based primary care for the older homebound Canadians. Part 1: Where we are now. *Canadian Family Physician* 59(3):237–240.

Stall N, Nowaczynski, Sinha SK. 2013b. Back to the future: Home-based primary care for older homebound Canadians. Part 2: Where we are going. *Canadian Family Physician* 59(3):243–245.

Stewart M, Sangster JF, Ryan BL, et al. 2010. Integrating physician services in the home: Evaluation of an innovative program. *Canadian Family Physician* 56(11): 1166–1174.

Williams CD. 1973. Health services in the home. *Pediatrics* 52(6): 773–781.

Wilson A, Parker H. 2003. Guest editorial: Intermediate care and general practitioners, an uncertain relationship. *Health and Social Care in the Community* 11(2):81–84.

Wong E, Stewart M. 2010. Predicting the scope of practice of family physicians. *Canadian Family Physician* 56(6):e219–e225.

CHAPTER 18

⌒∿⌒

Stewardship of Resources, Patient Information, and Data

Healthcare Resources

Virtually every nation struggles with the increasing cost of health care. In developed nations there has been a steady rise in healthcare costs, leading to considerable efforts to "bend the cost curve." Middle and lower income countries struggle to provide basic public health services to their populations and frequently lack the fundamental infrastructure to bring this about. The Commonwealth Fund keeps track of expenditures on the health and performance of 11 countries. Using a standard evaluation comparing healthcare quality, access, efficiency, and equity, as well as indicators of healthy lives such as infant mortality, the United States and Canada are ranked 11th and 10th of the 11 nations studied. At the top of the list in the 2014 were the United Kingdom, followed by Switzerland. In 2011 the United States spent \$8,508/ capita on health care, whereas the United Kingdom spent \$4,405/capita (Mossialos, Wenzl, and Osborn, 2014). Clearly, the United Kingdom received much better outcomes for considerably less cost. These kinds of international comparisons have spurred initiatives designed to improve the efficiency of health service delivery. Even within a single nation, there is considerable variation in the costs of medical care (Fisher, Bynum, and Skinner, 2009).

The reasons for rising healthcare costs are many and complex. Changing demographics, the increased availability of new and expensive technologies and treatments, patient and physician expectations, and defensive medicine all play a role in these costs. Physicians are sometimes viewed as "cost centers" in discussions about the economics of health care, as their clinical activity generates costs in investigations, medications, hospitalization, and follow-up visits.

Physicians are accountable not only to their patients, but also to society as a whole and have an obligation to take part in addressing healthcare costs. Typically these discussions, especially at the political level, avoid the term *rationing* and prefer *cost management* or *prioritizing*. The reality, however, is that rationing is not avoidable. Failure to address this results in inequitable allocation of resources, which itself carries a heavy ethical and even financial burden. Meeting the rising costs can be done by increasing the amount a nation spends on health, either privately or through government-sponsored insurance (and ultimately higher taxes), or by narrowing the boundaries of health care (Randall, 2000), reducing the range of what is covered. A third route, and one often preferred by policymakers, is to seek greater efficiency in the system. This avoids making difficult and contentious decisions while appearing to be doing something (Neumann, 2012).

The work of Starfield and others (Starfield, Shi, and Macinko, 2005; Macinko, Starfield, and Erinosho, 2009) has demonstrated that countries whose healthcare systems have a strong primary care sector deliver care that is less expensive and that produces better outcomes. Family physicians are important contributors to efficiency in care delivery. They provide comprehensive and continuing care close to the patient's home, institute preventive medicine, and ensure that the referral of patients to the more expensive secondary and tertiary levels of care is appropriate. In doing this, they keep things in proportion and protect their patients from "the zealous specialist" (Fox, 1960).

Nevertheless, improved quality and efficiency of care at all levels of the healthcare system, including primary care, remains a necessity. For the US health system, there has been a call for a "Triple Aim" (Berwick, Nolan, and Whittington, 2008), which consists of improving the experience of care, improving the health of populations, and reducing the per capita costs of health care. In observing the wide geographic variation in healthcare costs in the United States, Brody (2010) estimated that if physicians in high-cost areas ordered tests similar to physicians in low-cost areas, it would result in saving one-third of healthcare costs in that country without a loss of benefit to any patient. He recommended the development of a list of the top five diagnostic tests or treatments that are commonly ordered, but for which evidence of benefit to at least some major category of patients is lacking or weak, and suggested that physicians cease ordering them. This notion has been embraced more widely, and lists have been developed for many medical specialties, including family medicine, pediatrics, and internal medicine (Smith, 2011; Kuehn, 2012). It is recognized that educating physicians to avoid these tests and treatments is not sufficient, however. Patients also need to become aware that what has been commonly done in the past is not effective. The National Physician Alliance (NPA) offers free educational materials online for patients and physicians to aid in this. It is recognized that altering physician and patient behavior is much more complex, however. It involves system-level factors, such as the method of physician remuneration and favoring volume over value. The Choosing Wisely (www.choosingwisely.org/doctor-patients-lists) campaign was launched in 2012 and has become a worldwide movement intended to reduce unnecessary tests and procedures in medical care (Hudzik, Hudzik, and Polonski, 2014). Several commercial partners, including Consumer Reports, are aiding in the effort to keep the public informed about this movement.

In seeking health care that has high value and yet is conscious of costs, it is important to recognize that measuring costs alone is not sufficient. Measures that have high cost may provide high value and should be retained. Alternatively, low-cost measures may provide low value and should be stopped. Such calculations must take into account the "downstream costs," those that become evident much later. It may be that higher up-front costs of an intervention are more than compensated by later savings (Owens et al., 2011; Qaseem et al., 2012). A simple example of this in family practice is vaccine programs, whose attendant costs, including vaccine manufacture, distribution, storage, and administration, are more than paid for by reduced illnesses, hospitalization, and deaths later in time.

Undertaking cost–benefit analyses and calculations of value requires a great deal of expertise and time. It is not uncommon to describe a cost-effectiveness threshold when evaluating two beneficial interventions that differ in cost. The cost-effectiveness threshold describes how much a decision-maker is willing to pay for one additional unit of quality adjusted life years (QALY). Clearly such decisions are value judgments and will depend on who the decision-maker is. Such calculations are more relevant to policy-makers and healthcare planners. The necessary information for this type of calculation in family practice is generally not available. Calculations based on experience in the hospital setting are not transferable to family practice for a variety of reasons, including differences in disease prevalence, availability of resources, and need to respect patient values (over institutional or system values). Decisions are not generally made on the basis of precise mathematical computations but involve attitudes to risk and the personal value and meaning of health. Thresholds for treatment may be quite different for patients and physicians. For example, it was found that in evaluating the use of either warfarin or aspirin to prevent strokes in those with atrial fibrillation, patients required less reduction of stroke and were more tolerant of increased bleeding than were physicians (Devereux, Anderson, Gardner, et al., 2001). This study was done in a tertiary care site and needs to be replicated in community practice. The family physician's task is to present available options to patients in a way that they can understand, to help them clarify their own values, and to recognize and respect that their thresholds may vary over time and context.

Focusing on physicians' behavior is central to the idea of quaternary prevention (see Chapter 10, "The Enhancement of Health and the Prevention of Disease"). Adopted by WONCA, it aims to avoid over-medicalization of patients (Jamoulle, 2015), and this will also help to reduce unnecessary costs of health care.

Bringing about changes as recommended by guidelines or by the Choosing Wisely campaign requires the physician to change behavior in the examining room with patients. This is best accomplished through the patient-centered clinical method (see Chapter 9, "Clinical Method"). Epstein and colleagues (2005) found that physicians who scored low on measures of patient-centeredness ordered more diagnostic tests than those who scored higher, and this effect remained even after controlling for the shorter visit length characteristic of low-scoring physicians. Stewart, Ryan, and Bodea (2011) found that mean diagnostic tests in the 2 months following an index visit were substantially lower in those who scored in the highest quartile of a measure of patient-centeredness than physicians in the lowest quartile ($11.46 vs. $29.48). Clearly, encouraging a patient-centered approach, as well as producing better outcomes, must be a part of any initiative to reduce costs. It seems likely that the lower overall healthcare costs that Starfield observed in countries with strong primary care are, at least in part, mediated through the practice of patient-centered medicine.

PATIENT INFORMATION AND DATA

He is the objective witness of their lives . . . the clerk of their records. . . . It is an honorary position.
Berger (1967, p. 109)

. . . the record is the principal means to understand and monitor how the entire enterprise of medicine functions.
Reiser (2009, p. 103)

These two quotes represent the bookends of the evolution of the medical record in the last half of the twentieth century. The first relates to the role of a country general practitioner in 1950s Great Britain. The latter quote encapsulates the central importance occupied by the electronic health record (EHR)[1] in the twenty-first century.

As comprehensively detailed by Reiser (2009), the concept of a medical record of any kind was a project of the twentieth century and was initiated by hospitals to report to their funders. It received support for both educational and research reasons, but principally reflected the experience of the medical practitioner only. As more care providers became engaged in clinical care (such as nurses and medical social workers) and as laboratory and medical investigations became more numerous, there was a need to expand the record beyond just the observations of the physician. Organizing all of this information became a challenge, and in the 1970s the Problem-Oriented Medical Information System (PROMIS) was designed to facilitate communication across the range of care providers and to support clinical standards (Weed, 1971). Though developed in the hospital system, the PROMIS was adapted widely in family practice as well. As more people became involved in the care of patients, the record moved from being a medical record to a health record and assumed the role of integrator. Healthcare administrators and insurance carriers, whether private or government sponsored, are interested in costs, regulatory compliance, and quality, and thus have an interest in the practices and outcomes of the clinical world. Patients themselves are becoming more engaged in their health care and the content of their records. All of these changes have increased the expectations and directions in the development and evolution of the electronic health record.

The promise of information technology (IT) in health care goes beyond the health record and encompasses telemedicine, mobile devices, electronic appointments, social media, and so on. Attaching mobile devices to smartphones (e.g., blood pressure cuffs, glucose machines, ECG machines, ultrasound echocardiograms, and, of course, cameras) expands what is possible in point-of-care testing and patient self-monitoring (Cohn, 2013). Enthusiasts see this "disruptive technology" as important in driving down healthcare costs and improving the quality of health care. The uptake and range of uses of electronic records in primary care has received so much attention that it is sometimes used as a proxy for meaningful investment in this sector of health care.

Potential uses of health IT include personal medical records; personalized health reminders and follow-up; personal health, diet, and activity monitoring and motivation; pre-degree and continuing medical education; real-time clinical decision support; remote professional consultation and care; monitoring and advising of patients with chronic disease; quality assurance; performance assessment of providers and institutions; comparative outcomes research; matching of potential participants to clinical trials; monitoring for safety (or unanticipated benefits) of drugs, devices, diagnostic tests, surgery, and other treatments; enhanced peer-to-peer and professional–patient support; comparative health assessments across populations, communities, cities, and states; and public health surveillance for disease outbreaks, environmental risks, and potential bioterrorism (Fineberg, 2012). Others see the potential of replacing all or a major part of physicians' work, either by integrated IT systems alone or by use of lower cost healthcare workers supported by such systems (Khosla, 2012). Obviously, these are ambitious goals and are not easily attained.

Surveys of 10 countries in 2009 and again in 2012 found that uptake of electronic records in family and general practices increased, but varied between 41% and 98% of those surveyed. Capacity of those records for other functions (e.g., generating patient information, generating panel information, order entry management, and routine clinical decision support) and electronic exchange with other doctors was much lower (Schoen, Osborn, Squires, et al., 2012). The National Physician Survey of Canadian physicians in 2014 found that 42.2% of family physicians were using electronic records exclusively to enter and retrieve patient clinical notes. A further 37.5% were using a combination of paper and electronic charts for these purposes, suggesting that they were in a period of transition from paper to e-records (National Physician Survey, 2014). In the same survey, in response to the question "What electronic functions are you planning to use in the next two years?" the most common functionalities were entry and retrieval of patient notes, followed by medications taken by patients, and lab/diagnostic test results. Clearly, family physicians are not moving quickly in the direction of the vision outlined by enthusiasts.

Why might family physicians be reluctant to adopt this technology? A pan-Canadian study by Terry and colleagues (Terry, Stewart, Fortin, et al., 2014) examining this question found several themes: doubts remain about whether the benefits of electronic medical records (EMRs) had been adequately demonstrated; uncertainty about the optimal ways to implement EMRs into practice; continued tension between codified entry of information rather than free form entry (reflecting concern about losing the nuances or context of the patient encounter); and lack of agreement and understanding of data sharing. There is a need for further research in all these areas. Others have raised deeper concerns. As Reiser (2009) points out, computers are best at storing information and cannot, realistically, mimic a clinician's thinking given the subtle nature of human communication. Nevertheless, any technology, especially intellectual technologies, have profound effects on those who use them. "Every intellectual technology embodies an intellectual ethic, a set of assumptions about how the human mind works, or should work" (Carr, 2010, p. 45). Electronic records, more so than paper records, act as a filtering tool that dictates, sometimes overtly and sometimes covertly, what is to be recorded. There is realistic concern that what isn't required in the record will cease to take place in the encounter. The increased understanding of the neuroplasticity of the human brain provides a clue to how it is that our technologies shape us. "Whenever we use a tool to exert greater control over the outside world, we change our relationship with that world" (Carr, 2010, p. 212). The richness that characterizes the clinical encounter in family practice becomes shrunk to an alphanumeric code. There are also real concerns that as managers and governments continue to control healthcare costs, the EMR and the EHR will become a "prescriptive technology" closely tied to outside standards and remuneration (Franklin, 1999).

Adoption of EHRs in practice seem to be related to physician satisfaction with practice insofar as they are perceived as improving quality of care (Friedberg, Chen, Van Busum, et al., 2013). For physicians in this study, these benefits were perceived as potential at this time, and yet to be realized. On the other hand, the negative effects of EHRs were perceived to be more immediate and included poor usability, time-consuming data entry, interference with face-to-face patient care, inefficient and less fulfilling work content, inability to exchange health information between EHR products, and degradation of clinical documentation.

Many of the problems in the usage of EHRs will be addressed and improved upon. The generation of family physicians who started their careers with paper records and moved to electronic records (the digitally naïve) are giving way to the newer generation (the digitally native), who are more comfortable with the technology, and it is reasonable to expect that some of the problems cited earlier will lessen, but doubtless will be replaced by new ones. There are strong social, economic, and political forces involved in EHRs and the broader world of health IT. Among the social forces pertinent to health records is the rise of the "consumer" voice. Increasingly custodial stewardship of the medical record, in the past solely a physician role, is becoming a collaboration between physician and patient.

Family physicians must take care to be involved in the evolution of the technology and guide it in a direction that respects the values of the discipline. Reiser (2009) uses the example of the introduction of the stethoscope into medical practice and points out that it served to transform the relationship between the patient and the physician. The physician transferred attention from what patients were saying to the "sound produced by their organs." It was a distancing technology. Nevertheless, physicians incorporated the technology of the stethoscope (though it is being superseded by newer imaging technologies such as echocardiography) and learned to listen to the patient as well. The challenge for family physicians is to similarly incorporate the EHRs and other health technologies while continuing to listen to the patient.

BIG DATA

The increasingly widespread use of EHRs is generating massive amounts of data. As pointed out by Murdoch and Detsky (2013), some of this is quantitative (e.g., laboratory values), some is qualitative (e.g., text-based documents and demographics), and some is transactional (e.g., records of medication administered). The development of newer analytic techniques from computer sciences makes it possible to deal with disparate types of data. The uses of such data in health care might include generating new knowledge through computational techniques such as natural language processing applied to free-texts in medical records; knowledge dissemination by analyzing existing EHRs to produce a dashboard that guides clinical decisions; integrating personalized medicine into clinical practice; and linking traditional health data to other personal data, thus integrating the traditional medical model with social determinants of health. "The first information technology revolution in medicine is the digitization of the medical record. The second is surely to leverage the information contained therein and combine it with other sources" (Murdoch and Detsky, 2013, p. 1352).

SUMMARY

- Healthcare costs are rising, and family physicians must become engaged in identifying and reducing unnecessary tests and treatments.
- A strong primary care sector in health care reduces costs at a population level.
- Using the patient-centered clinical method helps to reduce costs at the individual level.
- The medical record has evolved from an *aide-memoire* for the physician to a health record whose contents are of interest to a much wider audience. It has become a collaboration between the physician and the patient.
- Secondary use of the information in EHRs needs appropriate oversight to protect the privacy of both patients and physicians, and physicians must be involved in developing and participating in this oversight (College of Physicians and Surgeons of Alberta, 2009).
- Family physicians, individually and through their associations and regulatory colleges, must be involved in ensuring appropriate use of the data emerging from EHRs and new health technologies in a way that benefits patients.
- Data and information are not the same as knowledge, and the role of the family physician and patient in generating knowledge and meaning in health and illness remains central in the patient–physician relationship (see Chapter 6, "Philosophical and Scientific Foundations of Family Medicine").

NOTE

1. In this chapter, Electronic medical record (EMR) refers to the electronic record of the physician's findings, investigations, and treatment. Electronic health record (EHR) refers to the electronic record of all providers involved in the patient's care, including the physician.

REFERENCES

Berger J, Mohr J. 1967. *A Fortunate Man.* New York: Pantheon Books, a division of Random House.

Berwick DM, Nolan TW, Whittington. 2008. The Triple Aim: Care, health and cost. *Health Affairs* 27(3):759–769.

Brody H. 2010. Medicine's ethical responsibility for health care reform: The top five list. *New England Journal of Medicine* 362(4):283–285.

Carr N. 2010. *The Shallows: What the Internet is Doing to Our Brains.* New York: W. W. Norton.

Cohn J. 2013. The robot will see you now: Is your doctor becoming obsolete? *The Atlantic:* March, 2013:59–67.

College of Physicians and Surgeons of Alberta. 2009. *Data Stewardship: Secondary Use of Health Information.* http://www.cpsa.ab.ca/Libraries/Res/Secondary_Use_of_Health_Information_-_Final_December_2009.pdf.

Devereaux PJ, Anderson DR, Gardner MJ, et al. 2001. Differences between perspectives of physicians and patients on anticoagulation in patients with atrial fibrillation: Observational study. Commentary: Varied preferences reflect the reality of clinical practice. *BMJ* 323:1218.

Epstein RM, Franks P, Shields CG, Meldrum MS, Miller KN, Campbell TL, Fiscella K. 2005. Patient-centered communication and diagnostic testing. *Annals of Family Medicine* 3(5):415–421.

Fineberg HV. 2012. A successful and sustainable health system: How to get there from here. *New England Journal of Medicine* 366:1020–1027.

Fisher ES, Bynum JP, Skinner JS. 2009. Slowing the growth of health care costs: Lessons from regional variation. *New England Journal of Medicine* 360(9):849–852.

Fox TF. 1960. The personal doctor: And his relation to the hospital. *The Lancet* 275 (7127): 743–760 (April 2).

Franklin U. 1999. *The Real World of Technology*, rev. ed. Toronto: Anansi.

Friedberg MW, Chen PG, Van Busum KR, et al. 2013. *Factors Affecting Physician Professional Satisfaction and Their Implications for Patient Care, Health Systems, and Health Policy.* Santa Monica, CA: RAND. http://www.rand.org/content/dam/rand/pubs/research_reports/RR400/RR439/RAND_RR439.pdf.

Hudzik B, Hudzik M, Polonski L. 2014. Choosing wisely: Avoiding too much medicine *Canadian Family Physician* 60:873–876.

Jamoulle M. 2015. Quaternary prevention: An answer of family doctors to overmedicalization. *International Journal of Health Policy Management* 4(2):61–64.

Khosla V. 2012. *Do We Need Doctors or Algorithms?* http://techcrunch.com/2012/01/10/doctors-or-algorithms/.

Kuehn BM. 2012. Movement to promote good stewardship of medical resources gains momentum. *Journal of the American Medical Association* 307:218.

Macinko J, Starfield B, Erinosho T. 2009. The impact of primary healthcare on population health in low- and middle-income countries. *Journal of Ambulatory Care Management* 32(2):150–171.

Mossialos E, Wenzl M, Osborn R, Anderson C. 2014. *International Profiles of Healthcare Systems.* The Commonwealth Fund, New York.

Murdoch TB, Detsky AS. 2013. The inevitable application of big data to health care. *Journal of the American Medical Association* 309(13):1351–1352.

National Physicians Alliance. http://npalliance.org/.

National Physician Survey. *2014 Results for Family Physicians*. http://nationalphysiciansurvey.ca/result/2014-results-family-physicians/

Neumann PJ. 2012. What we talk about when we talk about health care costs. *New England Journal of Medicine* 366(7):585.

Smith S. 2011. The "top 5" lists in primary care: Meeting the responsibility of professionalism. *Archives of Internal Medicine* 171(15):1385–1390.

Owens DK, Qaseem A, Chou R, Shekelle P. 2011. High-value, cost-conscious health care: concepts for clinicians to evaluate the benefits, harms, and costs of medical interventions. *Annals of Internal Medicine* 254(3):174–180.

Qaseem A, Alguire P, Dallas P, et al. 2012. Appropriate use of screening and diagnostic tests to foster high-value, cost-conscious care. *Annals of Internal Medicine* 156(2):147–149.

Randall F. 2000. Judgement and resource management. Chapter 5 in Downie RS, Macnaughton J (eds.), *Clinical Judgement: Evidence in Practice*. Oxford: Oxford University Press.

Reiser, SJ. 2009. *Technological Medicine: The Changing World of Doctors and Patients*. New York: Cambridge University Press.

Schoen C, Osborn R, Squires D, et al. 2012. A survey of primary care doctors in ten countries shows progress in use of health information technology, less in other areas. *Health Affairs (Millwood)* 31(12):2805–2816.

Starfield B, Shi L, Macinko J. 2005. The contribution of primary care to health systems and health. *The Millbank Quarterly*; 83(3):457–502.

Stewart MA, Ryan BL, Bodea C. 2011 Is patient-centred care associated with lower diagnostic costs? *Healthcare Policy* 6(4):27–31.

Terry AL, Stewart MA, Fortin M, et al. 2014. Gaps in primary healthcare electronic medical record research and knowledge: Findings of a pan-Canadian study. *Healthcare Policy* 10(1):46–59.

Weed LL. 1971. *Medical Records, Medical Education, and Patient Care*. Cleveland, OH: Press of Case Western Reserve University.

CHAPTER 19

✧

Practice Management

A family doctor's effectiveness depends not only on clinical skills, but also on managerial ability. Poor practice management can lead to poor patient care, public dissatisfaction, and demoralization of the doctor and his or her staff. This chapter will concentrate on the central management question of family practice: *the allocation of limited resources to meet the needs and demands for care in such a way as to respect the values of family medicine.* The word *limited* is used advisedly. Even in the most affluent societies, resources are insufficient to meet every need and every demand. Every family physician must, therefore, be involved in the process of assessing needs, establishing priorities, and allocating resources. A management process is illustrated in Figure 19.1 that is applicable to solo practitioners, group practices, and teams. As indicated on the flow chart, the process is a cyclical one, with feedback from the evaluation leading to a re-examination of objectives, priorities, and practice procedures.

FORMULATION OF OBJECTIVES

In the first instance, objectives are determined by the values of the practice and the expectations of the patients. Prominent among them will be the values of family medicine, such as accessibility of the doctor, availability of the service, personal care, continuity of care, and preservation of the patient–doctor relationship. Quality of clinical work and work satisfaction for the staff are values that all practices will share. To these may be added personal values, such as a satisfying personal and family life for the physician. Other objectives may relate more specifically to the prevention and management of

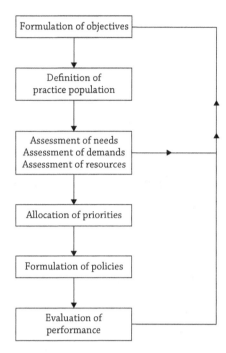

Figure 19.1:
The management process.

disease. The result will be a list of practice objectives, of which the following are examples:

1. Patients requesting appointments for acute problems will be seen on the same day. This immediately raises the question, "What is an acute problem?" Because policies will be implemented by the practice staff, they will need guidelines. For instance, in some practices of our acquaintance, a patient who calls about a breast lump is considered to have an acute problem and should be seen on the same day.
2. Patients requesting appointments for nonurgent problems will be seen within 2 weeks.
3. During office hours, patients will be seen by their personal physician.
4. Average time spent by patients in the waiting room will be no longer than 15 minutes.
5. Patients asking to speak to the doctor will receive a call from him or her on the same day.
6. All adult patients will have their blood pressure taken every 2 years.
7. Patients under treatment for hypertension or diabetes will be seen at least once every 3 months.

It will soon become apparent that some of these objectives are conflicting. How are patients with acute problems to be seen if all appointments for the day are filled by people with nonurgent problems? Should a patient see his or her own doctor if all that doctor's appointments are already taken, even if a partner is available? If objectives conflict, they must be put in some order of priority. It may, for example, be considered a higher priority for acute problems to be seen on the same day than for the patient always to see his or her own doctor.

One response to this conflict is advanced access or same-day booking systems that seek to balance patient needs with physician capacity. This approach came from the application of queuing theory and principles of industrial engineering as applied to the practice setting (Murray and Berwick, 2003; Mitchell, 2008). In this model, patients are offered an appointment with their physician on the same day, thus ensuring accessibility and continuity of care. This is consistent with the basic tenets of good family practice. To achieve this degree of organization requires commitment from the practitioner, but has been shown to be possible in many countries, including the United States (Murray, Bodenheimer, Rittenhouse, et al., 2003), Canada (Mitchell, 2008), and the United Kingdom (Pope et al., 2008), at times with local adaptations. Advanced access improves patient and physician satisfaction, reduces urgent care visits (O'Hare and Corlett, 2004), and improves patient care (Solberg et al., 2006). When objectives have been thus formulated, they are then made into practice policies. These will include the allocation of responsibilities among staff members. For example, what incoming calls does the receptionist pass on to the nurse or to the doctor? How many appointments are left free each day for acute problems? Who checks to see whether patients have had a blood pressure taken? Who is responsible for taking blood pressures? Who checks whether patients have come for follow-up visits? Under what circumstances may patients have repeat prescriptions? How are these to be authorized?

DEFINING THE PRACTICE POPULATION

Any assessment of needs requires a definition of the population for which the practice is responsible. In prepaid systems, this is readily available because patients register with the practice. Defining the population in fee-for-service systems is more difficult but is still eminently feasible. The list is compiled by going through the practice records and entering all patients who have used the practice regularly. Because more than 90% of a practice population attend at least once during a 5-year period, this list of patients who have attended does give an almost complete picture of the population at risk. Of course, the list will be inaccurate because it will contain some patients who have moved or changed doctors. However, the purpose of the list is management, not research, so a high degree of accuracy is not required. An alternative method, also feasible under the fee-for-service system, is to enter into a contract for continuing care when a new family joins the practice. Assessment of needs can be more refined if the defined population is listed in the form of an age–sex register. The compilation of a practice register by manual methods is a laborious and time-consuming procedure, and it must be emphasized that although it is a desirable objective, a practice register is by no means essential for the next stage of the process. Electronic health records have greatly simplified this step.

ASSESSMENT OF UNMET NEEDS

Two types of unmet needs[1] can be identified:

1. Needs of which the patient is unaware. It is well known that demands for service are not the same thing as an expression of needs. Community health surveys have shown the existence of many unmet needs, even when good primary care services are available. The following are common examples:
   a. Disabilities that elderly patients do not recognize as treatable disorders.
   b. Well-validated preventive procedures, the need for which may not be known to the patient, such as immunization, Pap smear, or hypertension screening.
   c. Mental illnesses such as depression, in which apathy or lack of insight inhibit the patient from seeking care.
2. Needs that the patient feels have not been met by the healthcare system.

Patient satisfaction, adequacy of preventive care, and unmet needs for common specific problems may be assessed by a brief questionnaire presented to a sample from each age group, drawn either from the practice records or from an age–sex register. The results enable the physician to identify specific areas in which the practice is failing to meet needs. Another method of assessment is to carry out periodic surveys of specific subgroups of the population that are felt to be at high risk of having unmet needs. Groups that may be at risk are the aged, single parent families, families of patients with chronic disabilities, and immigrant groups.

ASSESSMENT OF DEMANDS

Demands on resources can be divided into those generated by patients and those generated by the physician.

Patient-generated demands can in turn be divided into the following main categories:

Telephone consultations
Office visits for acute conditions
Office visits for nonurgent problems
Request for home visits
Office visits for preventive care
Requests for repeat prescriptions
Emergency and night calls
Visits for prenatal and well-baby care.

Physicians generate demand for their services by asking patients to make follow-up appointments and by calling them in for preventive procedures.

Demands can be readily assessed by doing periodic surveys of incoming telephone calls, requests for appointments, home visits, repeat prescriptions, and so on. Greater detail can be obtained by recording such information as problem label or diagnosis, drugs or other treatment prescribed, investigations ordered, or referrals made. For management purposes, it is not necessary to record this information continuously. It is quite sufficient to do it for all patients for a week at a time or for a sample of patients over a similar period.

ASSESSMENT OF RESOURCES

The resources of the practice include the physical plant, the communication system, the physicians, the staff, the attached personnel, and the hospital and community resources that can be deployed by the practice.

ALLOCATION OF PRIORITIES

Given the defined objectives of the practice, the needs of the practice population, and demands generated, it will be necessary to set priorities, as it will not be possible to do everything.

FORMULATION OF POLICIES

Policies need to be put in place to guide all involved in meeting the goals of the practice respecting the priorities. Such policies ensure stability in the way the business of the practice is conducted.

EVALUATION OF PERFORMANCE

The next stage is evaluation to determine whether or not the objectives have been achieved. Different types of evaluation are needed for different objectives. Donabedian (1966) has described three types: evaluation of structure, process, and outcome. Structure refers to the physical facilities and the qualifications of staff and is more relevant to external audit than the kind of internal evaluation we are discussing here. Outcome evaluation means the assessment of the results of care: recovery from illness or disability, relief of symptoms, functional capacity, and satisfaction with care. Although outcome is the ultimate criterion of good care, outcome evaluation poses certain problems. Outcome is often determined by factors that are outside the practice's control: social and economic conditions, for example. In chronic conditions such as hypertension, the outcome may be many years distant. Provided a process criterion can be related to a successful outcome, this is a satisfactory substitute for outcome evaluation. For example, it is reasonable to use the control of hypertension as a process criterion because this is known to prevent unfavorable outcomes of hypertension. For similar reasons, the proportion of the practice population screened can be used as a process criterion.

Most types of evaluation that are useful to the family physician are assessments of process. One exception is the assessment of satisfaction with care. Because results of treatment are known to be related to patient satisfaction, this is an important aspect of evaluation in family practice.

Three main strategies of evaluation are available to the family physician:

1. A direct approach to the patient.
2. Periodic assessments of practice procedures: documentation of incoming telephone calls, calculation of average time spent in the waiting room, and assessment of delay in obtaining appointments for acute and nonurgent conditions.
3. Audit of records. This can be used to monitor such aspects of performance as management, prescribing, referral, and use of investigations.

RECONSIDERATION OF OBJECTIVES AND POLICIES

Almost certainly, the evaluation will reveal that some objectives are not being achieved. Certain questions must, therefore, be asked:

1. Are the objectives realistic?
2. Can the demands be changed? We often tend to assume that the demands on a practice are a given. There are certainly limits to the degree they can be influenced. We should bear in mind, however, that there are two ways of

changing demand. Education of patients may affect not only the nature of demand but also its distribution. Instruction by booklets, videos of the self-management of simple problems, and group visits may reduce the demand for care for conditions such as upper respiratory infection. Prenatal and post-natal classes for mothers may reduce the number of calls for babies. Patient education by word of mouth or by practice brochure can reduce the number of inappropriate demands, such as out-of-hours calls for repeat prescriptions. Doctor-initiated demands are also subject to change by reviewing policies on follow-up visits and for preventive services. For example, should a physician see all recently hospitalized patients within 1 week of discharge, or can resources be used more effectively by utilizing other healthcare providers?

3. Are the resources of the practice being used to their maximum effect? How much time is being wasted? Is the doctor's time being used to the best advantage, or is it badly distributed? Is enough of the day being allocated to office appointments? Is time being wasted by poor patient flow, mislaid records, instruments not being readily available, or communication in the office being inefficient?

4. Are the staff members fully aware of the practice policies, and are they carrying them out? Being the first to receive incoming calls, the key staff person in the operation of the practice is the receptionist, who can only function effectively with a clear understanding of what is expected.

COMMON DEFECTS IN PRACTICE MANAGEMENT

1. Too many incoming calls for the number of telephone lines. Patients with acute problems may have difficulty getting through because of continuous busy signals.

2. Inadequate telephone answering services for out-of-hours calls. A commercially operated answering service may be inadequately supervised. There may be unacceptable delays between calls being received and relayed to the doctor.

3. Patients having to wait 2 or 3 days for appointments for acute conditions such as abdominal pain or urinary infection. In these circumstances, it is no wonder that patients use hospital emergency departments.

4. Patients unable to get through the barrier of the receptionist or nurse to speak to the doctor. This may be due to the receptionist's excessive shielding of the doctor from the demands of patients.

Unless the physician adopts a critical approach to the management of the practice, he or she may remain in complete ignorance of the existence of these deficiencies in his or her own practice.

TEAM-BASED PRACTICES

An interdisciplinary primary care (IPC) team consists of a group of professionals representing different disciplines working together under an arrangement to provide a range of health services to a population in the community (Dinh, Stonebridge, and Theriault, 2014). Such formal IPC teams are a feature of many initiatives to strengthen primary care in a number of countries, but often family physicians work in informal and loosely knit teams, and this will continue to be the norm in many places. Indeed, the traditional "core team" of physician–nurse dyad is able to provide excellent patient-centered care (Sinsky, Sinsky, Althaus, et al., 2010), and can be supplemented by other providers in the community according to patient need.

The move in primary care toward IPC teams is motivated by evidence that such organizations can improve the health of those with chronic conditions and risk factors and can offset costs in other parts of the healthcare system (Dinh and Bounajm, 2013). Others argue that such teams are a way of coping with physician shortages, but the evidence in this area is unclear (Grover and Niecko, 2013). There is hope that they will help address some of the factors that lead to burnout among family physicians (Sinsky, Willard-Grace, and Schutzbank, 2013).

When IPC teams reach a certain size, there is a danger that patients will have difficulty identifying one or two primary providers who they consider know them well. One solution to this is the use of "teamlets" that consist of a stable partnership of clinician and other provider who work together every day and share responsibility for the patients under their care (Bodenheimer, Ghorob, and Willard-Grace, 2014). This, of course, mirrors that traditional physician–nurse dyad mentioned earlier.

One challenge of IPC teams is maintaining the principles of family medicine. Teams can sustain patient-centeredness, by applying the principles of the patient-centered clinical method to the team (Stewart, Brown, Freeman, et al., 2014). This begins by ensuring that everyone on the team understands one another's scope of practice and individual strengths and experiences. This lays the groundwork for developing the shared language, culture, and philosophy of the team. There must be agreement on the goals of care, as well as communication (both formal and informal) and policies and procedures on how to reduce and deal with conflict. All of this requires a sharing of power, trust in one's colleagues, and being self-aware.

In patient-centered care, it is understood that patients share in the decisions that affect their individual care. On a team level, patients may share in the collective decisions of the practice through the mechanism of a patient advisory council.

Establishing and ensuring that IPC teams operate to their full potential requires fundamental changes in the way that many family physicians have practiced. In some versions of IPC teams, there is an emphasis on governance and administration that, if not aware of and responsive to the care providers' and patients' needs, runs the risk of evolving into a production model (Franklin, 1999) of health care. It is important that physicians and other direct care providers be involved in the governance and management of such teams. Family physicians must more consistently consider their practice and community on a population level and ask how the IPC team can improve the overall health of that population. Bringing together all healthcare providers during their basic education is desirable in fostering the attitudes necessary for success in working on such teams.

THE PATIENT-CENTERED MEDICAL HOME

The patient-centered medical home (PCMH) describes a way of organizing family practice, recognizing the importance of the principles of family medicine and the best practices of high-performing practices. There are eight characteristics of a PCMH (American College of Physicians, 2007):

1. Each patient has a personal physician who provides ongoing, comprehensive first-contact care for most health issues.
2. There is a physician-led team of individuals who collectively take responsibility for the ongoing needs of patients.
3. Care is based on a whole-person (holistic) model, taking responsibility for either providing care that encompasses all patient care needs across the life span or arranging for the care to be done by other qualified professionals.
4. The team will ensure that care is coordinated across the complexities of the healthcare system. Integration of care is ensured by practice registries, information technology, and exchange of information across the system.
5. Care is taken to ensure that patients receive the indicated care when and where they need and want it in a culturally and linguistically appropriate manner.
6. Quality and safety are a characteristic of the care provided.
7. Enhanced access is made available through open scheduling, expanded hours, and the use of other means of communication between the physician and the patient, such as patient portals.
8. A payment structure that supports and encourages this model of care.

There are more than 2000 recognized PCMHs in the United States. Other jurisdictions have developed models that demonstrate these same principles (Rosser, Colwill, Kasperski, et al., 2010).

THE IMPACT OF MANAGED CARE

Managed care is the term used for integrated systems for the provision of health services, such as health maintenance organizations (HMOs), preferred provider organizations (PPOs), and independent practice associations (IPA). *Managed care* is also used to denote the range of controls used by such organizations to control the practices of physicians and to limit the options of patients. Examples of such controls include entry to the system only through primary physician "gatekeepers," mandatory second opinion before elective surgery, formal utilization review, and mandatory approval of certain discretionary services.

Driven by the need for cost containment, managed care has become ubiquitous in the United States, with 90% of insured Americans reported to be in some form of managed care. Such plans are rapidly replacing the indemnity insurance plan as the predominant system for organizing and financing health care (Weiner and de Lissovoy, 1993). Under an indemnity insurance plan, the sponsor (e.g., an employer) purchased services through insurance companies that acted as intermediaries between purchaser and consumers. Consumers were free to choose providers of services, physicians practiced with few constraints, and insurance companies paid the bills. The insurance companies accepted the financial risk but could pass on any increases in cost to the sponsor in the form of higher premiums.

What distinguishes managed care plans is that there is a "party that takes responsibility for integrating and coordinating the financing and delivery of services across what previously were fragmented provider and payer entities" (Weiner and de Lissovoy, 1993, p. 97). The prototypical managed care institution is the HMO. Health maintenance organizations are committed to providing care for enrollees who prepay a premium. The organization assumes the financial risk and transfers some of this to the primary care physicians, who are often paid by capitation fee (a regular payment for each patient enrolled in their practice, irrespective of whether or not the patient has received services).

There are four types of HMOs. In a staff HMO, the physicians are paid mainly by salary. In a group HMO, a multispecialty group practice is the major source of care for enrollees. Network HMOs provide services to enrollees through two or more group practices. In an IPA, individual physicians or small group practices contract to provide care for enrollees. The primary care physicians may be paid by capitation or by fee-for-service with a risk-sharing provision. The physician may also treat patients outside the HMO on a fee-for-service basis.

In a preferred provider organization, consumers have the choice of using the preferred physicians who are members of the plan or physicians who are outside it. Benefits act as incentives for consumers to use the preferred physicians. The latter agree to managed care strategies and are usually paid a discounted fee. The physicians in the plan benefit by having patients channeled to them.[2]

Financial risk is defined as "variance in expenditure" (Weiner and de Lissovoy, 1993). The degree of variance depends on the number of enrollees and their health status. If numbers are small, one patient requiring expensive treatment can greatly increase the risk for the payer. Managed care organizations may transfer some or all of the risk to physicians. Primary care physicians, for example, may agree to a budget or capitation payment and take responsibility for the provision of all necessary services, including in-hospital and specialist care. Such transfer of risk can take place within government-funded services. In the British National Health Service, fund-holding practices are assigned capitation payments and are responsible for buying services from hospitals and specialist services. In the United States, Medicare payments are based on fees for diagnosis-related groups (DRGs). The fee paid is an average of all patients with the same diagnosis. When the physician's own income is included in the budget or capitation fee, a conflict of interest may clearly arise. The transfer of risk to primary care groups involves physicians in levels of management far beyond those experienced in private fee-for-service practice. This demands management skills and may add to the stress of practice. On the other hand, it can provide an opportunity for creative innovation in the provision of services.

Advances in information technology have made it possible for managers to maintain close surveillance of physicians' activities, including time spent with patients, prescribing costs, referral rates, and compliance with guidelines. If too rigid, these may have deleterious effects on physicians' morale, with negative consequences for patient care.

The term *managed competition* is used to describe competition between managed care plans in a market regulated by government. In the British National Health Service, for example, the government has created an internal market in which providers compete for contracts with payers.

NOTES

1. The systematic assessment of healthcare needs in the practice population, identification of community health problems, modification of practice procedures, and monitoring the impact of changes is known as community-oriented primary care (COPC) (Nutting, 1986; Wright, 1993). In the United States, COPC has been implemented mainly in not-for-profit primary care organizations. The application has thus far been limited in scope. Implementation difficulties include the cost of health surveys, the lack of epidemiological skills, and the problems of reallocating resources in organizations already working at full stretch.

COPC is said to require a new kind of hybrid practitioner with competencies in primary care, prevention, epidemiology, ethics, and behavioral science. As Toon (1994) has observed, these roles may be conflicting, leading to tensions in the individual physician and in the practice, especially if it is a small one. There are, however, some exemplars, notably Dr. Tudor Hart in his South Wales practice. In those organizations that have implemented COPC, there has been at least one physician with an unusual commitment to it (Nutting and Connor, 1986). Whether COPC can work successfully on a larger scale has yet to be demonstrated. Even if it proves to be impracticable in its present form, the principles could still be applied in different ways, such as by collaboration between a number of practices and a public health unit.

2. For an excellent guide to the often confusing nomenclature of managed care, see Razing a tower of Babel: A taxonomy for managed care and health insurance plans (Weiner and Lissovoy, 1993).

REFERENCES

American College of Physicians. 2007. Modified from: Joint principles of the patient-centered medical home, March 2007. http://www.acponline.org/advocacy/where_we_stand/assets/approve_jp.pdf.

Bodenheimer T, Ghorob A, Willard-Grace R, et al. 2014. The 10 building blocks of high-performing primary care. *Annals of Family Medicine* 12(2):166–171.

Donabedian A. 1966. Evaluating the quality of medical care. Part 2. *Millbank Memorial Fund* 44:166.

Franklin U. 1999. *The Real World of Technology.* Toronto: Anansi Press.

Grover A, Niecko LM. 2013. Primary care teams: Are we there yet? Implications for workforce planning. *Academic Medicine* 88(12):1827–1829.

Dinh T, Bounajm F. 2013. *Improving Primary Health Care Through Collaboration. Briefing 3: Measuring the Missed Opportunity.* Ottawa: The Conference Board of Canada.

Dinh T, Stonebridge C, Theriault L. 2014. *Getting the Most out of Health Care Teams: Recommendation for Action.* Ottawa: The Conference Board of Canada.

Mitchell V. 2008. Same day booking: Success in Canadian family practice. *Canadian Family Physician* 54:379–383.

Murray M, Berwick DM. 2003. Advanced access: Reducing waiting and delays in primary care. *Journal of the American Medical Association* 289:1035–1040.

Murray M, Bodenheimer T, Rittenhouse D, Grumbach K. 2003. Improving timely access to primary care: Case studies of the advanced access model. *Journal of the American Medical Association* 289(8):1042–1046.

Nutting PA. 1986. Community-oriented primary care: An integrated model for practice, research, and education. *American Journal of Preventive Medicine* 2(3):140.

Nutting PA, Connor EM. 1986. Community-oriented primary care: An examination of the U.S. experience. *American Journal of Public Health* 76(3):279.

O'Hare CD, Corlett J. 2004. The outcomes of open-access scheduling. *Family Practice Management.* www.aafp.org/fpm. February.

Pope C, et al. 2008. Improving access to primary care: Eight case studies of introducing advanced access in England. *Journal of Health Services and Research Policy* 13:33–39.

Rosser WW, Colwill JM, Kasperski J, Wilson L. 2010. Patient-centered medical homes in Ontario. *New England Journal of Medicine* 362: January 21.

Sinsky CA, Sinsky TA, Althaus D, Tranel J, Thiltgen M. 2010. "Core teams": Nurse-physician partnerships provide patient-centered care at an Iowa practice. *Health Affairs* 29(5):966–968.

Sinsky CA, Willard-Grace R, Schutzbank AM, Sinsky TA, Morgolius D, Bodenheimer T. 2013. In search of joy in practice: A report of 23 high-functioning primary care practices. *Annals of Family Medicine* 11(3):272–278.

Solberg LI, et al. 2006. Effect of improved primary care access on quality of depression care. *Annals of Family Medicine* 4:69–74.

Stewart M, Brown JB, Freeman TR, McWilliam CL, Mitchell J, Brown L, Shaw L, Henderson V. 2014. Team-centered approach: How to build and sustain a team. Chapter 13 in *Patient-Centered Medicine: Transforming the Clinical Method*, 3rd ed. London; New York: Radcliffe Publishing.

Toon PD. 1994. What is good general practice? Occasional paper 65. Royal College of General Practitioners.

Weiner JP, de Lissovoy G. 1993. Razing a tower of Babel: A taxonomy for managed care and health insurance plans. *Journal of Health Politics, Policy and Law* 18(1):75–103.

Wright RA. 1993. Community-oriented primary care. *Journal of the American Medical Association* 269(19):2544.

CHAPTER 20

୶

The Health Professions

Family physicians can gain the maximum benefit for their patients only if they understand the role of each of the health professions. As in medicine, these roles are changing. The purpose of this chapter is to summarize the current roles of health professionals who work in collaboration with family physicians.

NURSING

Nurses in the community work in a number of roles:

1. Home care nurses provide nursing care for patients at home with acute or chronic illness, or after discharge from hospital. On visits, they may provide dressings, injections, monitoring of blood pressure and temperature or other signs, bed or tub baths, treatment of pressure areas, rehabilitation exercises, or any other nursing service. Home nursing may be a single service offered on request from the family doctor or part of an integrated home care service. The best arrangement is for the family physician and home care nurse to work together as a team. Attachment of nurses to practices is a good way of attaining this. Home care nurses may have special training and qualifications in such areas as intravenous therapy, ostomy care, nursing for the terminally ill, newborn care, or geriatric nursing.
2. Public health nurses (health visitors) are concerned chiefly with health education, prevention of disease and disability, and rehabilitation. They may work in prescribed geographical areas or may be attached to a family group practice. In some areas, they are based in schools. Their responsibilities

include health education for pregnant mothers, either individually or in groups; postnatal visiting at home with guidance on infant care and feeding; anticipatory guidance in child development; family planning advice; preparation of patients and their families for hospitalization, and follow-up after discharge from the hospital; visiting patients with communicable diseases, including education for patient and family in preventing spread; guidance of patients with chronic disease; assessment of family function and home environment; assisting the physician by observation and appraisal of patients under care at home; and assessing the health status of elderly patients at home.

3. Midwives may work both in obstetric units and in the community, providing prenatal, intrapartum, and postpartum care in collaboration with obstetricians and family physicians.

4. Nurses as members of the primary care team. Increasingly, nurses and family physicians are working together as a team. The day-to-day working relationship can allow the roles of doctor and nurse to evolve according to the local context and their individual skills. The nurse may be available to patients with new clinical problems, and may be responsible for following up patients with chronic diseases such as diabetes and asthma, carrying out screening procedures, or counseling patients with special needs.

5. Specialized roles in nursing. Many nursing specialties have emerged in recent years. Some of these, such as intensive care and oncology nursing, do not have major involvement in primary care. Other specialist nurses work closely with family physicians. The success of shared care depends very much on the liaison role of nurses specializing in such fields as diabetes care and psychiatric nursing. Nurses specializing in palliative care often work closely with family physicians.

Nurses and physicians have a great deal to learn from each other. Physicians can learn from the special expertise of nurses and also from the different perspective that the discipline of nursing brings to patient care. As a member of a palliative care team, I learned from nurses how to assess a patient's level of pain and discomfort, and how important attention to the smallest detail is in the care of seriously ill patients. To be a helpful colleague to a nurse, a physician has to maintain the clinical diagnostic and therapeutic skills on which the nurse relies. If a palliative care nurse needs help with pain control, the physician will be helpful only if he or she is well informed. In many cases, the key role of the family physician will be to contribute his or her store of knowledge about patient and family, so that decisions about care are in accordance with the patient's values and preferences. For example, it may not be appropriate to mobilize multiple resources for a family that has always been very private and self-sufficient.

NURSE PRACTITIONERS

Nurse practitioners (NPs) or advanced practice nurses (APNs) are registered nurses with additional education and training. The scope of practice varies from one jurisdiction to another, but commonly includes the ability to order and interpret diagnostic tests, communicate diagnoses, prescribe pharmaceuticals, and undertake some procedures. Their approach emphasizes health promotion and the prevention of illness and injury. NPs have become mainstays in many primary care team arrangements, and their specific role will vary depending on the needs of the population served by the team, and the other team members and their specific skills. They may primarily deal with acute illnesses presenting to the clinic, or may engage in health promotion (e.g., smoking cessation), immunizations, monitoring of chronic diseases, or all of these activities. Working in collaboration with family physicians, NPs can greatly extend the services that are available to practice patients. In a randomized controlled trial involving a family health team network of family physicians, a nurse practitioner and a pharmacist visited, at home, 120 patients deemed by their family physicians to be at risk of having adverse health outcomes. A comprehensive medication review was undertaken and a tailored plan was developed with the patient and the family physician. Compared to baseline, the assessment of medication appropriateness 12 to 18 months later demonstrated significant improvements (Fletcher, Hogg, Farrell, et al., 2012).

The role of NPs continues to evolve, and in some locales, such as rural and remote areas, they work independently of physicians altogether. When working in collaborative arrangements with physicians, nursing brings a unique approach to patient care, and it is important that this not be lost as nurses move into new roles.

OCCUPATIONAL THERAPY

Occupational therapy uses activities to help patients regain lost function and develop their abilities. The activities range from everyday tasks, such as eating and dressing, to creative work and activities involving interpersonal relationships. Occupational therapists are skilled in assessing patients' capacity for work or activities of daily living and in prescribing programs to meet their needs. They have an important part to play in the rehabilitation of patients with such common problems as stroke, amputation, arthritis, multiple sclerosis, and mental disorder. Assessments in the home are particularly important in occupational therapy, for they may lead to appropriate changes in the physical layout of the home. Occupational therapists also work with disabled children to help them develop new skills.

PHYSIOTHERAPY (PHYSICAL THERAPY)

Physiotherapists are concerned with the assessment, maintenance, and improvement of bodily function. As with medicine, the view of bodily function as separable from mental function is giving place to a more organismic view of function as an expression of well-being of the whole person. An assessment based on this view includes an examination of the whole body as well as the part where symptoms are localized. It also includes attention to the patient's feelings and experiences, bodily flexibility, and breathing (Thornquist, 1992). Mental states are associated with bodily dysfunction, and physical therapy can improve mental well-being, even in schizophrenia (Roxerdal, 1985).

Physiotherapists are trained to be generalists. Some differentiation of role occurs, depending on the graduate's field of work. Most physiotherapists work in three areas: musculoskeletal disorders and injuries, neurological disorders, and cardiopulmonary disorders. Physiotherapists have a major role in rehabilitation. Some develop expertise in more specific fields, such as sports medicine.

Physiotherapists who work in primary care teams have excellent opportunities for the prevention of disability by early intervention and health education. Family physicians can also form useful links with physiotherapists who have special expertise in chronic pain, stress management (relaxation, breathing control), and manipulation.

MEDICAL SOCIAL WORK

The aim of social work is to help people improve their social functioning. Difficulties with social functioning may arise from acute or chronic physical illness, poverty, mental or physical handicaps, unemployment, or problems with relationships.

The following are all common social work functions: assessing the emotional and social components of illness; obtaining a social history to learn the patient's past behavior patterns and to relate these to current problems; identifying families who are at risk for mental and social breakdown so that preventive measures can be taken; assessing eligibility for assistance programs; establishing liaison with appropriate community resources; individual counseling, such as for unmarried mothers, isolated persons, and patients with problems of personality or relationships; and marital and family counseling for problems arising from relationships within the family.

Referrals to a social worker are especially helpful when problems with relationships are an important aspect of a patient's illness or when support from community resources is needed.

CLINICAL PSYCHOLOGY

Clinical psychologists offer a variety of methods for helping patients and families to identify and solve their problems. The approach taken by any particular psychologist will probably emerge from one of three psychological theories of personality development and human behavior: psychodynamic, behavioral, or humanistic. The main goal of those adhering to a psychodynamic orientation is to bring unconscious conflicts into awareness through exploratory and analytic or interpretative techniques. With the behavioral orientation, problems are approached with a view to correcting behavior patterns assessed either by the individual or by society as maladaptive. The humanistic approach focuses on the self-actualizing forces believed to be inherent in each individual that, when blocked, produce emotional distress or other symptoms of disrupted functioning. A fundamental aspect of this approach is that growth and change occur in the context of certain necessary relationship conditions: unconditional positive regard, genuineness, and empathic understanding.

Any of these therapeutic approaches can be applied to a wide variety of problems and symptoms, ranging from family dysfunction to psychophysiological symptoms, phobias, or other disruptions of functioning associated with anxiety, depression, or breaks from reality. Family physicians are often in the best position to assess the needs and capacities of the patient requiring psychological intervention, and therefore to match the patient with the most appropriate therapist and therapeutic approach.

In addition to providing psychotherapeutic services for the patients of family doctors, the clinical psychologist can serve as consultant to the family physician for a variety of purposes. First, the psychologist will often have some expertise in developmental psychology. Thus, the patient's symptoms or behaviors may be interpretable as a reflection of some developmental crisis. The psychologist can assist in putting the symptoms in perspective, acknowledging their adaptive as well as maladaptive functions. Second, the psychologist can work with the physician in sorting out organic from psychophysiological symptoms and as a consequence can minimize intrusive investigation, as well as suggest treatment or management strategies. In addition, the psychologist can facilitate the understanding and management of patients' problems in living when the patient will not accept a referral to the psychologist or some other allied professional. Finally, the psychological consultation can be useful in helping the physician to deal with problems in the patient–doctor relationship, and with difficult patients—for example, the nonadherent or superficially adherent patient, persons addicted to drugs or alcohol, or patients and their families who are in the process of dealing with illness or death.

BEHAVIORAL THERAPY

Behavioral therapy techniques developed by psychologists have proved useful in the treatment of such diverse conditions as chronic pain, depression, physical disabilities, addictions, psychophysiologic symptoms, and phobias (Bakal, 1979; Russell, 1986). The techniques can be broadly classified as conditioning, cognitive therapy, and relaxation training, and biofeedback. Besides being used by psychologists, these can also be used by physicians and physiotherapists.

Conditioning

Behavior is related in two ways to environmental stimuli. Respondent behavior is controlled by preceding stimulus events. An unconditioned stimulus produces a response by direct association, as when a dog salivates at the arrival of food. A conditioned stimulus produces a response by association, as when a dog salivates at the sound of a bell that has previously been paired with the arrival of food. Classical conditioning is the process of learning to respond to conditioned stimuli.

Operant behavior is affected by events following the behavior. If the behavior is followed by reinforcement, the behavior is increased, a process known as *operant conditioning*. Positive reinforcement is any event that increases the behavior that preceded it. Negative reinforcement occurs when a behavior is increased after withdrawal of a negative stimulus.

Conditioning is used in a number of ways to modify behavior. In counterconditioning, the fear or anxiety produced by the stimulus is replaced by an alternative learned response. A maladaptive behavior may be reduced by removing the reinforcement. For example, an overdependent patient who makes frequent demands for attention will be reinforced in this behavior if the physician responds to it by meeting every demand. If, on the other hand, he provides regular appointments and does not respond to demands between appointments, the behavior will cease to be reinforced and is likely to decrease in frequency. A patient with chronic pain who receives an analgesic on demand will be reinforced in his pain behavior. Regular analgesic medication at set times with no response in between will tend to reduce the behavior.

In aversive conditioning, the response is accompanied by an unpleasant stimulus, as in the administration of Antabuse (disulfuram) to alcoholics. Much of what we do to improve compliance with therapy is a form of conditioning. By removing unpleasant side effects, we reduce their aversive effects. To help patients to remember to take their medication, we try to associate it with certain cues, such as keeping the pill bottle by the toothbrush.

Often patients are unaware of the stimuli that produce symptoms or behavioral responses. Their awareness can be increased by asking them to keep a diary recording the events and sensations that precede or accompany the onset of a symptom. The patient thus develops self-knowledge, and the physician becomes aware of the stimuli that have to be either removed or responded to differently.

Cognitive Therapy

Cognitive therapy is based on the observation that conditions such as depression and chronic pain are maintained by thought processes such as inappropriate perceptions, interpretations, expectations, and coping responses. A depressed businessman may misinterpret certain cues as indicating that his business is on the rocks. A patient with chronic pain may have developed responses that actually increase the pain rather than relieving it. Cognitive therapy aims to teach the patient different ways of responding and coping.

Cognitive therapy is designed to provide the patient with a conceptual framework for understanding the nature of his or her problem. The patient learns a different way of coping with the problem. Instead of responding to physiological and psychological cues with a panic reaction or anxiety-producing thoughts, the patient uses them to trigger the coping responses for which he or she has been trained.

Relaxation Training

The relaxation response (Benson, 1975) is a physiological and psychological state in which there is decreased activity of the sympathetic nervous system, diminished muscle tension, and mental tranquility. It is induced by sitting or lying in a comfortable position, breathing deeply, systematically relaxing each muscle group in turn, emptying the mind of all thoughts, and repeating a sound or word over and over again. The technique is similar to the practice of meditative prayer practiced in all the major religions. The theory of relaxation training is that it counteracts the fight-or-flight arousal mechanism, which is an ineffective response to psychological stressors.

Biofeedback

Biofeedback is a technique for giving a person some control over physiological systems that normally function beneath the level of awareness. The method is that of control by negative feedback, an important principle of cybernetics and system theory. Physiological processes such as skin temperature, pulse rate, blood pressure, and skeletal muscle contraction are electronically monitored and displayed to the individual. Although biofeedback has been used successfully in conditions like recurrent headache, it is not clear that the relief of symptoms actually depends on the feedback mechanism. It may work by giving the patient a cognitive coping strategy. All the methods discussed here are ways of giving patients more control of their own bodies—one of the three conditions considered necessary for the placebo effect.

Case 9.5 provided an example of the application of behavioral therapy principles. In this case the principles were applied by the physicians and physiotherapist, without the involvement of a psychologist. The first physician was reinforcing the patient's panic reaction to chest pain by doing an ECG every time the patient came. The second physician helped to extinguish this behavior by arranging annual visits to a cardiologist and placing a moratorium on ECGs between these visits. The physiotherapist reduced the stimuli leading to panic reactions and reinforced behavior that increased the patient's activity. The family physician used cognitive therapy to help the patient to change her perception of what was happening to her. The doctor also reduced and then discontinued the medication, which was reinforcing the patient's belief in her invalidism.

DIETETICS (NUTRITION)

Two aspects of a dietitians's work of special importance to the family physician are nutrition education and dietary problems. The dietitian provides instruction to various groups in the community: pregnant women, mothers of young children, and elderly people.

The most common problems requiring dietary counseling are obesity, diabetes, hyperlipidemia, and digestive disorders. Individual or group counseling may be used. Nutritionists also have a key role in enteral and parenteral nutrition.

PHARMACY

With the declining use of mixtures, the role of the pharmacist has changed from dispensing medicines to advising both physicians and patients on the use of drugs. As a consultant to the physician, the pharmacist has an important role in advising on dosage, side effects, contraindications, and drug incompatibilities. For patients, the pharmacist interprets the physician's instructions on how drugs should be taken. In many communities, pharmacists are widely used by the public for advice on the treatment of common disorders such as colds, dyspepsia, and enteritis. The rapid development of drug therapy has increased the importance of communication between family physician and pharmacist. If the physician can identify the pharmacists who are filling most of his or her prescriptions, it is helpful if this communication can be at the personal level. Pharmacists are also playing important roles as members of interdisciplinary primary care teams. They assist in comprehensive medication reviews, starting new medications, and medication reconciliation of patients recently discharged from the hospital, as well as other functions.

CHIROPODY AND PODIATRY

Proper care of the feet, especially in individuals with diabetes, is an important part of comprehensive care. Monitoring and responding to early problems is essential to avoid complications such as the diabetic foot.

The title *chiropodist* is gradually being replaced by *podiatrist* depending on the country. In some jurisdictions they are legislatively distinct, with chiropodists having a narrower scope of practice. Podiatrists in many countries describe their scope of practice as including disorders of the foot, ankle, knee, leg, and hip.

THE TEAM CONCEPT

No one profession can meet all of patients' needs, hence the need to work together in teams. There are strengths, but also pitfalls, in team work. There are also misconceptions about what team work is. We distinguish three types of teams: core, greater, and ad hoc.

The *core team* is a team in which the members work together, day in and day out, closely integrated in the performance of a special task. Some common examples are the doctor–nurse teams that operate intensive care units, palliative care units, and family practices. In family practice, the team may include office nurses, public health nurses (health visitors), and home care nurses if they are based in the practice. By working closely together, the team members can develop a strong mutual understanding that can greatly enhance patient care.

To attain this, however, requires close attention to team morale and to communication between members. A group is a team only in name if it does not meet together frequently and regularly. Regular meetings should be held to discuss patients, but some meetings should also be devoted to team function and to the support of its members. Mutual respect is a key principle of team function, and this cannot be attained unless each member's views are listened to with respect. Being a member of a true team means being prepared to have one's actions and views challenged—sometimes a difficult thing for physicians to accept. Each team member has his or her own role, but roles do overlap, and there are many decisions in which different team members have a very legitimate stake. In deciding how to manage a patient addicted to tranquilizers, for example, or whether a patient with terminal cancer should be given an antibiotic for pneumonia, both nurses and physicians have much to contribute, even though the physician is the one who writes the prescription. Though decisions are discussed freely and openly, this does not mean that there is blurring of responsibility. Once the decision is arrived at, the responsibility for its implementation should be clearly assigned. Blurred responsibility and fragmentation of care are signs of a poorly functioning team. One of the most important responsibilities of the team leadership is the maintenance of morale, especially a team where there is a high level of work stress. The key to maintaining morale is the care and support given to each team member. When a team has urgent and difficult daily tasks to perform, it is all too easy for the welfare of team members to lose its priority. In a study of intensive care and palliative care teams, Vachon (1987) found that stress and "burnout" were much less frequent on teams where the welfare of members was the first priority of the leadership.

The *greater team* is the core team plus additional members who join the team for a specific function, but who are only involved when their services are needed. One of these members may perform the same function on several core teams as, for example, when a social worker in a health center works with several family practice nurse–physician teams. There is a similar need for team meetings, mutual respect, and open discussion. The relationship of these members with the team, however, is somewhat different in that they are less involved on a day-to-day basis and usually have their home in another administrative unit.

The *ad hoc team* is a team assembled for a particular patient and exists only for that patient. Case 9.6 was an example. The family physician brought together a cardiologist and a physiotherapist to work with the patient on her problem. It was not necessary for the team to meet; it was essential, however, for their activities to be coordinated and for a common purpose to be understood. Without leadership, the result would have been fragmentation of care. In the modern healthcare system, fragmentation is an all too common problem (for more on teams in family practice, see Chapter 19, "Practice Management").

REFERENCES

Bakal DA. 1979. *Psychology and Medicine: Psychobiological Dimensions of Health and Illness*. New York: Springer.

Benson H. 1975. *The Relaxation Response*. New York: Morrow.

Fletcher J, Hogg W, Farrell B, Woodend K, Dahrouge S, Lemelin J, Dalziel W. 2012. Effect of nurse practitioner and pharmacist counseling on inappropriate medication use in family practice. *Canadian Family Physician* 58(8):862–868.

Roxerdal G. 1985. *Body Awareness Therapy and the Body Awareness Scale: Treatment and Evaluation in Psychiatric Physiotherapy*. Goteborg: Department of Rehabilitation Medicine, University of Goteborg.

Russell ML. 1986. *Behavioral Counseling in Medicine*. New York: Oxford University Press.

Thornquist E. 1992. Examination and communication: A study of first encounters between patients and physiotherapists. *Family Practice* 9:195.

Vachon MLS. 1987. *Occupational Stress in the Care of the Critically Ill, the Dying, and the Bereaved*. Washington, DC: Hemisphere Publishing.

CHAPTER 21

֍

The Community Service Network

Family physicians are accustomed to thinking of themselves as part of the medical network, deploying the services of numerous specialists for the benefit of their patients. Their familiarity with the medical system arises from the hospital-centered education that is the norm in most medical schools. This educational environment, however, does not help them to understand that the physician is only one of many resources within the community for helping people to deal with their interrelated health and social problems. Unless family physicians have good lines of communication with these services and an awareness of what they have to offer, their effectiveness will be severely limited. The purpose of this chapter is to give a general description of the community service network. Although there are differences of detail between different jurisdictions, and between urban and rural communities, all advanced industrialized societies have support systems of the kind described here.

These services are important to family physicians in two ways. First, they can be a source of information about their patients. This applies especially to those two health services that are concerned with people's working lives: the school and industrial health services. Second, they can provide support and help of many different kinds. Family physicians starting in practice or moving to a new area should make every effort to learn about the local network of services, preferably by developing personal relationships with the people they will be dealing with regularly. The medical officer of health and his or her staff are particularly important for the family physician. It is important also to educate practice staff in the need to keep lines of communication open. Nothing is more infuriating for a nurse than to find that when he or she tries to speak to a family physician about one of the physician's patients, the route is blocked by an overprotective nurse or receptionist.

PUBLIC HEALTH

Public health and family physicians are natural allies in developing and maintaining systems for the prevention of illness and the promotion of health. Establishing and maintaining contact with the local Public Health Department is an important linkage between the family physician and the broader health care system. Very successful models have included a defined public health nurse (PHN) attachment to community practitioners, which enhances communication and establishes a continuum of care between family physicians and Public Health. The PHN becomes a member of the core team and provides in-home well-baby visits to new mothers, evaluation of the isolated elderly, and teen outreach programs.

Campos-Outcalt (2004) defines five functions that family physicians should fulfill as a part of the public health system: (1) implementing recommended preventive services guidelines in their practices; (2) serving as the front line of the surveillance system (e.g., as a sentinel physician); (3) appropriately referring to the Public Health Department (e.g., for prenatal classes or early child care classes); (4) accepting referrals from the Public Health Department (e.g., new patients who do not have a family physician); and (5) interacting constructively with the local health department. He goes on to suggest four levels of Public Health expertise, beginning with basic, and progressing through intermediate and advanced, to leadership. Each of these levels has defined knowledge and skills. All family physicians should have basic-level expertise; those engaged as sentinel clinicians should have intermediate-level knowledge and skills. Those who wish to be involved more deeply as consultants, medical directors, or to serve on Boards of Health require advanced knowledge and skills. Generally, those engaged in leadership roles have taken extra degree courses such as a master's in public health (MPH).

SERVICES FOR CHILDREN

All advanced societies have legislation to protect and safeguard the welfare of children. All have either official or voluntary bodies responsible for the welfare of children. These organizations deal with such matters as the following:

Investigations of allegations that children may be in need of protection
Counseling for family problems
Placing children in foster homes, group homes, or institutions
Supervision of children in care
Counseling for expectant unmarried mothers
Adoption

Prevention of childhood problems by community work and education in parenthood.

Day-care centers are an important source of help for families with preschool children, especially single-parent families. Not only can the children be assured of care by competent, trained workers, but parents themselves can also learn about childrearing.

Under this heading should be included services to parents and expectant parents: prenatal groups run by nurses, groups for young parents run by various social agencies, and self-help groups for parents with difficulties.

All societies have agencies for helping mentally and physically disabled children. These usually provide the parents and family doctor with a skilled assessment of the child, together with advice and support in his or her long-term care and education. Agencies also exist for aid to children with specific disabilities, such as blindness, deafness, cerebral palsy, muscular dystrophy, cystic fibrosis, and other conditions.

SCHOOL HEALTH AND GUIDANCE SERVICES

School health services were at first concerned mainly with the physical health of schoolchildren. As child health improved, attention shifted toward learning disabilities and behavior disorders that impair learning. Children may be referred to the health and guidance services either by a teacher or by the family doctor. Because school behavior problems often have their origins in family disturbance, the family is usually involved in the assessment. Information provided by the family physician may, therefore, be very helpful to the school. The prescription for the child may include special learning measures, family counseling, and drug treatment for attention deficit disorder.

The presentation of school learning and behavior problems to the family physician is an indication for consultation with the school. Investigation of the problem can then be planned jointly between the family doctor and educational services. It is important for the family physician to be aware of the services available within the school system in the area. These may include guidance, psychological services, speech therapy, and special education. Public health nurses are often attached to schools, and school physicians may be involved in the diagnosis and management of learning and behavior disorders.

INDUSTRIAL HEALTH SERVICES

All industrial societies have legislation governing industrial health and safety. Large industrial plants often have their own full-time industrial nurse, working either with or without a visiting medical officer, who is often a family physician. The medical officer is responsible for advising the company on the health and safety of the workforce, the prevention of industrial accidents and diseases, and the implementation of legislation on industrial health. The medical officer should communicate with the family physician when a patient is injured or taken ill at work, when the patient is returning to work after illness or injury, or when poor work performance or absenteeism is an early sign of illness.

Successful rehabilitation of a worker may depend on a graduated return to employment or a change of job within the same industry. In either case, collaboration with the industrial medical officer is important. Industrial nurses and medical officers often get to know workers very well and may be the first to identify signs of ill health. The first sign of alcoholism, for example, may be Monday morning absenteeism. Information provided by the industrial nurse may, therefore, be very important to the family physician. An industry may also have its own rehabilitation program for sick or injured workers.

Although communication with industrial health services is important, a word of caution is necessary about communication with employers. The family physician's responsibility is to the patient, not to the employer. Information about the patient should never be provided to the employer without the patient's written consent.

MENTAL HEALTH SERVICES

The earlier discharge of patients from psychiatric hospitals has not only placed more responsibility on the family physician, but also has created a need for more community services for the mentally ill. These include "halfway house" accommodation, rehabilitation workshops, follow-up visits, and group therapy by social workers. Special units for alcoholics and drug addicts exist in most communities, in addition to self-help groups like Alcoholics Anonymous.

Many urban communities also have crisis services based on the model of the Samaritans movement in Great Britain. People in despair can call a number where they will be able to talk to trained volunteers. Some services also provide face-to-face counseling for those in despair and contemplating suicide.

SERVICES FOR THE ELDERLY

All services in the home are important for the elderly—nursing, physiotherapy, occupational therapy. "Meals on Wheels" delivers nutritious hot meals. Day hospitals provide assessment, rehabilitation, recreation, and social activities.

Churches, service clubs, and volunteer organizations provide support services and arrange social activities. Geriatric units provide short-term admissions for patients so that their families can have a break.

HOME CARE SERVICES

Nurses, occupational therapists, physiotherapists, and podiatrists (chiropodists) all do home visiting. In some areas their services are integrated with homemaker services in a home care program. Integrated home care may be helpful for patients discharged from the hospital, for patients treated at home for acute or chronic illness, and for terminal illness.

SELF-HELP AND MUTUAL-HELP GROUPS

Many organizations exist for patients with specific diseases, such as cancer, multiple sclerosis, diabetes, arthritis, and chronic obstructive pulmonary disease (COPD). They may provide wheelchairs, walking aids, transportation, financial aid, support and counseling for families, visitors for patients after mastectomy, amputation, or colostomy, and education for patients and families.

Some provide group therapy and support, such as the various organizations that are available for people who are overweight. Others provide group support for the bereaved or for relatives of patients with disorders such as schizophrenia and developmental delay.

VOLUNTEERS

Besides the formal network of community services, there also exists in all communities a more informal system of volunteer services. Some of these are extensions of churches, service clubs, and other organizations. Some exist at the neighborhood level—good neighbors who rally round at times of crisis or need. Knowledge of these resources is very helpful to the family physician. In many communities, volunteer organizations exist to provide such services as delivering meals, visiting the isolated and lonely, transporting patients, and working on hospital units.

LOCATION OF BASIC SERVICES

A family physician new to a community will find workers administering government support programs in a courthouse, city hall, township office, or other government facility. Children's Aid Societies are a source of information on family and children's services. Libraries have government publications describing universal services, complete with addresses of branch offices.

REFERENCE

Campos-Outcalt D. 2004. Public health and family medicine: An opportunity. *Journal of the American Board of Family Medicine* 17:207–211.

CHAPTER 22

⌒⋎⌒

Consultation and Referral

One of the most important duties of family physicians is the deployment of all the resources of medicine and society for their patients. Without the continuing care and responsibility of the family doctor, uncoordinated care by fragmented specialties can be both wasteful and dangerous. Effective communication with colleagues—both in medicine and the other health professions—is therefore an essential skill of family practice. A failure of communication can be as harmful to the patient as a missed diagnosis or an error of treatment. The complexity of modern medicine carries with it the risk of divided responsibility, a situation fraught with danger. The system of communication described in this chapter is designed to eliminate divided responsibility and to clarify the lines of communication among colleagues.

In an Australian study, referral frequency in a single year was 10.6 per 100 encounters, most frequently to a specialist but also to allied health service, hospital, and emergency room. Specialist referral was at a rate of 7.7 per 100 encounters, with referral to orthopedic surgeons, ophthalmologists, surgeons, and gynecologists being the most common (Britt, Miller, Knox, et al., 2003). In the United States, 5.1% of office visits led to a referral, with surgeons and medical specialists accounting for over 76% of those consulted (Forrest, Nutting, Starfield, and Von Schrader, 2002). Over a 5-year period in 23 family practices and 29,303 patients in southwestern Ontario, there were 544,398 encounters. The mean number of referrals per practice in that time period was 2694, with an average of 2 referrals per patient (Thind, Stewart, and Manuel, 2012).

Utilizing data from the National Ambulatory Medical Care Survey and National Hospital Ambulatory Medical Survey from 1993 to 2009, Barnett and colleagues (2012) found that the probability of an ambulatory visit to a physician resulting in a referral to another physician increased from 4.8% to 9.3%. For primary care physicians, the increase was from 5.8% to 9.9%

(Barnett, Song, and Landon, 2012). The reasons for this increase are not clear, but it raises concerns about the contribution of referral rates to healthcare costs and quality of care.

CONSULTATION

In consultation, the doctor responsible for the patient asks a colleague for his or her opinion about the patient. The term *consultant* in this context means "a person who is consulted" and implies no particular office. The person consulted may be a specialist, a family physician, or a member of one of the allied health professions. Although the opinion will obviously carry weight, it is not binding. The patient is at no time under the care of the consultant; unless referral follows consultation, the physician requesting consultation remains in charge. Because of their respective roles in the healthcare system, most requests for consultation are from generalists to specialists. It is important to recognize, however, that other types of consultation do take place. A family physician may seek the opinion of another family physician who has a special area of interest and expertise. A specialist in another discipline may seek the advice of the patient's family physician after referral has taken place.

General practitioners, especially in rural or remote regions, have often had areas of special interests and skills (e.g., anesthesia, and operative obstetrics), which they have made available to colleagues. Such arrangements had no special designation, but were needed to meet medical demands in their area. This continues to be a need and is recognized as a necessary part of the training of rural generalist practice.[1] More recently, urban family physicians have developed areas of special interest and focused practices.[2] In the United Kingdom, general practitioners with special interest (GPwSI) are expected to maintain their community practices while offering additional services to colleagues. This is intended to reduce healthcare costs and unnecessary secondary care referrals; to improve skills and facilitate more effective management of patients in primary care; to improve care for patients by reducing delays; to improve access by keeping care close to home; and to enhance care by providing specialist-level care, taking into account a holistic approach to coexisting multimorbidities. Accreditation of these individuals takes into account competency frameworks as well as the needs of the locality (Royal College of General Practitioners, 2014). The College of Family Physicians of Canada (CFPC) distinguishes between family physicians with special interests (who maintain their community practice while offering consultations to colleagues) and those with focused practices (who do not maintain a community practice, but focus exclusively on an area such as emergency medicine, sports medicine, etc.). While the CFPC oversees accreditation for designated areas of special interest or focused practice (SIFP), there is at present no measurement of the local needs (College of Family Physicians of Canada, 2014).

Selection of the consultant most appropriate to the patient's needs is an important responsibility of the family physician. Case 9.5 gives an example of appropriate selection, where the attitude of the consultant played a crucial part in the patient's recovery.

A consultation may be formal or informal. Informal consultations are part of the daily language of medicine—on the telephone, in the corridor, or in the coffee room. Formal consultation is often a crucial episode in the patient's management. It should never be arranged or conducted in a casual manner. The following steps are necessary if the consultation is to be effective:

1. The physician requesting consultation should communicate directly with the consultant. In most cases, the communication should be in writing: either a letter, a note on the hospital chart, or a specially designed form sent by mail or electronic means. When the request is urgent, as in surgical consultation for an acute abdomen, a communication by telephone is an acceptable substitute. The ideal form of communication—rarely attainable any longer—is for the consultant and the doctor requesting consultation to see the patient together.

2. At a minimum, the letter requesting consultation should list all the significant problems of the patient, state the physician's main findings, the investigations that have been carried out, all medications that have been prescribed, and the purpose of the consultation. The possible reasons for consultation are many and varied: to help with a diagnostic puzzle, to advise on a specific course of treatment, to give an opinion on the significance of a test result or physical finding, or only to reassure the patient. Unless the consultant knows what question is being asked, he or she may waste time on unnecessary investigations and finish by answering the wrong question.

3. The reason for the consultation should be explained to the patient. It is important that the patient should not see consultation and referral as a rejection—a particular risk with psychiatric consultation.

4. The consultant should communicate back promptly (or telephone in urgent cases), giving his or her findings and opinion. If the consultant is unable to give an opinion, but thinks that another consultant would be appropriate, he or she should recommend this to the referring physician. The consultant should not refer the patient to another consultant himself or herself. Cross-consultations risk leaving the family physician out of the loop, causing fragmentation of care and lack of adequate follow-up on recommendations.

5. Finally, the consultation is not complete until it has been discussed with the patient by the family physician.

The patient's influence on the decision to refer appears to be high in most countries where it has been studied (The European Study, 1992; Little, Dorward, Warner, et al., 2004). A problem may occur when the patient requests a consultation. If physicians are unsure of themselves, they may interpret this as a lack of trust by the patient. Feelings of humiliation may lead the physician to refuse or resist the request or to agree to it with bad grace. A patient's request for another opinion should always be taken seriously, and it should be very exceptional not to agree to it readily. The situation can be avoided if the question of another opinion is first raised and discussed openly by the physician.

Failure to consult can often be traced to two causes: a failure by physicians to appreciate their own limitations, and a feeling that consultation and referral are a personal defeat. Our own observation of physicians is that a readiness to consult is usually a sign of maturity and self-confidence.

Problems may also arise when the referring physician disagrees with the consultant's opinion. In most medical schools, students are still taught mainly by specialists under conditions that tend to underemphasize the teacher's fallibility. When the young physician goes into practice, the authority vested in teachers becomes transferred to consultants. It then becomes very difficult to accept the fact that the consultant may be wrong, and even more difficult to take whatever steps may be required to protect the patient's interest. The fact is that when referring physician and consultant disagree, each has an equal chance of being correct. The special knowledge and experience of the consultant is balanced by the family physician's knowledge of the patient and his or her illness. Family physicians must, therefore, accept the possibility that consultants may be wrong. Two courses are open. First, the family physician can discuss the disagreement openly with the consultant. When there is no urgency, he or she may refer the patient back for a reconsideration. It is only fair that the consultant should have an opportunity to revise his or her opinion, perhaps in the light of new evidence. If this fails to resolve the issue, the family physician should then advise the patient of the disagreement and offer to obtain a third opinion if the patient so wishes. To reiterate a point made earlier, in consultation the referring physician remains fully responsible for the patient and must take whatever action is in the patient's interests. After referral, when responsibility for the patient is temporarily transferred, disagreements about the patient's care are more difficult to handle. The family physician's continuing responsibility, however, does require that he or she make any disagreement known, verbally and in writing, to the physician responsible for care. Another difficult problem for the family physician is a failure of rapport between patient and consultant. These situations require much tact and sensitivity (Case 22.1).

CASE 22.1

Following a lumpectomy for carcinoma of the breast, a 66-year-old woman in my practice (TRF) became extremely agitated and angry upon being told by her surgeon that she could go home. On doing routine hospital rounds, I encountered a woman who had closed herself up in her hospital room and refused to talk to anyone. By simply sitting and waiting for her anger to subside, it was possible to determine that staying an extra day in the hospital would alleviate some of her anxieties. This was communicated to the surgeon, who agreed to the extra stay. Weeks later, in talking about her feelings at the time, she recognized that she had the same feelings of vulnerability and anger as she had experienced many years earlier when her life was threatened by an intruder in her home. Close collaboration with the surgeon made it possible to manage a difficult situation and, subsequently, resulted in a deeper understanding of the patient's experience.

REFERRAL

Referral implies a transfer of responsibility for some aspect of the patient's care. For the family physician, the transfer of responsibility is never total, for he or she always retains an overall responsibility for the patient's welfare. Even if the patient is having major surgery in some distant medical center, the family physician should still be available to patient, family, and surgeon.

The division of responsibility between referring physician and specialist must be clearly defined. This is made easier by defining the different types of referral:

1. Interval referral. The patient is referred for complete care for a limited period. The referring physician has no responsibilities during this period except those described earlier. A common example is the referral of a patient for major surgery or a major medical illness. It is essential to good care that after referral only the specialist should prescribe treatment. The family physician should advise and comment, but not order treatment unless asked to do so. This situation may arise, for example, if a patient develops a respiratory infection, skin rash, or mental breakdown following surgery. In these circumstances it would be natural for the surgeon to ask for the family physician's advice as a consultant with special knowledge of the patient and skill in dealing with common disorders.

2. Collateral referral. The referring physician retains overall responsibility, but refers the patient for care of some specific problem. The referral may be long term, as for chronic glaucoma, or short term, as for counseling for a psychological or social problem.

3. Cross-referral. The patient is advised to see another physician, and the referring physician accepts no further responsibility for the patient's care. This may occur after self-referral by the patient or even after referral by a family physician. In either case, the practice must be condemned, because it is wasteful of resources, demoralizing for the patient, and alienating for the family physician. If a consultant feels that another specialist's opinion is required, he or she should so inform the referring physician before making any referral himself or herself.

4. Split referral. This takes place under conditions of multispecialist practice, when responsibility is divided more or less evenly between two or more physicians, such as one for the patient's diabetes, another for his ischemic heart disease. The danger of this type of care is that nobody knows who has overall responsibility for the patient.

The danger of fragmented care is the division of responsibility. This can all too easily lead to what Balint (1964) has called the "collusion of anonymity." This refers to decisions being made about a patient's management without a clear understanding of who is responsible for him or her. Although teamwork is necessary for good patient care, teams should not make decisions. It should always be clear who is responsible to the patient for clinical decisions.

UNDERSTANDING THE DECISION TO REFER

The decision to refer is complex and not well understood. It should be viewed as an intervention and studied just as any other intervention particularly with respect to outcomes. There are no widely accepted guidelines for referral, and it is driven more by physician practice patterns than anything else (Katz, 2012). In studies of referral, the term *referral* is used to denote both consultation and referral, as defined earlier. The referral rate is usually expressed as the number of referrals per 100 patient–doctor encounters (office or home). Studies on referral patterns have shown considerable variation among physicians. The 20% of physicians with the highest referral rates refer twice as many patients as the 20% with the lowest rates (Fleming, Cross, and Crombie, 1991; The European Study, 1992). No association has been found between referral rate and the age and social class mix of practice populations or the case mix among presenting patients. Two studies from the Netherlands have found distance from hospital (Gloerich, Schrijnemaekers, and van der Zee, 1989) and doctor's attitude toward defensive medicine (Grol et al., 1990) to be weakly associated with referral rates. A study in 15 European countries showed a strong inverse relationship between referral rates and number of patient–doctor encounters. Low-referring doctors saw more patients in the working week than high-referring doctors. Two studies have reported higher referral rates in doctors who had higher levels of confidence and diagnostic certainty (Reynolds, Chitnis, and Roland, 1991; Calman, Hyman, and Licht, 1992).

It is clear from these descriptive studies that referral is a very complex process and that it is important not to jump to conclusions about associations between referral rates and quality of care. A good deal of quantitative descriptive data has been amassed, and there is a move now to explore the issues by qualitative methods and to base research on some conceptual framework. Dowie (1983) interviewed 45 physicians and found a relationship between higher referral rates and doctors' lack of self-confidence and defensiveness about referral. Muzzin (1991a, 1991b, 1991c), who interviewed family doctors, consultants, and patients involved in 50 referrals, identified trust among physicians, consultants, and patients as the key to satisfactory referral. Bailey, King, and Newton (1994) applied an analytical framework to the referral decision in a study using both quantitative and qualitative methods. In the qualitative analysis, high referrers were more likely than low referrers to refer despite doubts about the usefulness of the referral (e.g., the effectiveness of treatment), and there was evidence of more uncertainty about decision-making among the high referrers. There was no evidence that referral rates were related to patient-centeredness.

THE INTERFACE BETWEEN PRIMARY AND SECONDARY CARE

Successful referral depends on good communication among primary physician, consultant, and patient, and good communication is a reflection of the degree of integration among the primary, secondary, and tertiary sectors of the health services. In studying communication problems across these interfaces, it is important to attend to all participants in the process: patients, referring physicians, consultants, nurses, administrators, and staff. Communication problems are rarely the fault of any one person or group. Any solution to the problem will probably need intervention at several points in the communication network.

A toolkit intended to improve communication between referring physicians and specialists has been developed (Canadian Medical Association, 2014). It emphasizes the need for some standardization of referral forms and processes.

Wood (1993) and Wood and McWilliam (1996) addressed problems of communication between family physicians and oncologists by qualitative studies of both groups. The identified problem was that patients were followed by the cancer clinic rather than being referred back, even for straightforward conditions such as stage I breast cancer.

The greatest source of dissatisfaction among family physicians was the failure of oncologists to assign them a specific role in follow-up care. Poor communication was identified as the key problem: difficulty of reaching the right consultant, several specialists following the same patient, not enough direct communication by telephone, and lack of information about discharge and follow-up plans. Family physicians also shared some feelings that inhibited their assertiveness in making a role for themselves: lack of self-confidence, fear of a loss of specialist support, inadequate knowledge, and fear of being blamed for not doing enough.

These responses provide an insight into how a problem in one component can affect the function of the entire system. Family physicians who lack self-confidence will tend to withdraw from cancer care, and the very act of withdrawal will reduce their experience and further impair their self-confidence. Their lack of self-confidence will probably be sensed by their patients, who will see cancer or surgical clinics as their source of care. The load on the cancer clinic will increase, and the clinic—believing that family physicians are not interested—might hire clinical assistants to help with the workload. Patients might receive subtle (if unintended) messages from the clinic that the family doctor is no longer involved in their care. That message can be conveyed simply by not mentioning the family physician.

The oncologists whom Wood interviewed viewed family physicians as very variable in their commitment to following up their cancer patients and in their knowledge of cancer therapy. Communication was often thwarted by lack of time, difficulty in contacting family doctors, and the rarity of a personal relationship. Oncologists were critical of family doctors for not sending information about tests done or illnesses occurring between visits to the clinic. They valued their relationships with their patients and felt a need to go on seeing some patients who were doing well. Both family physicians and oncologists expressed a wish for closer collaboration, and their suggestions for attaining this were very similar.

In a qualitative exploration of perceptions of potential recipients and GPs of shared care in oncology, there was support, especially among rural residents, for such arrangements, provided they could be assured that their GPs had received sufficient extra training. The GPs also had concerns about gaining the necessary knowledge and skills, especially with potentially small numbers of patients. They were concerned about lack of support from colleagues and the need for some organizational changes. Nevertheless, with proper preparation and support from oncologists, arrangements of this nature may help to provide good quality care closer to the patient's home (Hall, Samuel, and Murchie 2011).

At the present stage in the evolution of health services, some progress has been made in horizontal integration at the primary care level. The major challenge in many systems is vertical integration between levels. Information technology is providing new tools for removing some of the difficulties. For other difficulties, however, the route to integration lies in dialogue and mutual understanding among primary care physicians, consultants, patients, and others.

SHARED CARE

Problems in the communication between primary and secondary care has increased the interest in the different kinds of shared care. Shared care is defined as "the joint participation of hospital consultants and general practitioners in the planned delivery of care for patients with a chronic condition, informed by an enhanced information exchange over and above routine discharge and referral notices" (Hickman, Drummond, and Grimshaw, 1994, p. 447).

Hickman et al. (1994) suggested a taxonomy of shared care systems that had six categories by questionnaire surveys:

1. Electronic mail, which requires a common database with multiple access points for all participating doctors and nurses;
2. Computer-assisted shared care, in which patients are recalled by a central database either to general practice or to hospital and an agreed data set collected for entry onto a central computer;
3. Shared record cards, which can be either patient-held or posted back and forth between generalist and specialist;
4. Liaison meetings, used most frequently in mental health and drug dependency;
5. Regular communication by letter or standard record sheets (basically a manual version of computer-assisted shared care);
6. Community clinic, where a consultant or specialist nurse conducts clinics in primary care.

Greenhalgh (1994) reviewed shared care for diabetes, commenting that the establishment of a successful shared care system is a complex exercise in change management.

She stresses the need for general practitioners to take ownership of the system. Some form of structured care is necessary. This means registering patients at the time of diagnosis, recall, reminders, and regular review.

A review of the literature on shared care identified that communication continues to be a problem (Hampson, Roberts, and Morgan, et al., 1996). The evidence is mixed on whether shared care improves outcomes in the management of chronic diseases (Smith, Allwright, and O'Dowd, 2008) and is plagued by poor quality (Ontario Health Technology Assessment, 2012).

Frequent audits should be mandatory for all shared care systems, and the effects of the system on other parts of the practice should be noted. As requirements change over time, the system will also have to change. Until recently, general practitioners were not expected to manage type 1 diabetes mellitus (T1DM). The increased use of insulin for T1DM and T2DM is beyond the reach of the endocrinologists, and it is becoming the standard of care for family physicians to institute and manage insulin therapy (see Chapter 14, "Diabetes").

Improved collaboration between family physicians and psychiatry and mental health has been an area of active development since the mid-1990s. Shared care is one element of the goal of improving the integration between care providers. Kates and Craven (2011) define what both mental health providers and family physicians need to do to arrive at more integrated care. Mental health providers need to

Understand the demands of primary care (the fast pace, the frequent interruptions, the unpredictability);

Be respectful of and adapt to the environment and routines of the primary care setting;

Be clear about the limitations of what they are able to and not able to offer;

Allow time for case discussions and case reviews with the family physician, as well as seeing new patients;

Make these case discussions brief and relevant, with as much practical, how-to information as possible;

Chart (legibly) in the continuing medical record (electronic or paper) before leaving the office;

Provide clear and concise treatment plans, with contingencies built in for failure to respond and for crises.

Family physicians need to

Attempt to find serviceable space for the visiting psychiatrist or mental health worker;

Be willing to spend time reviewing cases;

Be willing to discuss patient problems and implement advice rather than refer everyone to the visiting psychiatrist or mental health worker;

Follow through on treatment plans once care is handed back;

Champion this approach with other primary care staff.

Together the psychiatrist and family physician need to

Meet periodically to evaluate the collaborative program and make any necessary adjustments;

Determine which patient populations and/or mental health problems are the priorities for collaborative care;

Work out how appointments will be made, charts pulled, notes written, reports dictated, and so on;

Meet at the start of each day to review who is coming in (for the family physician and mental health team), what their care needs may be, and how, if necessary, each could help the other;

Meet periodically to review how the model is working.

E-CONSULTS AND ENHANCED TELEPHONE CONSULTS

The widespread availability of electronic means of communication and electronic health records has made possible e-consultations. An e-consultation consists of a web-enabled system that supports processes to improve communication between family physicians and specialists. It can range from simply written communication, written communication with attached photographs, or video communication. It has the advantage of reducing wait times to obtain a specialist opinion, and enhances the family physician's confidence. A Mayo clinic study estimated that e-consults could avoid 1800 specialty consultations, thus reducing direct costs by $450,000 annually (Homer, Wagner, and Tufano, 2011). This does not include the savings in time and travel costs to the patient. Primary care practitioners report better access for nonurgent issues and shorter wait times for arranging a new appointment for specialty opinion (Hamo, Paavola, Carlson, et al., 2000). The Champlain BASE (Building Access to Specialists through e-consultation) reported success in implementing an e-consult service across a variety of specialties and primary care providers (PCPs). Among 59 PCPs, there were 406 e-consultations to 16 specialty services. The service was perceived as highly beneficial to providers and patients in more than 90% of cases and avoided a traditional referral in 43% of cases (Keely, Liddy, and Afkham, 2013).

The need for a completely secure electronic communication that protects patient privacy can be problematic and a potential barrier to more widespread use of e-consults in some parts of the world.

Timely and prompt telephone advice with dedicated system infrastructure is another variation to enhance availability of specialist advice. The Rapid Access to Consultative Expertise (RACE) in the province of British Columbia provides ease of accessibility and is more sustainable due to an organized rotation schedule for specialists on call.

NOTES

1. We wish to acknowledge Dr. Jill Konkin for bringing this to our attention.
2. General/family practitioners with special interests are individuals with extra train-
    ing in a medical area (e.g., dermatology, minor surgical procedures) who provide
    consultations for the patients of colleagues, while maintaining their own general
    practice. A related phenomenon are those trained in general/family practice who
    have focused exclusively on another field (e.g., hospitalist care, sports medicine,
    palliative care). They do not provide care for defined community-based practice.
    There is some concern that the latter may represent a turning away from generalist
    practice, potentially further fragmenting care of patients.

REFERENCES

Bailey J, King N, Newton P. 1994. Analyzing general practitioners' referral decisions.
    II. Applying the analytical framework: Do high and low referrers differ in factors
    influencing their referral decisions? *Family Practice* 11(1):9.
Balint M. 1964. *The Doctor, His Patient and the Illness*. London: Pitman Medical.
Barnett ML, Song Z, Landon BE. 2012. Trends in physician referrals in the United
    States 1999–2009. *Archives of Internal Medicine* 172(2):163–170.
Britt H, Miller GC, Knox S, Charles J, Valenti L, Henderson J, et al. 2003. *General
    Practice Activity in Australia 2002–03*. Canberra: Australian Institute of Health
    and Welfare.
Calman NS, Hyman RB, Licht W. 1992. Variability in consultation rates and practitio-
    ner level of diagnostic certainty. *Journal of Family Practice* 35(1):31.
Canadian Medical Association. 2014. Streamlining *Patient Flow From Primary to
    Specialty Care: A Critical Requirement for Improved Access to Specialty Care*.
    http://policybase.cma.ca/dbtw-wpd/Policypdf/PD15-01.pdf. College of Family
    Physicians of Canada, Section of Family Physicians with Special Interests or
    Focused Practice (SIFP). Project Update. http://www.cfpc.ca/uploadedFiles/
    Directories/Sections/SIFP%20Progress%20Update%20(FINAL%20ENG%20
    July%205%202013).pdf.
Dowie R. 1983. *General Practitioners and Consultants: A Study of Out-patient Referrals*.
    London: King Edwards Hospital Foundation.
The European Study of Referrals from Primary to Secondary Care. 1992. Report to
    the Concerted Action Committee of Health Services Research for the European
    Community. Occasional paper 56. Royal College of General Practitioners.
Fleming DM, Cross KW, Crombie DL. 1991. An examination of practice referral rates in
    relation to practice structure, patient demography, and case mix. *Health Trends*
    23:100.
Forrest CB, Nutting PA, Starfield B, Von Schrader S. 2002. Family physicians' refer-
    ral decisions: Results From the ASPN Referral Study. *Journal of Family Practice*
    51(3):215–222.
Gloerich ABM, Schrijnemaekers V, van der Zee J. 1989. Referrals in sentinel practices.
    In: Bartelds AIM, Francheboud J, van der Zee J, eds. *The Dutch Sentinel Practice
    Network: Relevance for Public Health Policy*. Utrecht: NIVEL.
Greenhalgh PM. 1994. Shared care for diabetes: A systematic review. Occasional Paper
    67. Royal College of General Practitioners.

Grol R, Whitfield M, De Maeseneer J, et al. 1990. Attitudes to risk taking in medical decision making among British, Dutch, and Belgian general practitioners. *British Journal of General Practice* 40:134.

Hall SJ, Samel LM, Murchie P. 2011. Toward shared care for people with cancer: Developing the model with patients and GPs. *Family Practice* 28(5):554–564.

Hamo K, Paavola T, Carlson C, Viikinkoski P. 2000. Patient referral by telemedicine: Effectiveness and cost analysis of an intranet system. *Journal of Telemedicine and Telecare* 6(5):320–329.

Hampson JP, Robers RI, Morgan DA, McGhee SM, Hedley AJ 1996. Shared care: A review of the literature. *Family Practice* 13(3):264–279.

Hickman M, Drummond H, Grimshaw J. 1994. A taxonomy of shared care for chronic disease. *Journal of Public Health Medicine* 16(4):447.

Homer K, Wagner E, Tufano J. 2011. Electronic consultation between primary and specialty care clinicians: Early insights. *The Commonwealth Fund Issue Brief* pub. 1554, vol. 23.

Kates N, Craven M. 2011. Improving collaboration between mental health and primary care services. In: Goldbloom DS, Davine J (eds), *Psychiatry in Primary Care: A Concise Canadian Pocket Guide*. Toronto: Canadian Mental Health Association.

Katz MH. 2012. How can we know so little about physician referrals? *Archives of Internal Medicine* 172(2):100.

Keely E, Liddy C, Afkham A. 2013. Utilization, benefits, and impact of an e-consultation service across diverse specialties and primary care providers. *Telemedicine Journal and e-Health* 19(10):733–738.

Little P, Dorward M, Warner G, Stephens K, Senior J, Moore M. 2004. Importance of patient pressure and perceived pressure and perceived need for investigations, referral, and prescribing in primary care: Nested observational study. *BMJ* 328:444.

Muzzin LJ. 1991a. Understanding the process of medical referral. Part 1: Critique of the literature. *Canadian Family Physician* 37:2155.

Muzzin LJ. 1991b. Understanding the process of medical referral. Part 2: Methodology of the study. *Canadian Family Physician* 37:2377.

Muzzin LJ. 1991c. Understanding the process of medical referral. Part 3: Trust and choice of consultant. *Canadian Family Physician* 37:2576.

Ontario Health Technology Assessment Series. 2012. Specialized community-based care: An evidence based analysis. *Ontario Health Technology Assessment Series* 12(20).

Rapid Access to Consultative Expertise (RACE). http://www.raceconnect.ca/.

Reynolds GA, Chitnis JG, Roland MO. 1991. General practitioner out-patient referrals: Do good doctors refer more patients to hospital? *British Journal of Medicine* 302:1250.

Royal College of General Practitioners. *GPs with a Special Interest (GPwSI) Accreditation.* http://www.rcgp.org.uk/clinical-and-research/clinical-resources/gp-with-a-special-interest-gpwsi-accreditation.aspx.

Smith SM, Allwright S, O'Dowd T. 2008. Does sharing care across the primary-specialty interface improve outcomes in chronic disease? *American Journal of Managed Care* 14(4):213–224.

Thind A, Stewart M, Manuel D, Freeman T, Terry A, Chevendra V, Maddocks H, Marshall N. 2012. What are wait times to see a specialist? An analysis of 26,942 referrals in Southwestern Ontario. *Healthcare Policy* 8(1):80–91.

Wood ML. 1993. Communication between cancer specialists and family doctors. *Canadian Family Physician* 39:49.

Wood ML, McWilliam CL. 1996. Cancer in remission: Challenge in collaboration for family physician and oncologists. *Canadian Family Physician* 42:899.

CHAPTER 23

༄

Alternative or Complementary Medicine

Alternative, complementary, or unconventional medicine[1] (CAM) is the name given to those medical practices not usually available in mainstream institutions and not usually taught in medical and other professional schools. Although seemingly ambiguous, this definition reflects the history of the relationship of these practices to mainstream medicine, which, after all, only delineated itself scarcely 150 years ago. Those practices outside the mainstream were designated *alternative*, but as some of them achieve greater acceptance they are considered complementary to conventional medicine and, in some instances, may be fully accepted as mainstream. However, the vagueness of this definition does lead to problems in a number of areas. Some practices that are alternative in one country may, by reason of history and custom, be included in the professional sector of another. Homeopathy in North America is generally considered nonconventional, but in the United Kingdom it enjoys greater acceptance and is best described as spanning the folk and professional sectors of health care. Osteopathy in the United States has a status similar to that of conventional medical doctors. Midwives in many countries have crossed the boundary from alternative to professional sector and provide a significant proportion of maternity care. Such "crossovers" undoubtedly influence both the former "alternative" practices and mainstream medicine.

Even in countries with the most advanced systems of medical care and the most effective technology, the use of alternative medicine is widespread. Using data from the National Health Interview Survey and comparing trends across three points in time (2002, 2007, 2012), it was found that one in three Americans used some form of CAM[2] in the year prior to the survey. The most popular complementary health approach across all three time points was nonvitamin, nonmineral dietary supplements (e.g., fish oil, probiotics, prebiotics, melatonin, all of which increased, and echinacea, garlic, ginseng, ginkgo, and saw palmetto, all of which decreased over the three time periods). Mind/body approaches such as yoga, tai chi, and qi gong increased in use from 6.7% of respondents in 2002 to 10.1% in 2012. More than 95% of respondents used complementary health approaches as an adjunct to conventional medicine rather than a replacement (Clarke, Black, and Sussman, 2015). Using the same surveys, it was found that 11.6% of children aged 4–17 used complementary approaches (Black, Clarke, and Barnes, 2015).

Widespread use of alternative therapies has been found in other countries as well. In a systematic review of 12-month prevalence studies across 15 countries, estimates of use ranged from 26% in the United Kingdom to 76% in Japan. Visits to alternative practitioners varied from 12% in Canada to 27% in Australia (Harris, Cooper, and Relton, 2012). Comprehensive summaries of CAM are available (Zollman, Vickers, and Richardson, 2008) and the National Center for Complementary and Integrative Health of the National Institutes of Health maintains a current website.

In considering why there is so much interest in CAM, one study in the United States found that those who utilized CAM felt it aligned more with their values and beliefs toward health and life. They tended not to reject conventional medicine, but combined it with CAM (Astin, 1998). For several reasons, family doctors should be well informed about alternative medicine. They should be in a position to advise patients who wish to use alternative therapies. Some unconventional therapies are known to be effective for certain conditions; some are potentially dangerous if used without a diagnostic assessment; some remedies are toxic, and others may interact with medically prescribed drugs; many therapies are harmless and, although not supported by good evidence, may give comfort to the patient. Because many alternative practitioners are not members of self-regulating professional bodies, the public has very little protection against charlatans. Family doctors may be in a position to protect patients from harm or exploitation, especially if they have knowledge of local providers. The help that a family doctor can give will be enhanced if there is openness between doctor and patient and if the doctor is perceived as unbiased.

The concurrent use of multiple healthcare systems, alternative and conventional, is viewed as a return to the medical pluralism that characterized health practices before what is now known as conventional medicine established hegemony. Biomedical professionals, whether they know it or not, frequently share the care of their patients with unconventional approaches. Over the past 20 years, the discourse on CAM in the medical literature has changed from examining the differences of various CAM practices and conventional medicine to discussing how CAM can be integrated with usual practice (Jonas, Eisenberg, Hufford, et al., 2013).

Family medicine has often served as a portal for the entry of CAM practices into mainstream medicine. Many family physicians combine acupuncture and conventional medicine, for example. *Integrative medicine* explicitly exists at the boundary of conventional medical practice and CAM. This relationship should not be surprising, considering the overlap in the values shared by both. Family medicine, like some of the CAM practices, emphasizes the diagnosis of the patient, not only a disease, seeking to understand the biological, psychological, and social dimensions and their interactions. Even when a patient's health belief system exists outside the mainstream, the family physician affirms its importance if it advances the health of the patient. Like some CAM practices, family medicine emphasizes the development of a cooperative relationship with patients. That there is such an overlap in values has been attributed to the common roots of general practice and some CAM practices in the humoral medicine of Hippocrates (Greaves, 2003). Greaves argues that alternative medicine is a continuation of humoral medicine, which emphasizes the need for balance within the body and its parts and recognizes the strong relationship between mental and physical processes. When the biomedical model became dominant in the mid-nineteenth century, humoral medicine and its practitioners were relegated to the "alternative" category. General practice, although part of conventional medicine, never fully severed its roots in the former humoral tradition.

ALTERNATIVE TO WHAT?

Unconventional therapy is defined in terms of its opposite: conventional or mainstream medicine. However, there are different ways in which a therapy can be unconventional. Conventional medicine has a number of levels. Its foundation, as in all sciences, is a set of assumptions about what the world is like. These assumptions are neither questioned nor made explicit (Kuhn, 1967). They may take the form of metaphors, such as the metaphor of nature as a machine. At another level, medicine has theories that can be tested experimentally for their coherence and truth. On the practical level, therapies are derived from theories and are subject to testing for their effectiveness. When medicine is at its best, all these levels are congruent with each other. Assumptions are reasonable, theories have stood up to empirical testing, and therapies derived from the theories shown by clinical trials to be effective. Often, however, this is not the case. Therapies that should work in theory do not work in practice; a therapy derived from an inadequate theory may prove to be very effective. The strength of modern medicine is its insistence that a therapy should prove itself experimentally, however well founded its theory.

Some unconventional medicine is an alternative at all these levels. Traditional Chinese medicine is based on a worldview totally different from that of Western medicine. Its theory of disease is at variance with Western science. On the other hand, acupuncture can be evaluated by clinical trial and can be adopted by mainstream medicine without subscribing to the theory from which it is derived. Chiropractic theory has no empirical foundation, but chiropractic manipulation is effective for certain conditions. Hypnosis was for a long time rejected by mainstream medicine because of its theory of animal magnetism. Now, hypnosis is recognized as an effective therapy in some circumstances, and the theory of animal magnetism has been abandoned. Some alternative paradigms and theories have deep roots in the tradition of Western medicine. The various movements in medicine that come under the term *holistic*, for example, have roots in the Hippocratic tradition.

In medical education there has been an increasing recognition of the need to include some exposure of medical students to CAM (Wetzel, Kaptchuk, Haramati, et al., 2003). In a survey of medical schools in the United States, it was found that among 53 responding institutions (out of 73), most provided only a minimal amount of contact hours. Topics that tended to be emphasized were acupuncture (76.7%), herbs and botanicals (69.9%), meditation and relaxation (65.8%), spirituality/faith/prayer (64.4%), chiropractic (60.3%), homeopathy (57.5%), and nutrition and diets (50.7%) (Brokaw, Tunnicliff, Raess, et al., 2002). A small survey of medical students in the United Kingdom found that 54% had received lectures on CAM (Ho, Chan, Bewley, et al., 2013).

CATEGORIES OF ALTERNATIVE MEDICINE

Alternative medical practices come in a bewildering variety. The British Medical Association Report listed 116 therapies. Most of these fall into one of the following categories:

1. Ancient medical traditions such as traditional Chinese medicine (TCM), Ayurvedic, and traditional Iranian medicine (TIM), which represent a complete paradigm, theory, and range of therapeutic practices.
2. Shamanistic healing in traditional societies that retain their links with the past. Although using herbal medicines, the shaman is distinguished by an initiation that is believed to confer power over the spirit world. The healing process often involves altered states of consciousness and includes members of the patient's family and community.
3. Folk medicine: lore handed down through generations, often about medical properties of plants. Some modern drugs and practices had their origins in folklore—for example, smallpox vaccination, quinine, digitalis, ergotamine, colchicine.

4. Alternative paradigms and practices with recent roots in Western societies: homeopathy, osteopathy, chiropractic, anthroposophic medicine, naturopathy.
5. Nutritional therapies, ranging from herbal medicines to dietary regimes.
6. Body therapies, including many kinds of massage.
7. Spiritual healing, either within the mainstream religions or by individuals claiming to have special powers.
8. Individual therapies, either borrowed from other traditions or developed autonomously: acupuncture, biofeedback, hypnotherapy, meditation, imaging.

The availability and use of these different therapies vary from one country to another. In the United States, osteopathy has become so close to conventional medicine that osteopaths are often regarded as equivalent to medical doctors. Chiropractic is prominent in the United States and Canada, and in several Canadian provinces chiropractic services are covered by Medicare. Naturopathy is widespread in Germany. Homeopathy is practiced by significant numbers of medical doctors in several European countries.

One useful taxonomy of unconventional healing practices is provided by Kaptchuk and Eisenberg (2005). In this taxonomy, there are two very broad divisions: CAM and parochial unconventional medicine. The largest division, CAM, is then subdivided into professional systems (chiropractic, acupuncture, homeopathy, naturopathy, massage, and dual-trained physicians), popular health reform (mega-vitamins, nutritional supplements, botanicals, macrobiotics, organic food, vegan diet), New Age healing (esoteric energies, crystals and magnets, spirits and mediums, reiki, qi gong), mind/body (Deepak Chopra, Bernie Siegel, Course in Miracles, Silva Mind Control, biofeedback, hypnosis, guided imagery, relaxation response, cognitive-behavioral therapy), and non-normative (chelation, antineoplastons, pleomorphic bacteria cancer therapy, iridology, hair analysis). Parochial unconventional medicine has three divisions: ethno-medicine (Puerto Rican spiritualism, African-American rootwork, Haitian voodoo, Hmong practices, Mexican-American *curonaderismo*), religious healing (Pentecostal churches, Catholic charismatic renewal, Christian Science), and folk medicine practices (copper bracelets for arthritis, chicken soup for the common cold, red string for nosebleed). To this taxonomy some would add a category called the popular sector, which includes self-medication, advice from pharmaceuticals, advice from family, friends, and self-help groups (Helman, 2001).

COMMON ALTERNATIVE PRACTICES

The frequency with which alternative medicine is used makes it advisable for family doctors to have a basic knowledge of the common practices, their claims, their benefits, and their risks. Some of them are better thought of as complementary to conventional medicine, rather than alternative to it. Evaluating the usefulness of various CAM therapies is difficult for the practitioner due to the relative lack of high-quality evaluative studies. This is to some extent rooted in the different epistemologies of many CAM practices and conventional medicine. The latter places highest value on randomized control trials and replicability, and is rooted in a reductionist framework. CAM practitioners would argue that a broader framework is necessary and credence given to different types of knowledge if we are to fully understand and help our patients. Most family physicians would agree. There are useful references available for the practitioner, and some of these are listed at the end of the chapter. Websites have the advantage of being more frequently updated and easier to access than textbooks.

Manipulation

Spinal manipulative therapy (SMT) is commonly employed in the treatment of back and neck pain. One mechanism of pain relief, common to manipulation, acupuncture, massage, and transcutaneous electrical nerve stimulation, is thought to be the release of enkephalin by the selective stimulation of mechanoceptors.

A systematic review of 20 randomized controlled trials (RCTs) involving manipulation and mobilization, including studies from chiropractic, manual therapy, or osteopathic for acute low back pain, found the quality of evidence low to moderate. SMT was no more effective than inert interventions, sham SMT, or when added to another intervention. Given the small number of studies, the authors recommended that more studies be done and that patient preference, safety, and cost be taken into account (Rubinstein, Terwee, Assendelft, et al., 2012).

In a review of 39 RCTs, it was found that spinal manipulation was more effective in alleviating pain and improved the ability to perform everyday activities when compared to sham treatments but was no more effective than conventional medical therapies (Assendelft et al., 2004). Massage therapy, when combined with exercise education, may have short term benefits for subacute and chronic low back pain (Furlan, Giraldo, Baskwill, et al., 2015).

For chronic low back pain, there is high-quality evidence that SMT is no better than other treatments in reducing pain or improving function (Rubinstein, Middelkoop, Assendelft, et al., 2011).

The main contraindications to manipulation are rheumatoid neck, basilar insufficiency (drop attacks, vertigo) vertebral myelopathy, coagulation disorders, including patients on anticoagulants, and any vertebral disease carrying a risk of spinal cord compression (osteoporosis, spinal metastases).

Homeopathy

Introduced in Germany by Hahnemann in the late eighteenth century, home-opathy[3] was in strong disagreement with the prevailing allopathic medicine, with its purgings and bleedings. It is based on the theory that like cures like, that ailments are cured by minute doses of the drug that in larger doses produces the same symptoms. An individual diagnosis and regimen is established for each patient. Homeopathic remedies are made by serial dilutions and shaking (succussion), a process thought to increase the potency of the drug.

Because serial dilutions may remove all traces of the drug, any effects of homeopathic medicines cannot be explained in terms of current medical knowledge. A meta-analysis of 89 randomized or placebo-controlled clinical trials published in 1995 found an overall positive effect with an odds ratio of 2.45 in favor of homeopathy (Linde et al., 1997). It appears, therefore, that the results cannot be explained in terms of the placebo effect. These results have been disputed and remain controversial (Hahn, 2013).

Naturopathy

Naturopathy focuses on the healing powers of the body—the ancient medical principle of *vis medicatrix naturae*. The aim of therapy is to strengthen the patient's own powers of healing by attention to diet, rest, relaxation, and by use of stimuli to activate the healing process. The diagnosis is made of a patient, not of a disease—an interesting parallel with premodern medicine, when diagnosis often had the same connotation.[4]

Naturopaths view health as having three components: structural, biochemical, and emotional. The diagnosis is made after a long history and physical assessment. Naturopaths are generalists who use a wide variety of therapeutic modalities, including nutrition, homeopathy, botanical medicine, hydrotherapy, massage, manipulation, and traditional Chinese medicine.

By focusing on the "host," naturopathy follows an ancient medical principle, one that has been neglected by modern medicine. Medical doctors may adopt some of the naturopathic principles while continuing to use the conventional approach to diagnosis and treatment (Boon, 1996).

Herbal Medicine

Medicines prepared from plant materials are used in many traditional societies and in ancient systems of medicine such as the Chinese. They are now widely consumed in Western countries in the form of teas, powders, tablets, or capsules. They may be bought over the counter in pharmacies or prescribed by an herbalist after an assessment of the patient. Because the medicines are prepared from plants, they contain a mixture of substances rather than a single active ingredient.

In Canada, one in 10 people is reported to be taking some form of natural medicine, including herbal remedies. The most popular herbs are garlic, echinacea, ginseng, alfalfa, and devil's claw root (Institute for Clinical Evaluative Studies [ICES], 1996).

It is not possible here even to summarize the properties of the many herbs in common use. Good reference sources are available and may be kept in the practice library.[5] Because of the possibility of toxic properties and interaction with prescribed drugs, the physician should know if the patient is taking herbal medicines. This information is unlikely to be volunteered. Most herbs are harmless when taken in the recommended dose, following the guidelines in Box 23.1. The fact that some herbs are toxic need not be used to scare patients into avoidance of all herbal remedies.

Because herbal remedies are derived from plants, many people believe incorrectly that they can have no harmful effects. Not only are there some well-known toxic effects of specific herbs, but preparations sometimes contain potentially toxic additives that are not listed on the label. Patients should be advised, therefore, to obtain their medications from qualified professional herbalists or from ethical manufacturers (see Box 23.1).

Box 23.1

ADVICE FOR PATIENTS ON THE USE OF HERBAL PRODUCTS

If you are going to take herbs, see a practitioner formally trained in botanical medicine.

Buy herbal remedies from trusted and reliable sources. Avoid herbs in which the purity and quality are suspicious, especially imported herbs.

Most herbs, like drugs, should be avoided during pregnancy and lactation and should not be given to small children.

Consider drug/herb interactions.

Start with low dosages and beware of the dosages: two pills from the same bottle may have completely different strengths.

To avoid possible chronic effects, do not use herbal remedies for long periods.

If you are unwell, discontinue use immediately and seek medical advice.

Reproduced with permission from Getting Acquainted with Herbs: Weeding Fact from Fiction, in Informed: Information for Medical Practitioners from the Institute for Clinical Evaluative Sciences in Ontario (ICES) 1996: V2(2):2.

Some herbs are hepatotoxic and may cause either acute hepatic necrosis or chronic hepatitis and cirrhosis (see Box 23.2). A number of herbs contain the hepatotoxic pyrrolozidine alkaloids. Renal failure has been reported in women receiving Chinese herbal medicine at a weight-loss clinic (ICES, 1996). Amygdalin (Laetrile), used for cancer, may cause cyanide poisoning.

Herbal medicine may interact with orthodox drugs. Taking ginseng and a monoamine oxidase inhibitor may cause headache and insomnia. Psyllium-seed products can decrease the absorption of lithium. Evening primrose oil, when taken with phenothiazines, may increase the number of seizures. Garlic increases the effect of warfarin. Licorice may upset control of hypertension by causing hypo-kalemia and salt retention. Karela, used in curries, can destabilize diabetic control by causing hypoglycemia. Lily of the valley contains cardiac glycosides and can potentiate digitalis. Horse chestnut, ginger, and ginkgo can potentiate coumadin (Penn, 1986; Ernst, 2005). Other drugs with these properties are described in the sources listed at the end of this chapter.

Nutrition

After years of neglect, nutrition is now assuming greater importance in medical education, practice, and research. Cancer of the breast, colon, and pancreas appears to be associated with the high-fat, low-fiber diet in Western countries. Individuals at high risk for cardiovascular disease on a Mediterranean diet (low consumption of meat and meat products; high consumption of

---

Box 23.2
SOME HEPATOTOXIC HERBS

Chaparral
Comfrey
Germander
Mistletoe and skullcap
Margosa oil
Maté tea
Gordolobo yerba tea
Pennyroyal
Jin by huan

Reprinted with permission from Koff RS. 1995. Herbal hepatotoxity: Revisiting a dangerous alternative. Journal of the American Medical Association 273(6):502.

vegetables, fruits, nuts, legumes, fish, and olive oil), when compared to those on a low-fat diet, experienced a 30% relative risk reduction in stroke, heart attack, death from cardiovascular disease, or death from any cause after 5 years (Estruch, Ros, and Salas-Salvado, 2013). The number needed to treat (NNT) for this group is 1 in 61 with no known harms to the diet. There is now much public interest in the potential role of diet in preventing or even arresting cancer. Conventional dietary advice now is emphasizing the reduction of refined carbohydrates in the diet, with the World Health Organization (WHO) recommending that they represent less than 10% of total daily caloric intake, but lowering to less than 5% as a goal. For an average-sized adult, 5% of total recommended caloric intake would represent 25 grams or 6 teaspoons of sugar (WHO, 2014).

Outside conventional practice and research, claims have been made for dietary therapies in the form of complete nutritional regimens or the intake of megadoses of vitamins. The macrobiotic diet consists of whole grain cereals, vegetables, and fruits, but no animal products. Vitamins and other elements may be added. There is some evidence that this diet may increase survival in advanced pancreatic and prostate cancer (Carter et al., 1993). Conventional nutritionists have considered the macrobiotic diet inadequate, and it is certainly not sufficient for children. However, older patients do not have the same needs, and it may be this feature of the diet that can slow the growth of a tumor while maintaining normal tissue (Wiesburger, 1993). Because we have little else to offer many patients with advanced cancer, we have reason to support those who wish to try the macrobiotic diet, though the evidence so far does not justify using it as a standard therapy. Those using megadoses of vitamins, however, should be warned about the toxic effects of high doses of vitamins A and D.

The upsurge of interest in nutritional aspects of disease and the discovery of a scientific basis for some unconventional therapies may lead to a new era of nutritional therapies based on both biochemical research and clinical trials.

Hypnosis

After being rejected by orthodox medicine for many years, hypnosis is now accepted as a therapy for certain conditions and as a way of inducing analgesia and anesthesia. Its main therapeutic uses are for anxiety states, phobias, chronic pain, addictions, and post-traumatic stress disorders. It should be practiced only by physicians, psychologists, and dentists who are in a position to use it as part of a comprehensive management plan after a full clinical assessment. The effect of hypnosis is not so much to remove the symptoms as to enhance the patient's control over his or her reactions.

Meditation

Meditation, a practice in the major spiritual traditions, is now used as a therapeutic method. Medicine has borrowed the technique, without absorbing the
doctrines with which it is associated. The essence of meditation is the concentration of attention on what is going on at the present moment in our minds
and bodies. Anyone trying to do this for the first time is surprised by how difficult it is to keep the attention focused. One's mind is constantly wandering
from one thought and feeling to the next. By systematically reducing tension in
the body, attending to one's breathing, and constantly bringing the mind back
to a single point of attention, a state of calmness and relaxation is induced.
Relaxation produces physiological changes (the relaxation response) and a
decrease in arousal (Benson, 1975). Meditation is taught as a way of reducing
stress and anxiety and as a response to chronic pain (Kabat-Zinn, 1990).

Acupuncture

Acupuncture, based on the principles of traditional Chinese medicine, is practiced in China and other parts of Asia but to a lesser extent in other parts
of the world. In Western countries, a modified form is practiced, based on
a scientific explanatory model rather than the Chinese theory of meridians.
Its main application is for pain relief in musculoskeletal disorders, joint pain,
and chronic headache (Ernst, 2005). Provided proper aseptic techniques are
observed, there is little risk, though some cases of internal injury have been
reported (British Medical Association, 1986).

Integrative Medicine

Dissatisfied with the dominant paradigm of medicine, some physicians have
developed an approach to practice based on traditional principles of Western
medicine: a respect for the *vis medicatrix naturae*, a diagnosis of the individual
patient as well as the disease, attention to the whole context of illness, and the
formulation of a regimen for each patient as a way of restoring and maintaining health. Returning to these basic principles does not mean rejecting the
conventional approach to diagnosis and treatment whenever this is appropriate. Many of the values of integrative medicine are consistent with the values of family medicine represented in the patient-centered approach (Maizes,
Rakel, and Niemiec, 2009).

    Some of the alternative therapies described earlier may be included
in holistic practice. It is likely that we will see increasing interchange
between mainstream and alternative medicine, with serious attempts to

validate alternative practices empirically. There are increasing numbers of scientific journals devoted to the subject, for example, *The Journal of Alternative and Complementary Medicine*, and a major textbook on the topic (Rakel, 2007).

NOTES

1. There is no universally agreed-upon name for what has been called alternative, complementary, or unconventional medicine. The term *complementary* seems to be replacing *alternative*. It has the advantage of conveying the relationship between mainstream medicine and other healing practices.
2. For this survey, the definition of CAM included acupuncture; Ayurveda; biofeedback; chelation therapy; chiropractic care; energy healing therapy; special diets (including vegetarian and vegan, macrobiotic, Atkins, Pritikin, and Ornish); folk medicine or traditional healers; guided imagery; homeopathic treatment; hypnosis; naturopathy; nonvitamin, nonmineral dietary supplements; massage; meditation; progressive relaxation; qi gong; tai chi; or yoga.
3. For additional reading, see the chapter on homeopathy by Heather Boon in *Nonprescription Drug Reference for Health Professionals*, premier edition (Ottawa: Canadian Pharmaceutical Association, 1996).
4. Naturopaths are licensed in Ontario, Manitoba, Saskatchewan, and British Columbia, and in the latter are covered by Medicare. Licensed naturopaths must complete a 4-year full-time graduate program at the Canadian College of Naturopathic Medicine or one of the three naturopathic colleges in the United States.
5. For example, the *British Herbal Pharmacopoeia* and a similar publication used in Germany, the *Nonprescription Drug Reference for Health Professionals*, published by the Canadian Pharmaceutical Association; and *The Desktop Guide to Complementary and Alternative Medicine: An Evidence Based Approach*, ed. Edzard Ernst (Mosby, 2001).<AU: Please add place of publication.>

REFERENCES

Assendelft WJJ, Morton SC, Yu EI, et al. 2004. Spinal manupulative therapy for low back pain. *Cochrane Database of Systematic Reviews*, Issue 1.

Astin JA. 1998. Why patients use alternative medicine: Results of a national survey. *Journal of the American Medical Association* 279:1548–1553.

Boon H. 1996. Canadian naturopathic practitioners: The effects of holistic and scientific world views on their socialization experiences and practice patterns. Ph.D. dissertation, Faculty of Pharmacy, University of Toronto.

Benson H. 1975. *The Relaxation Response*. New York: Morrow.

Black LI, Clarke TC, Barnes PM, et al. 2015. *Use of Complementary Health Approaches among Children Aged 4–17 Years in the United States: National Health Interview Survey, 2007–2012*. National health statistics reports; no 78. Hyattsville, MD: National Center for Health Statistics.

British Medical Association (BMA). 1986. *Alternative Therapy: Report of the Board of Science and Education*. London: British Medical Association.

British Medical Association (BMA). 1993. *Complementary Medicine: New Approaches to Good Practice.* London: BMA.

Brokaw JJ, Tunnicliff G, Raess BU, Saxon DW, 2002. The teaching of complementary and alternative medicine in U.S. medical schools: A survey of course directors. *Academic Medicine* 77(9):876–881.

Carter JP, Saxe GP, Newbold V, et al. 1993. Hypothesis: Dietary management may improve survival from nutritionally linked cancers based on analysis of representative cases. *Journal of the American College of Nutrition* 12:209.

Clarke TC, Black LI, Sussman BJ, et al. 2015. *Trends in the Use of Complementary Health Approaches among Adults: United States, 2002–2012.* National health statistics reports; no 79. Hyattsville, MD: National Center for Health Statistics. 2015.

Ernst E. 2005. The evidence for or against common complementary therapies. In: Lee-Treweek G, Heller T, Spurr S, MacQueen H, Katz J, eds., *Perspectives on Complementary and Alternative Medicine: A Reader.* London; New York: Routledge.

Estruch R, Ros E, Salos-Salvado J, et al. 2013. Primary prevention of cardiovascular disease with a Mediterranean diet. *New England Journal of Medicine* 368(14): 1279–1290.

Furlan AD, Giraldo M, Baskwill A, Irvin E, Imamura M. Massage for low-back pain. Cochrane Database of Systematic Reviews 2015, Issue 9. Art. No.: CD001929. DOI: 10.1002/14651858.CD001929.pub3.

Greaves D. 2003. *The Healing Tradition: Reviving the Soul of Western Medicine.* Oxford; San Francisco: Radcliffe Publishing.

Hahn RG. 2013. Homeopathy: Meta-analyses of pooled clinical data. *Forschende Komplementarmedizin* 20: 376–381.

Harris PE, Cooper KL, Relton C, Thomas KJ. 2012. Prevalence of complementary and alternative medicine (CAM) use by the general population: A systematic review and update. *International Journal of Clinical Practice* 66:924–939.

Helman CG. 2001. *Culture, Health and Illness.* New York: Arnold.

Ho D, Chan K, Bewley S, Bender DA. 2013. Evidence-based medicine and complementary and alternative medicine teaching in UK medical courses: A national survey of the student experiences. *Focus on Alternative and Complementary Therapies* 18(4):176–181.

Institute for Clinical Evaluative Sciences in Ontario. 1996. Getting acquainted with herbs: Weeding fact from fiction. *Informed* 2(2):1.

Jonas WB, Eisenberg D, Hufford D, et al. 2013. The evolution of complementary and alternative medicine (CAM) in the USA over the last 20 years. *Research in Complementary Medicine* 20(1): 65–72.

Kabat-Zinn J. 1990. *Full Catastrophe Living: Using the Wisdom of your Body and Mind to Face Stress, Pain and Illness.* New York: Bantam Doubleday Dell.

Kaptchuk TJ, Eisenberg DM. 2005. A taxonomy of unconventional healing practices. In: Lee-Treweek G, Heller T, Spurr S, MacQueen H, Katz J, eds., *Perspectives on Complementary and Alternative Medicine: A Reader.* London; New York: Routledge.

Koff RS. 1995. Herbal hepatotoxity: Revisiting a dangerous alternative. *Journal of the American Medical Association* 273(6):502.

Kuhn TS. 1967. *The Structure of Scientific Revolutions.* Chicago: University of Chicago Press.

Linde K, Clausius N, Ramirez G, et al.1997. Are the clinical effects of homoeopathy placebo effects? A meta-analysis of placebo-controlled trials. *Lancet* 350:834–843.

Maizes V, Rakel D, Niemiec C. 2009. Integrative medicine and patient-centered care. *EXPLORE: The Journal of Science and Healing* 5(5):277–289.

National Center for Complementary and Integrative Health, https://nccih.nih.gov/.

Penn AG. 1991. Adverse reactions to herbal medicines. In: Shekelle PG, Adams AH, Chassin MR, et al. *The Appropriateness of Spinal Manipulation for Low-Back Pain.* Santa Monica, CA: RAND.

Rakel D (Ed). 2007. *Integrative Medicine*, 2nd ed. Philadelphia: Saunders, Elsevier.

Rubinstein SM, Terwee CB, Assendelft WJJ, et al. 2012. *Spinal Manipulation Therapy for Acute Low-Back Pain.* Cochrane Database of Systematic Reviews. DOI: 10.1002/14651858.CD008880.pub2.

Rubinstein SM, Van Middelkoop M, Assendelft WJJ, et al. 2011. *Spinal Manipulative Therapy for Chronic Low-Back Pain.* Cochrane Database of Systematic Reviews. DOI: 10.1002/14651858.CD008112.pub2.

Wetzel MS, Kaptchuk TJ, Haramati A, Eisenberg DM 2003. Complementary and alternative medical therapies: Implications for medical education. *Annals of Internal Medicine* 138(3):191–196.

Wiesburger JH. 1993. Guest editorial. A new nutritional approach in cancer therapy in light of mechanistic understanding of cancer causation and development. *Journal of the American College of Nutrition* 12(3):205.

World Health Organization. 2014. *WHO Opens Public Consultation on Draft Sugar Guideline.* http://www.who.int/mediacentre/news/notes/2014/consultation-sugar-guideline/en/

Zollman C, Vickers A, Richardson J, eds. 2008. *ABC of Complementary Medicine*, 2nd ed. Oxford: Wiley-Blackwell.

Useful WebsitesMedline plus-Alternative Medicine. A service of US National Library of Medicine and the National Institutes of Health.

National Center for Complementary and Alternative Medicine. https://nccih.nih.gov/

PART IV

Education and Research

CHAPTER 24

Continuing Self-Education

Each case has its lesson—a lesson that may be, but is not always, learnt, for clinical wisdom is not the equivalent of experience. A man who has seen 500 cases of pneumonia may not have the understanding of the disease which comes with an intelligent study of a score of cases, so different are knowledge and wisdom.

Sir William Osler (1905, p. 169)

Any observer of physicians cannot help noticing the wide variation in their capacity for self-education. At one end of the scale is the physician who learns something, however little, from every patient and every illness. At the other is the physician who continues to make the same errors time after time, year after year, with little intellectual or personal growth. What is the difference between them? The good learner, it may be said, will be an assiduous reader of journals and will be seen often at postgraduate courses, thus keeping abreast of medical progress. This may be true, but our observation is that the bad learner may also be a reader of journals and a frequent attendee of courses. The difference between them is that the good learner has grasped the truth that the main source of development as a physician lies not in some distant center of learning but in the day-to-day experience of his or her own practice. Hours spent listening to lectures or bent over medical journals will be of little help unless the physician has reflected deeply on his or her own experience. To say this is not to underrate the value of these modes of learning. Both of them have an important place in the continuing education of the physician, but they are not sufficient in themselves.

It is helpful to consider different kinds of knowledge (Eraut, 1994; Epstein, 1999):

Prepositional knowledge: this consists of facts, theories, concepts, and principles. This is acquired in formal training programs prior to assuming practice and to most (but not all) continuing professional education. Reading programs and courses are ways that the practitioner can keep up to date with developments in the field. Most major medical journals are available in online format, which facilitates refreshing this type of knowledge.

Personal knowledge: this knowledge is only acquired through experience (Polanyi, 1962). This begins in the pre-qualification period and continues throughout practice. To learn from experience, physicians must obviously know what their experience is. They should know the outcome of their actions, both in the short term and in the long term. They should have some standard against which to measure their performance and must have the capacity for accepting criticism and, if necessary, making changes in methods of practice. Information on the physician's methods of practice and their outcome should be available in the practice records. Too often, however, it is hidden in the records. The information has to be not only available but also accessible. It is not enough for physicians to base their actions on the last two or three cases seen; they should be able to review all their cases of diabetes, hypertension, otitis media, depression, or whatever condition is being studied. The electronic medical record has made this much easier to attain. When physicians review their cases, they will have some questions in mind. How did the patients present? What were the early symptoms? Could the diagnosis have been made earlier? Did the treatment achieve its objectives? They will also be judging their results against certain standards. Two kinds of standards may be used: empirical and normative. Empirical standards are derived from statistical averages obtained from similar settings. These enable the physician to compare activities such as prescribing, referral, or follow-up with those of other physicians. Normative standards are derived from traditional sources of orthodox medical standards. When medical audit is used as an educational process, it is best for the physician or the group to begin by defining their own standards for the specific problem or disease being studied. The development of these standards is an educational process in itself because it involves a review of the literature, a review of empirical data, and often discussions with consultants. Once the standards are defined, the records are then reviewed and data collected. Almost certainly, the results will show that the physician's performance falls short of his or her own standards. The physician or group must then decide whether the standard is realistic; if it is, they should take steps to improve their performance. Repeat of the audit after an interval will show whether the required changes have occurred.

Process knowledge: this type of knowledge refers to knowing how to undertake a procedure or do a task. Physicians who wish to learn a particular skill— such as reading ECGs or doing sigmoidoscopies—can arrange to spend time in a clinical center where they will gain this experience.

Know-how: this refers to knowing how to get things done, such as organizing appropriate referrals, obtaining necessary investigations, and community supports for patients.

Teaching is a valuable learning experience because it forces the teachers to examine their own methods of practice. Research, too, is valuable in that it explores areas of family medicine in depth.

SELF-KNOWLEDGE AND MINDFULNESS

Important change requires critical self-knowledge. As Popper and McIntyre (1983) have observed, we learn from our errors. Without self-knowledge, however, we have a great capacity for hiding our errors from ourselves, especially those arising from countertransference. Belonging to a group of colleagues that meets regularly to discuss each other's experience can be both a support and an opportunity for learning about ourselves. The more secure that members of the group feel with each other, the more they will feel able to confide in each other. Problem-based small group learning is an increasingly popular way for family physicians to learn, not only new medical information, but also from one's colleagues. In the past, family physicians have been slow to realize how much they have to learn from each other.

Mindfulness means that one attends to the ordinary events of life and work in a non-judgmental way. Many philosophical and religious traditions recommend practices of mindfulness as a way of linking cognition, memory, and emotion. "The goals of mindful practice are to become more aware of one's own mental processes, listen more attentively, become flexible, and recognize bias and judgments, and thereby act with principles and compassion" (Epstein, 1999, p. 835). Epstein describes the characteristics of mindful practice. It involves active observation of oneself, the patient, and the problem, as well as critical curiosity, adoption of a beginner's mind, humility, and presence, as well as other characteristics. It also involves learning emotional self-regulation, and such skills as emotional debriefing after a challenging patient, and taking time to relax outside work. Attending mindfully to one's own needs may help avoid "burnout" in practitioners (Bodenheimer and Sinsky, 2014) and may help avoid faulty thinking and hence errors in diagnosis (Groopman, 2007).

For family physicians, being well informed and up to date is necessary but not sufficient. Good family practice depends also on relationships, and the maturing of a family physician is a matter of educating the emotions as well as the intellect. Learning in this sense is often a matter of going through some personal change. Learning to be patient-centered is a case in point. This is not simply a question of learning some communication skills or following a set of rules. Practicing patient-centered medicine is a different way of being a physician, and unless this change has taken place, no technique will be effective. Work of this nature involves, at some level, a conversation with grander, more eternal, essential parts of ourselves, ". . . the consummation of work lies not only in what we have done, but who we have become while accomplishing the task" (Whyte, 2001, p. 5).

REFERENCES

Bodenheimer T, Sinsky C. 2014. From triple to quadruple aim: Care of the patient requires care of the provider. *Annals of Family Medicine* 12(6):573–576.

Eraut M. 1994. *Developing Professional Knowledge and Competence*. Philadelphia: Falmer Press, Taylor & Francis.

Epstein RM. 1999. Mindful Practice. *Journal of the American Medical Association* 282(9):833–839.

Groopman J. 2007. *How Doctors Think*. Boston; New York: Houghton Mifflin.

Osler W. 1905. On the educational value of a medical society. In: *Aequanimitas with Other Addresses to Medical Students, Nurses and Practitioners of Medicine*. Philadelphia, PA: Blackiston's Son.

Polanyi M. 1962. *Personal Knowledge: Towards a Post-Critical Philosophy*. Chicago: University of Chicago Press.

Popper K, McIntyre N. 1983. The critical attitude in medicine: The need for a new ethics. *British Medical Journal* 287:1919.

Whyte D. 2001. *Crossing the Unknown See: Work as a Pilgrimage of Identity*. New York: Riverhead Books.

CHAPTER 25

Research in Family Practice

Two hallmarks of any discipline, such as family medicine, are the definition of a body of knowledge and an active area of research (McWhinney, 1966). The knowledge base of family practice is rooted in a unique clinical world. Since its inception as an academic discipline in the latter half of the twentieth century, research in family medicine has greatly expanded this knowledge base. Research methods have expanded and been adapted to the world of the practitioner. This chapter describes how general practice has contributed to medical knowledge in general, as well as to knowledge pertinent to daily practice. It also discusses some of the methodological issues raised by research in the discipline.

A BRIEF HISTORY OF THE PROGRESS OF RESEARCH IN FAMILY MEDICINE

Although medicine should be regarded mainly as a science-based technology, it is founded on a descriptive body of scientific knowledge accumulated by physicians over the centuries. Like other sciences, medicine has developed two interrelated conceptual systems: an observational schema to classify its subject matter, and an experimental schema to describe the origins and destinies of these categories. The observational schema is our system for classifying diseases; the experimental schema tests our theories about how these diseases are caused and how they evolve over time.

The methods used in building our observational schema are those of the naturalist: observing, recording, classifying, analyzing (Ryle, 1936). The physician observes the natural phenomena of illness in the same way that the field naturalists observe the flora and fauna of their neighborhoods. Many of the early physician-scientists were naturalists in this broad sense. The country doctor Edward Jenner (1749–1823), for example, was made a member of the Royal Society for his discovery of how the female cuckoo invades another bird's nest (usually a hedge sparrow's) and makes room for her offspring by throwing the young sparrows out of their nest.

Jenner was in practice in the eighteenth century, a time when general practice was beginning to take form, under the name of *surgeon apothecaries*. His greatest discovery was vaccination for the prevention of smallpox. At least as early as the eighteenth century, healthy children were exposed to smallpox because the mortality (10%), was much less than the mortality during an epidemic. Those who recovered from smallpox were immune for the rest of their lives.

The concept of immunization, therefore, started with two proto-ideas (Fleck, 1979): one was the idea of immunity after survival from smallpox (this idea was general in the population); the other was the idea of immunity after smallpox in dairy workers in rural areas. Jenner began to study the illnesses of cows, taking an artist with him onto the farms, so he could have accurate drawings of cowpox pustules. Then, for the first time, the concept reached the mind of a scientist (Jenner) with proven powers of observation and the determination to pursue his investigation in the face of skepticism and ridicule.

Twenty years passed before Jenner carried out his crucial experiment. A boy was inoculated in a gazebo in his garden, first with material from a cowpox pustule, then later with smallpox. He was ready to submit his paper for publication. Jenner had many followers, but also many critics. Many of these failed to replicate this experiment. They had inoculated material from a pustule, but not from a smallpox pustule. How fortunate that Jenner was such a meticulous observer. In other hands, the whole project might have been abandoned—dismissed as another old wives tale.

William Withering (1741–1799) was similar to Jenner in many ways. He was trained in Shropshire by a surgeon, then went to study medicine in Edinburgh and to graduate as an MD. Back in Shropshire, he set up practice and worked as a physician in the Staffordshire Infirmary. Like Jenner, he became interested in a plant that a "wise woman" of Shropshire had told him was good for the dropsy. Withering knew that Leonard Fuchs (1501–1566) used the foxglove and, being a distinguished botanist, was able to put Digitalis on a scientific footing. His study of dosage and of side effects was very important in the use of Digitalis. Jenner and Withering were able to use their skills in observing, recording, classifying, and analyzing, to advance the progress of medicine.

Perhaps the greatest example of the naturalist method in general practice was the Scottish general practitioner James Mackenzie. There is much to learn from his work and we will therefore describe it in some detail.

Mackenzie was born in Scotland in 1853, graduated from Edinburgh in 1878, and soon afterward entered general practice in Burnley, a cotton-manufacturing town in Lancashire. It was there, during the following 20 years, that he carried out the studies that were to lay the foundations of modern cardiology.

Like so many before and after him, Mackenzie was mystified by his inability to diagnose so many of the illnesses he encountered in general practice. His medical education had not prepared him to deal with the illnesses of general practice. Blaming himself for his lack of knowledge, he searched the textbooks for answers—but in vain. The knowledge he sought did not exist. In his book, *The Future of Medicine* (1919, p. 64), Mackenzie wrote,

> . . . from the patient's statement can be acquired information that is absolutely essential to the recognition of disease, especially in the early stages. It would not be exaggerating to say that the failure of medicine to detect disease in its early stage is due to the fact that the sensations of patients have never been adequately investigated. Even when I had recognized the importance of this mode of investigation I found the greatest difficulty in eliciting the sensations, and in understanding the mechanism of their production . . . there is in the patient's sensations a field of enormous value . . .

Mackenzie bequeathed to us two principles of clinical research. The first was "record your patient's symptoms." The second was "follow your patient indefinitely." By the study of your patients' symptoms, you will learn their meaning ("wait and see"). By following your patients, you will learn the prognosis of their diseases. How can we follow our patients if they leave our practice? With our patient's cooperation, we can arrange to follow them for a confidential report on their health.

One of MacKenzie's discoveries was auricular paralysis (now called atrial fibrillation). He described the discovery in a letter to a friend.

> I had been watching a patient with mitral stenosis since 1880, as I was trying to find out when the mitral stenosis appeared, and the changes that occurred in its development. This patient had shown for many years a presystolic murmur, pulsation in the jugular vein and in the liver, due to the systole of the auricle. The heart had been regular . . . except for the occasional extra-systole. In 1898 she suddenly became very ill with breathlessness, cyanosis and a weak, rapid, irregular pulse. After some weeks the heart slowed down, and records taken showed a complete disappearance of all signs of auricular activity, and in place of a negative venous pulse there was now a positive venous pulse, and on auscultation the presystolic murmur had disappeared and the pulse had now become persistently irregular. (Mackenzie, 1919, p. 104.)

This account of Mackenzie's discovery of paralysis of the auricle shows what a single practitioner, following a single patient, can achieve by careful observation. There is no reason that a general practitioner should not do this today, either with single patients or with series of patients, collected because of their similarity to each other.

The example shows that discoveries may not appear all at once. A discovery that comes "out of the blue," perhaps when physicians are not thinking of their problem, may require a combination with another idea. Sometimes the person who brings the ideas together is not the person who makes the original discovery.

Mackenzie managed without complicated statistics: counting was all he needed. Nor did he need randomized controlled trials. Clearly they have their important uses, but they also have their drawbacks, especially for general practitioners. They are very expensive, so much so that only a few of those eligible can be accommodated. Because they are expensive, they have to be shortened, often too short to adequately test the efficacy of a new drug or treatment. There is still room for observational studies. If our journals reject all but randomized controlled trials, patients will miss the benefits of those discoveries which, otherwise, will never be brought to light.

It is ironic that Mackenzie became famous for something that he regarded as an incidental aspect of his work: his invention of the polygraph. Then, as now, both public and profession were more impressed by gadgets than by the clinical observations without which they would have been useless. His disciples, the new generation of cardiologists, embraced the new technology but, to Mackenzie's disappointment, failed to appreciate the importance of prolonged clinical observation to discover the natural history of disease. Mackenzie was by no means opposed to investigative medicine or the use of the laboratory; on the contrary, he made frequent use of both. But he never wavered in his belief that the basic science of medicine is clinical observation, and that general practice is the best place to learn the natural history of disease.[1]

There is, unfortunately, very little evidence that Mackenzie's example is being followed today. It is rare to read a description of clinical observations made over a long period of time by the author herself. More commonly, the author has extracted data from records made by other physicians, often not the result of disciplined observations. If there is systematic follow-up at all, it is usually for a short period of time.

Many reasons could be given for this neglect of our traditional methods. Ours is a restless and impatient age. To wait 10 years before publishing one's results would earn few grants and little credit in a medical school. Some physicians may think that the last word has been written on the natural history of disease. Yet we still fall into traps because of our ignorance.

When we encounter a disease we do not recognize, we should ask ourselves if it might be one of those diseases that are forgotten. Ludwick Fleck had taught us how long it may be before a scientific idea becomes a fact—perhaps centuries. "Thoughts pass from one individual to another, each time a little transformed" (Fleck, 1979, p. 39). A "thought collective" is a "community of persons mutually exchanging ideas or maintaining intellectual interactions . . ."

providing "the special 'carrier' for the historical development of any field of thought." (p. 68).

Before there can be a scientific fact, there must be an agreement with societal assumptions. "The futility of work that is isolated from the spirit of the age is shown strikingly in the case of that great herald of excellent ideas Leonardo da Vinci, who nevertheless left no positive scientific achievement behind him" (Fleck, 1979, p. 45).

Alexander Fleming is a case in point. The *Penicillium notatum* that grew by accident on his Petri dish, and killed the staphylococci, might have been thrown away. Fleming had for many years been in search of such an antibiotic. He published his finding, but was ignored. The chemists he worked with were unable to produce a mold that would remain constant in the human body. Eventually, Fleming and his work were forgotten for 12 years. In the early years of the World War II, Florey, an Australian medical scientist, formed a team in Oxford with Chain, a German chemist, and brought Fleming's work back from oblivion. After 12 years, Chain supplied the process that Fleming's work required.

"The great field for new discoveries," wrote William James, "is always the unclassified residuum. Round about the accredited of every science there ever flows a sort of dust cloud of exceptional observations, of occurrences minute and irregular and seldom met with, which it always proves more easy to ignore than to attend to" (James, 2007, p. 299). There is no greater field for the unclassified residuum than general practice.

Since the inception of national colleges of family/general practice following World War II, followed by training programs and academic departments, journals devoted to family medicine have increased in number. There are now 19 journals focusing on family/general practice or primary care just in English. As the knowledge base of family medicine has increased, textbooks have increased in number as well; as of 2012, there were more than 400 in English alone. In the early decades of academic family medicine, journal articles focused on themes such as the care of families and their problems; theoretical frameworks in family health; methods to study families and their effects on health; as well as original research in family and health (Culpepper and Becker, 1987). These themes were quite suitable and necessary for a new discipline engaged in defining itself. As academic family medicine has matured and expanded, so, too, have the volume and scope of the research enterprise, encompassing all aspects of clinical practice, epidemiology of practice, research methods, education, and theory.

TYPES OF RESEARCH
Observational

Any study that intends to document and communicate experience is an observational study. Several types of observational research can be identified. First are studies of the natural course and outcome of illness: the illness studied may be a well-defined disease category, such as herpes zoster, or a symptom, such as headache. Strictly speaking, the natural history of illness means the outcome of the illness when untreated. When the illness is highly responsive, it is no longer possible to study the true natural history. There are still, however, many diseases that are not greatly modified by treatment. There is also much to be learned from the study of diseases that are responsive to therapy. The action of the treatment on the disease may be to produce a new form of the disease that has its own natural history. In otitis media, for example, the treatment of the acute illness with antibiotics was followed by the emergence of serous otitis. In this kind of study, the denominator is the total number of patients with the disease or symptom. In a study of headache, for example, the denominator is all patients presenting with headache, and the numerator is different subgroups of this population with special features associated with particular outcomes.

The second type of observational research involves studies of incidence and prevalence. Information about the incidence and prevalence of symptoms and diseases is used by family physicians in estimating diagnostic probabilities. Studies in general practice have corrected some of the erroneous information on incidence and prevalence that have arisen from studies on selected populations. Incidence and prevalence are usually expressed as rates per thousand of the population at risk. The incidence rate is the number of new cases of the problem or disease seen per thousand of the population in 1 year. The prevalence rate is the total number of cases per thousand of the population at one point in time (the point prevalence) or in the course of a period of time (the period prevalence). For acute illness, the incidence rate is the more useful figure; for chronic illness, the prevalence rate is more useful. Care must be taken in extrapolating incidence and prevalence figures from family practice to the general population. One practice may not be representative of the total population. A more representative population can be obtained, however, by using a large number of practices. Because the recording of incidence depends on whether or not the patient consults, episodes of illness not presented to the family physician will be excluded. Incidence and prevalence studies in family practice are based on the number of patients consulting for the disease or problem in question (the consultation rate). Several types of denominator are used to calculate this rate. In registered practices, the practice population can be used; in practices with no registered population, the denominator may be the number of patients consulting during the year, a population arrived at by counting the practice records or the number of office visits during the year. None of these denominators is entirely satisfactory. The registered practice population may include people who have left the area but have not registered with a new doctor; a population obtained by counting practice records excludes people at risk who have never consulted, and may include some patients who have moved; patients consulting in 1 year are only about 70% of the total practice population.

Nevertheless, incidence and prevalence studies in family practice do give a much more complete picture of illness than studies done in hospitals, which rarely have a denominator population. Many examples of incidence and prevalence studies could be cited. Some of these have been done by individual practitioners, such as Hodgkin (1978) and Bentsen (1970). Others have been combined studies, such as the British National Morbidity Study carried out by the Royal College of General Practitioners, the National Ambulatory Care Study in the United States, and the National Morbidity and Interventions in General Practice Survey conducted by the Netherlands Institute of Primary Care.

Determination of the sensitivity, specificity, or predictive value of symptoms or tests make up the third type of observational research. To determine these values, certain data must be collected. The sensitivity of a symptom or test is the percentage of all people with the disease who have the symptom or positive test:

$$\text{Sensitivity} = \frac{\text{True positives}}{\text{All people with the disease}} \times 100$$

Suppose that we wanted to discover the sensitivity of palpable spleen in the early stages of infectious mononucleosis. We would need to record in every case the presence or absence of a palpable spleen. The result would then be calculated as follows:

$$\text{Sensitivity} = \frac{\text{Patients with palpable spleen and infectious mononucleosis}}{\text{All patients with infectious mononucleosis}} \times 100$$

The positive predictive value of a symptom or test is the percentage of people with the symptom or positive test who have the disease, that is, who are true positives:

$$\text{Predictive value} = \frac{\text{True positives}}{\text{All positives}} \times 100$$

Suppose that we wanted to discover the predictive value of sinus tenderness for acute sinusitis in patients with headache. We would need to record the presence or absence of sinus tenderness in every patient with headache. We would also have to ensure that sinus tenderness was elicited and recorded

Table 25.1. CROSS-SECTIONAL STUDY

	CHD	No CHD	Total
Non-immigrants	10	90	100 (10%)
Immigrants	40	160	200 (20%)

in the same way by all observers and that sinusitis was diagnosed according to uniform criteria. The result would be calculated as follows:

$$\text{Predictive value} = \frac{\text{Allpatients with sinus tenderness and s inusitis}}{\text{All patients with sinus tenderness}} \times 100$$

Observational Studies with an Analytic Component

These studies, sometimes called explanatory, attempt to shed light on the etiology of illness or the efficacy of treatment through the use of comparisons. For example, a study of coronary heart disease (CHD) may show that coronary disease appears to have a higher prevalence in people who have moved into the area than in non-immigrants. To demonstrate that the observed significance is not due to chance, we must do a comparison study. Two methods are available. First, in a cross-sectional study, a random sample of the practice population would be surveyed at one point in time. Suppose that 10% of natives and 20% of immigrants had coronary heart disease (Table 25.1).

A χ_2 test applied to these figures would show that the difference is significant at the $P = 0.05$ level. Second, in a case–control study, for every case of CHD a control, matched for age and sex, would be chosen. Both would be asked their origins (Table 25.2).

Experimental Studies

Much of medical research is now devoted to the development and evaluation of tools and methods—preventive, diagnostic, and therapeutic. The prototype

Table 25.2. CASE–CONTROL STUDY

	Non-immigrants	Immigrants	Total
CHD	10	40	50
No CHD	20	30	50

A χ_2 test applied to these figures would show that the difference is significant at the $P = 0.05$ level.

of this research is the randomized controlled trial (RCT). At one time, it was thought that effective therapeutic methods would be deducible from the theory of disease developed by experimental medicine. The results soon showed that our theoretical knowledge is incomplete. New diagnostic methods and therapies may be derived from scientific theory, but they still require testing empirically. The RCT was developed for this purpose.

Much progress has been made in the description and development of the diagnostic, therapeutic, and preventive methods of family practice. In many instances, this process has involved the formalizing of skills that had long been practiced at the intuitive level. One result has been a theory of family practice designed to explain the family physician's approach of diagnosis, therapy, and prevention. The early chapters of this book are an attempt to expound this theory.

For the evaluation of its methods, family medicine uses the technique of the RCT. It is also applicable to the organizational tools of family practice: record-keeping systems, management systems for case finding or for controlling chronic disease, and functions of the healthcare team. Drugs require testing in family practice as well as in hospitals. Because the patient population is so different, it may be misleading to extrapolate from one population to another. For example, there have been very few trials of antidepressants in family practice.

Pragmatic Trials

Carefully controlled trials are important for establishing the efficacy of an intervention, but there is a great difference between whether a treatment works under the ideal conditions of an RCT and whether it works in the world of practice. Our patients rarely look like the patients in controlled trials, as they frequently have many of the characteristics such as older age and multimorbidity that would have excluded them from such studies. Under the pressures and distractions of daily life, patients forget to take medications as they are prescribed and often are on other forms of alternative medicine that may alter the pharmaceutical effects of prescribed drugs. Pragmatic trials are controlled trials designed to inform decisions in everyday practice. They are essential in determining the effectiveness of an intervention; whereas RCT trials determine efficacy, pragmatic trials determine effectiveness. Pragmatic trials research plays an important role in family medicine, but presents significant challenges (Godwin, Ruhland, Casson, et al., 2003). Standards on the reporting of pragmatic trials have been developed (Zwarenstein, Treweek, Gagnier, et al., 2008).

Qualitative Research

Science produces generalizations by making abstractions[2] from the world of concrete experience. The problem is that the higher the level of abstraction, the more the rich texture of the world of experience is flattened out and rendered unrecognizable. This applies especially when the things abstracted are only those that can be quantified.

In the preface to *The Varieties of Religious Experience*, William James (1958) wrote, "a large acquaintance with particulars often makes us wiser than the possession of abstract formulas, however deep." A large part of medical knowledge is made up either of particulars or of generalizations at a low level of abstraction.

This is the knowledge gathered over years of observation in the form of case histories or series of cases. Much of it was made useful without quantification, or with quantification of a very elementary kind.

This way of contributing to medical knowledge is still valid. When family physicians see the results of some quantitative studies done in family practice, they are sometimes struck by how little they reflect the actual experience of being a family doctor. Perhaps it is a bald statement of results of a morbidity study, no doubt very useful at the planning level, but so far from the concrete world as to have very little application to day-to-day practice.

The same applies to many behavioral studies. The generalization "communication difficulties increase with cultural distance" is probably of less value than the observation that feelings like anger and gratitude are not openly expressed by Aboriginal North Americans. Of course, the power of generalization is sacrificed when knowledge is more concrete. The latter item of knowledge is useful only to physicians who care for Aboriginal patients. To take another example, it has been shown that self-perception is directly related to control in juvenile diabetics: the worse the self-perception, the worse the control. A less abstract item of information is that many juveniles are so ashamed of their diabetes that they try to hide it from their friends. Which of these items is more helpful to a physician counseling a juvenile diabetic?

Some of the most important questions facing family medicine are very unlikely to be answered by research that involves a high level of abstraction and quantification. A method must be found that preserves the richness and explores the meaning of the family practice experience. How, for example, do family physicians work with families? How do patients experience illness? Qualitative research methods have been developed to answer questions about the meaning of experience.

Family medicine is not alone in trying to find its way in research. The human sciences generally are engaged in the same debate, prompted by the aridity of so much of the work done by the experimental method. The human sciences differ from the natural sciences in some fundamental ways. For one thing, human events do not repeat themselves in exactly the same way. This does not mean that we cannot learn from studying human events. It does mean, however, that understanding rather than prediction is the objective in human research. One cannot study persons like objects. The very act of studying people changes them by altering their perceptions of events and of themselves.

In a controlled trial of a system for detecting and managing hypertension in general practices, the control practices changed almost as much as the experimental practices. Both were performing much differently at the end of the study than at the beginning. This does not mean that the results were of no value. The purpose of human research is often to produce change. It does suggest, however, that the experimental method has limited value in human affairs. It is this capacity for change that makes prediction invalid: whatever is predicted as a result of human research can be deliberately rendered void by the subjects themselves.

Randomization of human subjects is often impossible. Controlled trials of educational projects are made difficult because students selecting a new program are compared with students not selecting it. One can never then be sure that differences are due to the program and not due to the personal factors that led students to choose it. Again, this does not mean that educational research is of no value. In medical education, there are many examples of carefully designed demonstration models from which much has been learned.

Qualitative research is concerned with the meaning of actions and events.[3] There are no empirical tests for establishing meaning. Engel (1980) gives, as an example of human research, the gesture of "giving up." This gesture can be observed, described, and recorded, but its meaning cannot be deduced from the observation. It is not that we cannot establish the meaning; it is that we have to use other methods. We may find the meaning by entering into a dialogue with the patients about their feelings, we may do it by studying the context of the gesture in a number of patients, or we may understand the meaning intuitively because this act of communication is part of our own language; or we may use all these ways of understanding the gesture. Having verified the meaning in this way, we have made a valuable contribution to knowledge, even though it may not be applicable to the whole human race. Other cultures may have different gestures for giving up.

Qualitative research is intensive and time-consuming. The depth required in person-to-person interviews limits the number of people who can be interviewed. Those who have been educated in conventional quantitative methods sometimes ask how it is possible to generalize from such small samples. The answer is that the purpose of qualitative research is not to generalize but to enrich understanding. A study based on in-depth interviews with 19 patients with multimorbidity found that they generally held positive attitudes toward their life and endeavored to maintain their autonomy to the maximum extent. Emotionally they oscillated between anxiety and strength and tended to take a critical approach to medication (Loffler, Kaduszkiewicz, Stolzenbach, et al., 2012). Such studies makes us aware of the different ways our patients experience multiple chronic illnesses and enlarges our understanding, even though the findings cannot be generalized to everyone.

There is no antithesis between quantitative and qualitative research. Which method is chosen depends on the question asked. The same study may include some questions answerable by quantitative, others by qualitative, methods.[4]

VALIDATION IN THE HUMAN SCIENCES

In the search for a different research paradigm, we face the same problems of validation as other human sciences. Empirical science has well-established criteria of validation. What are the criteria in human science? How do we know that the changes we have made are responsible for the outcomes observed? How do we know that in explaining and interpreting human events we are not deceiving ourselves? In this review of means of validation in human inquiry, we are indebted to Reason and Rowan (1981), who describe eight processes of validation:

1. Personal preparation by the investigator. As Schumacher (1977) observed, the understanding of the knower must be adequate to the thing known. One cannot understand a psychological state without the capacity to experience it, or understand a social situation without entering into the experience of those involved. Preparation of this kind requires self-knowledge and the ability to deal with countertransference.
2. Systematic interpersonal development by the co-investigators, with the same purpose of enhancing self-knowledge.
3. Having one member of the investigator group whose role it is to act as devil's advocate by challenging conclusions reached by the group. This is a protection against self-deception by the whole group.
4. The cyclical process of testing, revising, and retesting one's conclusions, often many times (the hermeneutic cycle). This includes feeding back the results to the subjects and refining them in the light of their comments. Conclusions are suspect if they do not make sense to the subjects of the study.
5. Putting together knowledge from different levels of knowing. Gregory Bateson (1979) remarked that extra depth is given to knowledge by juxtaposing descriptions obtained in different ways. Developing different modes of human inquiry does not mean abandoning more orthodox modes.
6. A systematic effort by the investigators to refute their own conclusions.

7. Putting together the conclusions with other evidence from different sources and different methods of inquiry, a validation criterion known as triangulation.
8. A thorough description of the context of the inquiry (thick description).

Much remains to be done in working out modes of inquiry that will do justice to the rich texture of family practice. The process does not necessitate abandoning more conventional modes of inquiry. We will still continue to use experimental and quantitative methods for their proper reasons. We encourage a greater balance among the methods and methodologies in family practice research.

CLINICAL DISCOVERIES

Seeing illness in its earliest stages, family physicians are in an excellent position for making new clinical discoveries. These may begin as observations, insights, or hunches, which can develop over time into important new findings. Physicians practicing full-time are rarely in a position to carry the necessary research to a conclusion. Clinical discoveries do not begin as research. They are not planned in advance like traditional forms of research, such as those in university departments. They arise in the course of practice. Clinical discoveries are iterative. A certain clinical observation attracts the physician's attention. He or she takes notes and looks out for other cases, with each case adding more information. As time goes on, the observations coalesce, and the physician may have an intuitive insight. Such insights are often not the result of logic: they are, perhaps, a key observation that has been overlooked by others. Roentgen's discovery of X-rays is a case in point. His finding had been ignored by many others. Alexander Fleming's discovery was a single observation: the accidental effect of mold in a Petri dish containing bacterial culture. His paper was published, but ignored. James Mackenzie was attracted, early in his career, by the significance of the pulsations in the jugular pulse. Mackenzie wrote, "Others had studied the subject before, and, beyond recognizing some of its features, left the matter as one of no practical importance. On the other hand, I used it as a stepping stone for a further advance, and by this means the mechanism of regular heart action was revealed" (Mackenzie, 1919, p. 128).

In Mackenzie's time, there were no journals of family medicine. He was, however, able to publish his discoveries step by step in the existing medical journals. Now there are many peer-reviewed journals of family medicine and general practice. Many articles on research have been published, but very few from practicing physicians reporting their discoveries. It has been suggested that the editors and reviewers are judging these discoveries by the criteria of traditional research.

The *Annals of Family Medicine* (McWhinney, 2008; Stange, 2008) has now introduced a new category called *Clinical Discoveries*, which will be reviewed and evaluated according to four criteria: plausibility, support from the basic sciences and appropriate literature, clarity of concepts, and reproducibility of the procedures.

CHALLENGES AND RESPONSES TO DOING RESEARCH IN FAMILY PRACTICE

Research in family medicine has faced significant hurdles, but responses to each challenge have been forthcoming. Individual practitioners generally have small numbers of any given clinical entity, and this makes statistical analysis difficult. One response to this has been the emergence of practice-based research networks (PBRNs), which are groups of family physicians and practices that work together to answer questions arising in practice and to implement evidence-based quality improvements. The template for this development is Sir James McKenzie's Institute for Clinical Research, now with more support than was present at that time (Sullivan, Hinds, Pitkethly, et al., 2014). The Agency for Healthcare Research and Quality (AHRQ) in the United States has devoted funds to support PBRNs, and as of 2013, there were 161 registered in that country. The Agency provides a resource center with a bibliography of papers published from PBRNs and holds an annual conference (http://pbrn.ahrq.gov/).

PBRNs are receiving more attention from funding bodies (Westfall, Mold, and Fagnan, 2007). Such PBRN networks have been developed in the Netherlands, Canada, Australia, the United Kingdom, and elsewhere. Another development has been the large amounts of data emerging from EHRs (see Chapter 18, "Stewardship of Resources, Patient Information, and Data"), which have facilitated the gathering of health information from large patient populations that can support research and quality improvement initiatives.

In the past, family physicians have entered practice with little or no formal training in research. There are now numerous fellowships and graduate courses available that have trained new generations of researchers for family medicine and primary care. The graduate studies program of the Department of Family Medicine at Western University offers training leading to either a master's or a PhD degree, and makes it available in a mixed on-site and online format. This enables family physicians from around the world to increase their knowledge and skills while continuing to provide care in their community.

As mentioned, much of scientific research involves a process of abstraction, sometimes leading to conclusions that seem distant from their practice population. Qualitative methods and mixed methods research have become more common and help to address this issue. The Oxford Health Experiences

Research Group (http://www.phc.ox.ac.uk/research/health-experiences) is an example of how research has broadened to take into account the subjective experiences of individuals coping with health issues.

For many practitioners, the relevance of research as published in the major medical journals has seemed remote. The reality is that the more common diseases are the least studied (de Melker, 1995). Randomized controlled trials generally lack external validity. Pragmatic trials help to bridge the gap between what may be shown to work in carefully controlled clinical trials and what actually works in the real world of practice. Case reports and case series are receiving more attention now than in the recent past, and these often speak more clearly to the practitioner (Pimlott, 2014). There are now journals specifically dedicated to case reports (Kidd and Hubbard, 2007).

Another ongoing challenge has been obtaining funding. However, recent funding developments have been favorable to family medicine research. There are sources of funding for PBRNs. In addition, there are now specific funding streams for primary care research within national institutes. Three examples are the Australian Primary Health Care Research Institute, the Community-based Primary Health Care Team Initiative of the Canadian Institutes of Health Research, and the School for Primary Care Research in England. Also, there are funding agencies whose mandate for research fits well with the goals of family medicine research, such as the mandate for applied research (Netherlands Institute for Health Services Research [NIVEL], the Institute of Health Services and Policy Research in Canada, the National Institutes for Health Research in the UK), and the mandate for patient-oriented research (the Patient-Centered Outcomes Research Institute [PICORI] in the US and Strategic Patient-Oriented Research [SPOR] in Canada).

Family physicians may doubt that their work has anything to contribute to medical research, but with wider understanding of the true impact of research (Dunikowski and Freeman, 2015), it becomes clearer that this is far from true. Policymakers and funding bodies are requiring researchers to be more accountable and to explain how their research has a social impact (Lancet, 2014). Family medicine research is well placed to take advantage of this development.

No longer are family physicians only receivers of knowledge from other branches of medicine. Over the past 50 years they have expanded a unique base of knowledge relevant to the discipline and have contributed to the larger enterprise of medicine. Family medicine research has emphasized, among other topics, the importance of context, both proximal (e.g., family, occupation) and distal (neighborhood, environment) on health and illness; the importance of the subjective experience of illness; attention to marginalized populations; healing as distinct from curing; and the patient-centered clinical method.

NOTES

1. Mackenzie's philosophy of medicine and medical education are expressed in his book *The Future of Medicine* (1919). William Pickles's *Epidemiology in Country Practice* (1939) and John Fry's *The Catarrhal Child* (1961) are also excellent examples of descriptive research in general practice.
2. For a fuller discussion of abstraction, see Chapter 6.
3. For descriptions of qualitative research methods, see Liamputtong L, *Qualitative Research Methods*, 4th ed. (Oxford: Oxford University Press, 2012).
4. For examples of qualitative research in this book, see Veale, p. 24–25; Miller, p. 56–57; Jones and Morrell, p. 256; Woodward, p. ; Muzzin, p. 453; Dowie p. ; Bailey et al., p. 453; and Wood, p. 453–454; Woodward, Broom, and Legge, p.

REFERENCES

Bateson G. 1979. *Mind and Nature: A Necessary Unity*. New York: E. P. Dutton.

Bentsen BG. 1970. *Illness and General Practice*. Oslo: Universitetoforlaget.

Culpepper L, Becker L. 1987. Family medicine research: Two decades of developing its base. In: Doherty WJ, Christianson CE, Sussman MB, eds., *Family Medicine: The Maturing of a Discipline*. New York: The Howarth Press.

de Melker RA 1995. Diseases: The more common the less studied. *Family Practice* 12(1):84–87.

Dunikowski L, Freeman T. 2015. The impact of family medicine research (accepted for publication).

Engel G. 1980. The clinical application of the biopsychosocial model. *American Journal of Psychiatry* 137:535.

Fleck L. 1979. *Genesis and Development of a Scientific Fact*. Chicago: University of Chicago Press.

Fry J. 1961. *The Catarrhal Child*. London: Butterworths.

Godwin M, Ruhland L, Casson I, et al. 2003. In primary care: The struggle between external and internal validity. *BMC Medical Research Methodology* 3:28.

Hodgkin K. 1978. *Towards Earlier Diagnosis in Primary Care*, 4th ed. Edinburgh: Churchill Livingstone.

James W. 1958. *The Varieties of Religious Experience: The Gifford Lectures on Natural Religion Delivered at Edinburgh in 1901–1902*. New York: New American Library.

James W. 2007. *The Will to Believe and other Essays in Popular Philosophy*. Cosimo Classics, New York.

Kidd M, Hubbard C. 2007. Introducing Journal of Medical Case Reports. *Journal of Medical Case Reports* 1:1.

Loffler C, Kaduszkiewicz, Stolzenback C-O, et al. 2012. Coping with multimorbidity in old age-a qualitative study. *BMC Family Practice* 13:45. doi: 10.1186/1471-2296-13-45

Mackenzie J. 1919. *The Future of Medicine*. London: Oxford University Press.

Mair A. 1973. *Sir James Mackenzie, M.D., General Practitioner, 1853–1925*. Edinburgh: Churchill Livingstone.

McWhinney IR. 1966. General practice as an academic discipline: Reflections after a visit to the United States. *Lancet* 19:419.

McWhinney IR. 2008. Assessing clinical discoveries. *Annals of Family Medicine* 6(1):3–5.

Pickles WN. 1939. *Epidemiology in Country Practice*. Bristol: John Wright.

Pimlott N. 2014. Two cheers for case reports. *Canadian Family Physician* 60(11):966

Reason P, Rowan J. 1981. Issues of validity in new paradigm research. In: Reason P, Rowan J, eds., *A Source Book of New Paradigm Research*. Chichester, UK: John Wiley.

Ryle J. 1936. *The Natural History of Disease*. London: Oxford University Press.

Schumacher EF. 1977. *A Guide for the Perplexed*. New York: Harper and Row.

Stange KC. 2008. Clinical discoveries: A new feature of the Annals. *Annals of Family Medicine* 6:175–176.

Sullivan F, Hinds A, Pitkethly, et al. 2014. Primary care research network progress in Scotland. *European Journal of General Practice* 20:337–342.

Westfall JM, Mold J, Fagnan L. 2007. Practice-based research: "Blue Highways" on the NIH roadmap. *Journal of the American Medical Association* 297(4):403–406.

Zwarenstein M, Treweek S, Gagnier JJ, et al. 2008. Improving the reporting of pragmatic trials: An extension of the CONSORT statement. *BMJ* 337:a2390.

INDEX

Lung cancer, 285
Lymphosarcoma, 119

Macbeth (Shakespeare), 157
Mackenzie, J, 227, 267, 482–484,
    493, 494
Macrobiotic diet, 470
Macrolides, 301, 302
Macular degeneration, 148
Maintenance ceremonies, 204, 205
Maintenance stage of change, 277
Malaysia, 345
Malpractice litigation, 258, 287, 394
Malterud, K, 273
Mammograms, 280
Manageability, 272
Managed care, 10–12, 27, 33
    defined, 426
    practice management and, 426–427
Managed competition, 427
Manipulation, spinal, 466
Manitoba Longitudinal Study on
    Aging, 272
Matthews, D, 193
Mayans, 313–314
Mayo Clinic, 457
Mays, JB, 325–326
Mazonson, PD, 273
McCormick, J, 283
McDaniel, S, 179
McGuire, L, 111
McIntyre, N, 479
McNamara, Robert, 30
McWhinney, IR, vii, ix–x, 42, 49, 50, 51,
    52, 74, 79, 138, 156, 157, 161,
    183, 192, 194, 197, 199, 220, 258,
    259, 314–315, 328, 393, 404
McWilliam, CL, 453–454
Meals on Wheels, 444
Meaning, 174
Meaningfulness, 272
Mechanic, D, 38, 42
Medalie, JH, 62, 74, 115, 298
Medawar, P, 30–31
Medical knowledge, 131–134
Medically unexplained symptoms (MUS),
    108–109, 179–180
Medical social work, 433
Medicare, 399, 402, 427, 465
Medicine

epistemology of, 131
    paradigm change in, 107–108
Meditation, 464, 465, 471
Mediterranean diet, 349
Meeting the Challenges of Family Practice
    (Willard), 8
Meglitinides, 350
Melatonin, 462
Membership of the Royal Colleges of
    Physicians (MRCP), 49
Mental health, 4, 152, 379, 420
    community services for, 444
    shared care and, 456–457
    social support and, 115–116
    stress and, 114
Mental level of being, 132, 133
Metabolic syndrome, 347
Metamessages, 180
Metaphors, 177, 463
Metformin, 350, 355
Methyxanthines, 304
Mexican Americans, 465
Mexico, 342
Meyer, RJ, 61
Middlemarch (Eliot), 6
Midwives, 6, 431, 461
Migraine headache, 113, 126
Miller, FJW, 57
Miller, WL, 204–205
Millis, JS, 8
Milnacipran, 316
Mind-body relationship
    anomalies and, 110–112
    complementary/alternative medicine
        and, 462
    diabetes treatment and, 349
    dualistic view of, 21–22
    symptoms and, 175
    therapeutic implications of unity,
        112–116
Mindfulness, 25, 158, 164, 170n 2,
    479–480
Mirtazeapine, 331
Mitral valve prolapse (MVP), 140,
    267–268
Moclobemide, 331
Moerman, DE, 117
Mohr, J, 170
Monoamine oxidase inhibitors (MAOIs),
    331, 469